Vitamin D
in Dermatology

Vitamin D
in Dermatology

edited by
KNUD KRAGBALLE
Marselisborg Hospital
and University of Aarhus
Aarhus, Denmark

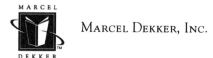
MARCEL DEKKER, INC.　　　　　　　NEW YORK • BASEL

ISBN: 0-8247-7704-2

This book is printed on acid-free paper.

Headquarters
Marcel Dekker, Inc.
270 Madison Avenue, New York, NY 10016
tel: 212-696-9000; fax: 212-685-4540

Eastern Hemisphere Distribution
Marcel Dekker AG
Hutgasse 4, Postfach 812, CH-4001 Basel, Switzerland
tel: 41-61-261-8482; fax: 41-61-261-8896

World Wide Web
http://www.dekker.com

The publisher offers discounts on this book when ordered in bulk quantities. For more
information, write to Special Sales/Professional Marketing at the headquarters address
above.

Current printing (last digit):
10 9 8 7 6 5 4 3 2

PRINTED IN THE UNITED STATES OF AMERICA

Preface

Rapid progress in the understanding of vitamin D action has led to a consideration of the potential application of vitamin D therapy to a range of diseases not previously envisioned. One of these new avenues of research is represented by the skin and its diseases, particularly psoriasis. The goal of this book is to bring the basic science and clinical dermatology together in an up-to-date volume.

The classic view of vitamin D action as a hormone limited to calcium metabolism and bone homeostasis has undergone extensive revision. The new spectrum of vitamin D activities includes important effects on cellular proliferation, differentiation, and the immune system. This information has resulted in the investigation of vitamin D therapy for a variety of skin diseases. The need for vitamin D analogs with a more favorable therapeutic profile has created another large and complex area of vitamin D research. This book provides a current picture of vitamin D research in investigative and clinical dermatology.

All the chapters are written by authors who are experts in their respective areas of vitamin D research, and I am grateful to them for their willingness to contribute to this book. I would also like to express my thanks to the Marcel Dekker staff and my secretary Mrs. Jette Nivaa for their diligence, expertise, and patience in helping me complete this work.

Knud Kragballe

Contents

Contributors

Ole Baadsgaard, M.D. Department of Dermatology, Gentofte Hospital, University of Copenhagen, Hellerup, Denmark

Daniel D. Bikle, M.D., Ph.D. Departments of Medicine and Dermatology, University of California, San Francisco, and Veterans Affairs Medical Center, San Francisco, California

Lise Binderup, Ph.D. Biological Research, Leo Pharmaceutical Products, Ballerup, Denmark

John F. Bourke, M.B., B.Ch., B.A.O., F.R.C.P.I., M.D. Department of Dermatology, South Infirmary–Victoria Hospital and University College Cork, Cork, Ireland

Martin J. Calverley, M.A., Ph.D. Department of Pharmaceutical Research, Leo Pharmaceutical Products, Ballerup, Denmark

Carsten Carlberg, Ph.D. Institut für Physiologische Chemie I, Heinrich-Heine-Universität Düsseldorf, Düsseldorf, Germany

Tomas Norman Dam, M.D. Department of Dermatology, Marselisborg Hospital, University of Aarhus, Aarhus, Denmark

Charles R. Darley, M.D., F.R.C.P. Department of Dermatology, Brighton Health Care NHS Trust, Brighton, England

Erik Fink Eriksen, M.D., D.M.Sc. Department of Endocrinology, Aarhus Amtssygehus, University Hospital of Aarhus, Aarhus, Denmark

Karsten Fogh, M.D., Ph.D.   Department of Dermatology, Marselisborg Hospital, University of Aarhus, Aarhus, Denmark

Masami Fukuoka, M.D.   Pharmaceutical Research Department, Teijin Institute for Bio-Medical Research, Tokyo, Japan

Henning Glerup, M.D., Ph.D.   Departments of Endocrinology and Metabolism, Aarhus Amtssygehus, University Hospital of Aarhus, Aarhus, Denmark

Erik R. Hansen, M.D.   Department of Dermatology, Marselisborg Hospital, University of Aarhus, Aarhus, Denmark

David J. Hecker, M.D.   Department of Dermatology, Mount Sinai Medical Center, New York, New York

Michael F. Holick, Ph.D., M.D.   Section of Endocrinology, Nutrition, and Diabetes, Department of Medicine, Boston University School of Medicine, Boston, Massachusetts

Philippe G. Humbert, M.D., Ph.D.   Department of Dermatology, University Hospital St. Jacques, Besançon, France

Stefania Jablonska, M.D.   Department of Dermatology, Warsaw School of Medicine, Warsaw, Poland

Sewon Kang, M.D.   Department of Dermatology, University of Michigan Medical Center, Ann Arbor, Michigan

Anne-Marie Kissmeyer, M.Sc. Pharm.   Department of Pharmacokinetics and Metabolism, Leo Pharmaceutical Products, Ballerup, Denmark

Michael R. Klaber, M.A., M.B., F.R.C.P.   Dermatology Department, Royal London Hospital, London, England

Keiji Komoriya, Ph.D.   Pharmaceutical Research Department, Teijin Institute for Bio-Medical Research, Tokyo, Japan

John Koo, M.D.   Psoriasis Treatment Center and Department of Dermatology, University of California–San Francisco Medical Center, San Francisco, California

Knud Kragballe, M.D. Department of Dermatology, Marselisborg Hospital, University of Aarhus, Aarhus, Denmark

Andrzej W. Langner, M.D. Department of Dermatology, Medical University of Warsaw, Warsaw, Poland

Mark Lebwohl, M.D. Department of Dermatology, Mount Sinai School of Medicine, New York, New York

Slawomir Majewski, M.D. Departments of Dermatology and Venereology, Warsaw School of Medicine, Warsaw, Poland

Jack Maloney, M.D. Department of Dermatology, University of California–San Francisco Medical Center, San Francisco, California

Rebecca S. Mason, M.B., B.S., Ph.D. Department of Physiology and Institute for Biomedical Research, University of Sydney, Sydney, New South Wales, Australia

Masayuki Nishimura, M.D. Nishimura Dermatology Office, Usa, Oita, Japan

Tomohiro Ohta, Ph.D. Pharmaceutical Research Department, Teijin Institute for Bio-Medical Research, Tokyo, Japan

Jörg Reichrath, M.D. Department of Dermatology, University of the Saarland, Homburg, Germany

Hiroaki Sato, M.Sc. Pharmaceutical Research Department, Teijin Institute for Bio-Medical Research, Tokyo, Japan

Jørgen Serup, M.D., D.M.Sc. Dermatological Research Department, Leo Pharmaceutical Products, Ballerup, Denmark

Lone Skov, M.D., Ph.D. Department of Dermatology, Gentofte Hospital, University of Copenhagen, Hellerup, Denmark

Henrik Sølvsten, M.D., Ph.D. Department of Dermatology, Marselisborg Hospital, University of Aarhus, Aarhus, Denmark

Wadim Stapór, M.D. Department of Dermatology, Medical University of Warsaw, Warsaw, Poland

Peter M. Steijlen, M.D.   Department of Dermatology, University Hospital Nijmegen, Nijmegen, The Netherlands

Peter C. M. van de Kerkhof, M.D.   Department of Dermatology, University Hospital Nijmegen, Nijmegen, The Netherlands

Niels K. Veien, M.D., Ph.D.   The Dermatology Clinic, Aalborg, Denmark

1

Molecular Mechanisms of Action of Vitamin D

Carsten Carlberg
Institut für Physiologische Chemie I, Heinrich-Heine-Universität Düsseldorf, Düsseldorf, Germany

I. INTRODUCTION

The biologically active form of vitamin D, $1\alpha,25$-dihydroxyvitamin D_3 (VD), is an important nuclear hormone with pleiotropic physiological function, such as maintenance of calcium and phosphate homeostasis, bone formation, and cellular growth [1]. Moreover, VD can induce cellular differentiation and apoptosis [2] in addition to immune-suppressive effects [3]. VD is a lipophilic molecule that easily passes cellular membranes and enters the nucleus, where it binds with high affinity (K_d approximately 0.1 nM) to the nuclear VD receptor (VDR). VDR is rather ubiquitously expressed and also found in the skin [4,5], i.e., skin is a VD target tissue. Vitamin D, the precursor of VD, is either taken up systemically directly through diet or, interestingly, can be synthesized in the skin from 7-dehydrocholesterol, indicating that the term *vitamin* was not ideally chosen. Synthesis of vitamin D requires energy from ultraviolet (UV) radiation at an approximate wavelength of 300 nm, therefore restricting endogenous production of vitamin D to daylight hours. Two subsequent enzymatically controlled hydroxylation reactions at carbon atoms 25 and 1, mainly performed in the liver and the kidney, respectively, lead to the hormonally active form, VD. However, keratinocytes also express a 1α-hydroxylase, so that they are able to produce VD [6]. In this way UV radiation increases in a paracrine fashion the VD concentration in the skin, which appears to explain observations that exposure to sunlight improves psoriasis; this has been known for a long time [7].

VDR is a member of a superfamily of structurally related nuclear receptors that can act as ligand-inducible transcription factors [8]. Thus the VD nuclear hor-

1

mone directly modulates transcription of those genes that have a functional binding site for the VDR in their regulatory region. Moreover, VDR appears also to have indirect, mostly transrepressive effects on gene regulation through other nuclear receptors and general transcription factors. Moreover, rapid actions of VD are known, but they are simply too fast (1–5 min) to be mediated through transcription of VD target genes. These "nongenomic" actions have been suggested to be mediated via membrane receptors [9]. The mechanisms by which VD-mediated membrane signaling occurs, still remain relatively unmasked, as a gene for a putative membrane receptor has not yet been isolated, in contrast to the respective cloning of the VDR a decade ago [10]. Interestingly, VDR does not appear to be exclusively located in the nucleus [11], which allows speculation that membrane-associated VDR may mediate (possibly through modulating the activity of a kinase such as protein kinase C) nongenomic actions of VD [12,13].

Taken together, VD and skin appear to be closely linked, i.e., skin is one of the important VD target tissues. The nuclear hormone VD is a direct regulator of gene expression and the mechanisms of gene regulation through VDR-containing protein-DNA complexes, also referred to as nuclear VD signaling, is the major theme of this chapter. The understanding of VD signaling is important for a most effective design and application of VD analogs for the therapy of skin disorders such as psoriasis [14].

II. THE NUCLEAR RECEPTOR SUPERFAMILY

The nuclear receptor superfamily is one of the largest families of transcription factors that can be classified into several subclasses [15–17] (Figure 1). Class I con-

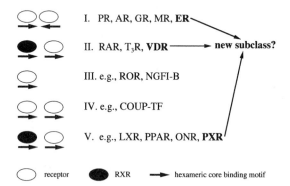

Figure 1 The nuclear receptor superfamily. The five subclasses of the nuclear receptor superfamily are schematically depicted by naming their members (in the case of the orphan receptor families only representative examples) and their characteristic interaction with DNA.

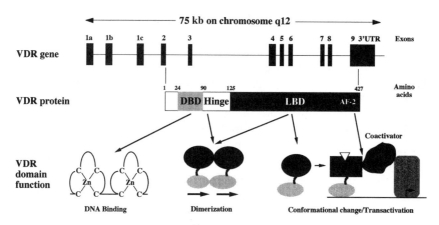

Figure 2   The VDR. Schematic representation of the exon structure of the VDR gene and of location of the DBD and LBD within the primary protein structure and of the main functions of these domains.

sists of the nuclear receptors for the steroid hormones, such as estrogen, progesterone, glucocorticoids, mineralocorticoids, and androgens (ER, PR, GR, MR and AR, respectively), which are commonly referred to as the classical nuclear hormone receptors. Class II consists of the VDR and the receptors for the thyroid hormone 3,5,3′-triiodothyronine (T_3) and the vitamin A–derivative all-*trans* retinoic acid (RA), named T_3R and RAR, respectively. The natural ligands for the eight nuclear receptors of classes I and II were already known as nuclear hormones prior to cloning of their cognate receptors. Although the ligands are in part very different in their structure, their respective nuclear receptors are structurally related: they all contain a highly conserved DNA binding domain (DBD) of 66–70 amino acids, which is formed by two zinc-finger structures, and a moderately conserved carboxy-terminal ligand binding domain (LBD) of 250–300 amino acids that is composed of approximately 12 α-helices. The DBD and the LBD are separated by a hinge region that is thought to allow free rotation of the two domains relative to each other (Figure 2). In addition to the eight established nuclear receptor gene families, the typical nuclear receptor structure has also been found in over 30 vertebrate transcription factor gene families. These transcription factors lacked a cognate ligand at the time of their discovery and were therefore referred to as "orphan" nuclear receptors [18]. Consequently, intensive screening for possible ligands for these orphan receptors started [19], resulting in the initial reports identifying 9-*cis* RA as a ligand for the retinoid X receptor (RXR) [20,21]. The orphan members of the nuclear receptor superfamily can be subclassified into those that (1) bind DNA as a monomer (class III), (2) form homodimers (class IV), and (3) form heterodimers with RXR (class V) (Figure 1).

III. CLASSIFICATION OF THE VDR WITHIN THE NUCLEAR RECEPTOR SUPERFAMILY

According to amino acid sequence homology and response element preference, the VDR has been grouped together with T_3R and RAR as a member of class II of the nuclear receptor superfamily. The latter two receptor families have been investigated more intensively than the VDR, thus theoretically extending many principles of actions that have been found for T_3R and RAR to the VDR. However, on the level of the ligand structure, the secosteroid VD has greater similarity with the classical steroid hormones such as estrogen, than with T_3 or RA. ER is the only classical nuclear receptor that shares the preference for the core binding motif consensus sequence RGKTCA (R = A or G, K = G or T) with VDR and is also capable of recognizing response elements that are formed by direct repeats (DRs) of these motifs [22]. Moreover, VDR and ER appear to be functionally linked, as they demonstrate some parallel as well as antiparallel effects on the control of bone mineralization and growth arrest, respectively [23,24]. Additionally, the very recent cloning a VDR-related receptor, referred to as pregnane X receptor (PXR), was reported [25]. This receptor appears to be the mammalian homologue of the *Xenopus laevis* orphan nuclear receptor (ONR), which was identified by using the cDNA of human VDR as a probe [26]. Both PXR and ONR form heterodimers with RXR and bind, such as VDR-RXR heterodimers, preferentially to DR3-type response elements. ONR did not generate very much follow-up investigative interest, and therefore a ligand has not yet been identified for this receptor. In contrast, PXR is activated by pharmacological concentrations of the GR ligand dexamethasone as well as progesterone and its derivatives [25]. Although it is not clear whether these compounds are the natural ligands to PXR, it is interesting to note that steroids have been found to activate a nuclear receptor that heterodimerizes with RXR and binds to DR-type response elements. Taken together, these observations hint that a new subclass of the nuclear receptor superfamily— grouping VDR, ER, and PXR together—could be considered, which would thus provide a link between classes I and II (Figure 1).

IV. THE VDR GENE

The human gene for the VDR spans over 75 kb of DNA on human chromosome 12 [27] (Figure 2). The 12 exons that make up the VDR gene are transcribed into an mRNA of 4800 nucleotides that encodes for a protein of 427 amino acids [10]. In contrast to T_3Rs [28] and RARs [29], only one VDR gene has been identified thus far. VDR is one of the most compact members of the nuclear receptor superfamily, which is primarily due to the very short amino-terminal region of only 23 amino acids. The amino-terminal region of some members of the nuclear receptor superfamily has been described to contain a constitutive transactivation domain, referred to as AF-1 domain [30]. Moreover, this region appears to act as amino-terminal extension of the DBD that modulates the response element selectivity of different amino-terminal variants of the RORα orphan nuclear receptor [31]. Comparable functions are not known for the amino-terminal region of the VDR, but, interestingly, the only known allelic variation of the VDR gene that affects the translated region has been described in this compact region. It was found that in nearly half of the human population, the first three amino acids of the VDR are not translated, but alternatively a methionine located at position 4 is used as translation start. However, the possibility of a significant functional difference between the 424 or 427 amino acid forms is not yet clear.

V. HORMONE RESPONSE ELEMENTS

An essential prerequisite for mediating transactivation by a nuclear hormone is location of the respective ligand-activated nuclear receptor close to the basal transcriptional machinery. This is initially achieved through specific binding of the nuclear receptor to DNA binding sites, referred to as hormone response elements (HREs), located in the regulatory regions of primary hormone responding genes. HREs are ideally composed of hexameric core binding motifs with the consensus sequence RGKTCA or, in the case of the classical steroid receptors PR, GR, MR, and AR, with the consensus sequence RGGASA (S = C or G). The affinity of monomeric VDR to a single core binding motif is not sufficient for the formation of a stable protein-DNA complex, which is typical for most nuclear receptors. Thus, VDR requires formation of homo- and/or heterodimeric complexes with a second partner receptor in order to allow efficient DNA binding. These dimeric receptor complexes are usually formed on an arrangement of two core binding motifs that can be in three relative orientations: as direct repeats, palindromes (Ps, also referred to as inverted repeats) and inverted palindromes (IPs, also referred to as everted repeats) [32]. On DR-type response elements, the DBDs of the two partner receptors bind asymmetrically to each other, whereas on P- and IP-type response elements the two DBDs are symmetrically arranged. Throughout evolution, the classical steroid receptors appear to have selected a rather simple recognition code of their response elements; they all bind as homodimers to P3-type response elements, i.e., to palindromic arrangements with three spacing nucleotides (Figure 1). In contrast, the distance between the core binding motifs has been developed as a major distinguishing feature for specific recognition of individual response elements for the other dimer-forming members of the nuclear receptor superfamily. In 1991 Umesono and coworkers [33] reported an ingenious, simple code for the interaction of VDR, T$_3$R, and RAR with DNA called the 3-4-5 rule. According to this rule, the class II-type members of the nuclear receptor superfamily preferentially bind to DR-type response elements that differ only in the number of their spacing nucleotides; therefore DR3-type structures are VD response elements (VDREs), DR4-type structures are T_3 response elements, and DR5-type structures are RA response elements. Shortly after this fundamental report, it was found that VDR, T_3R and RAR preferentially form heterodimeric complexes with RXR [34,35]. Moreover, it was suggested that RXR always assumes the 5'-motif position within these heterodimeric complexes [36,37]. These biochemical observations could be confirmed by x-ray crystallography of T_3R-RXR heterodimers [38]. Studies using the DR3-type VDREs from the mouse osteopontin and the rat osteocalcin gene have demonstrated binding of the VDR to the 3'-position [39,40], but surprisingly, binding of the VDR to the VDRE of the chicken carbonic anhydrase II has been found to apparently occur at the 5'-position [39].

VI. VD RESPONSE ELEMENTS

The first VDRE was reported in the human osteocalcin promoter [41,42], which has a DR6-type structure and was later found to be overlaid by a binding site for the AP-1 transcription factor [43] (Figure 3). Moreover, in accordance with the 3-4-5 rule [33], a third core binding motif downstream of the DR6-type structure was interpreted as a part of a DR3-type structure [44]. In the rat osteocalcin gene promoter a DR3-type VDRE was identified that was also overlaid by an AP1 binding site [45]. Subsequent studies defined a third core binding motif upstream of the DR3-type structure, which was interpreted as being part of an IP9-type VDRE [40]. These studies collectively indicate that the first two identified VDREs appeared to be complex structures each consisting of three core binding motifs and an AP-1 site and could therefore be considered as "complex" VDREs. Other complex VDREs have also been identified in the genes for mouse, rat and human fibronectin (DR6-type structures overlaid by a CREB binding site) [46], in the rat bone sialo protein gene (DR3-type structure overlaid by an inverted TATA-box), in the rat and human 24-hydroxylase (CYP24) gene (three core binding motifs, with 3 and 6 nucleotides in distance) [47,48], in the mouse c-*fos* gene (three core binding motifs each with a 7 nucleotide intervening distance overlaid by a CTF binding site) [49], and in the human tumor necrosis factor α gene (three core binding motifs with 7 and 12 nucleotides in distance) (unpublished). Simple VDREs have also been identified and extensively reported (Figure 3). These VDREs are apparently composed of only two core binding motifs. Several examples of simple VDREs fit into Umesonos 3-4-5 rule and have a DR3-type structure such as the VDREs for mouse and pig osteopontin [50,51], rat atrial natriuretic factor (ANF) [52], chicken carbonic anhydrase II [39], and chicken PTH [53] genes. These VDREs can be collectively classified as type I simple VDREs. Simple

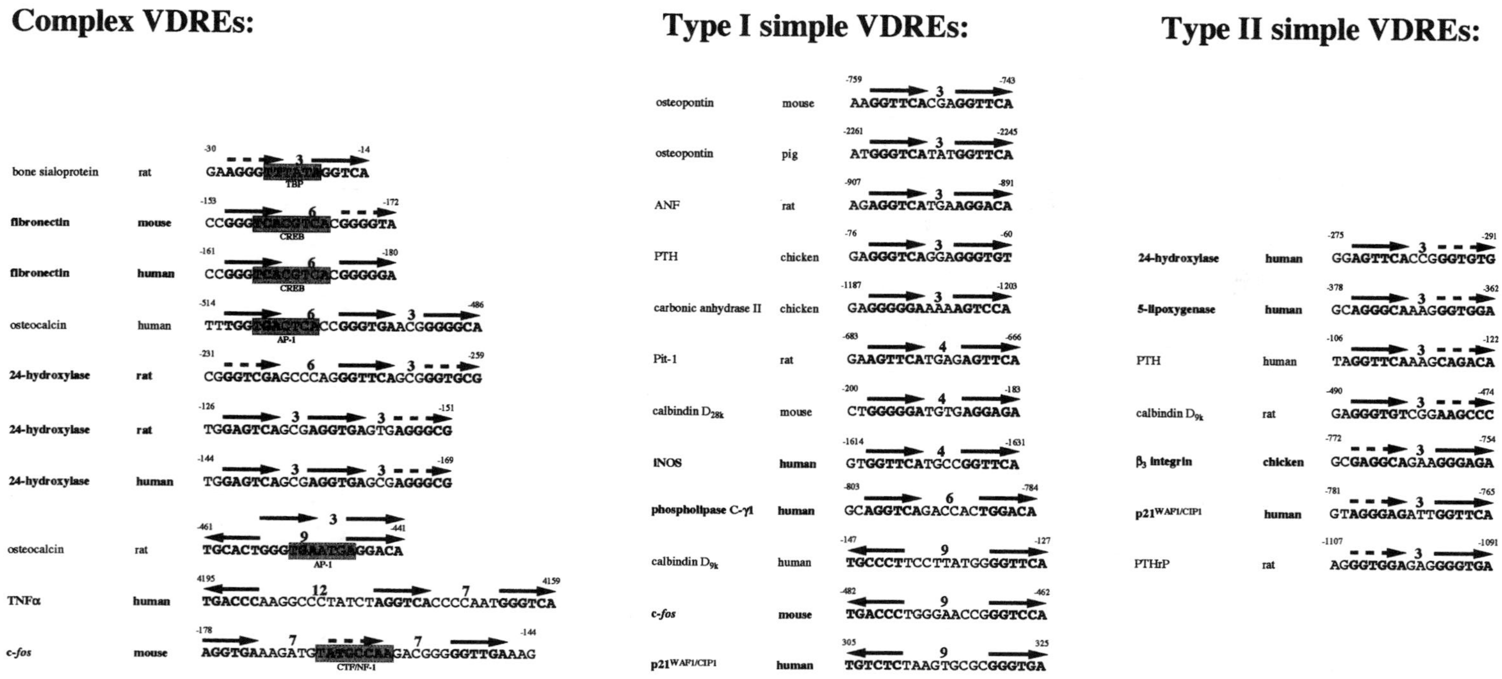

Complex VDREs:

Type I simple VDREs:

Type II simple VDREs:

Figure 3 VDRE list. The core sequence of the presently known VDREs are given, small numbers indicate the position of these sequences within the respective genes. Hexameric core binding motifs are indicated in bold and their relative orientations are indicated by arrows. Binding sites for nonreceptor transcription factors are indicated by gray boxes. VD-responding genes that are expressed in the skin are labeled in boldface.

DR3-type VDREs have also been found in the human p21$^{WAF1/CIP1}$ [54], human 5-lipoxygenase (unpublished), human PTH [55], rat calbindin D$_{9k}$ [56], rat CYP24 [57], rat PTH-related protein [58], and chicken β_3 integrin [59] genes (Figure 3). However, the sequence of at least one of the core binding motifs of these VDREs was found to be rather cryptic; i.e., it deviates in two or more nucleotides from the RGKTCA consensus sequence. In contrast to the consensus type I simple VDREs, the latter sequences can be classified as type II simple VDREs. Further examples of type I simple VDREs include VDREs that have DR4-, DR6-, and IP9-type structures and have been identified in the rat Pit-1 [60], human inducible NO synthase (iNOS) (unpublished), mouse calbindin D$_{9k}$ [61] (all DR4-type), human phospholipase C-γ1 [62] (DR6-type), human calbindin D$_{9k}$ [40], mouse c-*fos* [63], human, and mouse p21$^{WAF1/CIP1}$ (unpublished) genes (all IP9-type). A gene with a functional VDRE is a primary VD responding gene; i.e., its mRNA transcription is modulated within a few hours after treatment with VD. All above-mentioned VDRE-containing genes are therefore primary VD-responding genes. However, most of them are cell-specific and not expressed in the skin. So far only the genes p21$^{WAF1/CIP1}$, iNOS, β_3 integrin, fibronectin, phospholipase C-γ1, 5-lipoxygenase, TNFα, c-*fos,* and CYP24 are know as primary VD responding genes in keratinocytes. (indicated in bold in Figure 3). Moreover, in activated T cells that participate in inflammatory reactions of the skin interleukin-2 is known to be downregulated by VD (see Section XII).

VII. THE ROLE RXR AND 9-*CIS* RA IN VD SIGNALING

In vitro studies like gel shift assays and protein-protein interaction tests like the two-hybrid system suggest that the main dimerization partner of the VDR is RXR. The RXR family consists of three genes, but in skin RXRα was found to be the most abundant RXR subtype [64]. The formation of VDR-RXR heterodimers can be obtained on all proposed natural VDREs, but in some cases (e.g., [54]) only at receptor concentrations that would be sufficient to bind any unrelated DNA sequence. Consequently, the current widely accepted model of VD signalling is based on the assumption that all transcriptionally active VDR molecules are complexed with RXR. In fact, RXR appears to have a central role in a vast variety of nuclear signalling processes, as more than half of all nuclear receptors, including many orphans, heterodimerize with RXR [65]. RXR can be activated by 9-*cis* RA, therefore this retinoid may theoretically influence all of these signaling pathways. However, within these different heterodimeric complexes, RXR appears to assume different conformations. When complexed with the PPAR and NGFI-B orphan receptors, for example, it can be activated by 9-*cis* RA [66,67], whereas when complexed with T$_3$R and RAR, for example, it appears to be silent—i.e. 9-*cis* RA cannot activate the dimeric receptor complex. When T$_3$R-RXR or RAR-

RXR heterodimers are already activated by T_3 or all-*trans* RA, 9-*cis* RA is able to further enhance this activation. VDR-RXR heterodimers appear to react similarly: when VDR is not activated, 9-*cis* RA achieves only minor activation of the complex, but it is able to enhance the response after VD stimulation [40,68]. However, the molecular ratio of VDR:RXR appears critical for this synergistic action between VDR and RXR. In the case of limiting RXR concentrations all RXR interacting receptors create a transrepressive effect that can result in a reduction or even inversion of the synergistic effect [40,69]. In vitro experiments with bacterially expressed receptor proteins suggest that 9-*cis* RA destabilizes the VDR-RXR heterodimer [70] and functional studies were interpreted as supporting this observation [71,72]. However, in vivo studies on CYP24 gene activation supported the view of synergistic or at least additive effects of VD and 9-*cis* RA [73,74]. Moreover, the ligand-dependent allosteric interaction between VDR and RXR has recently been demonstrated in an in vitro study [68].

VIII. ALTERNATIVE VD SIGNALING PATHWAYS

Most of the current nuclear VD signaling models are dominated by the idea that the VDR can act as a heterodimer only with RXR on a DR3-type VDRE. If these models hold true, they imply that the pleiotropic action of VD is mediated essentially by a uniform protein-DNA complex. This would also mean that the molecular basis of a desired sharper profile of VD analogues has to be understood on this single type of heterodimer-DNA complex. Therefore, alternatives have been investigated. The first indication came from studies on the repressive potential of the orphan nuclear receptor chicken ovalbumin upstream promoter transcription factor (COUP-TF) on nuclear VD signaling as well as other hormone signaling pathways [75,76]. The mechanisms of this interference appear to be via competition between VDR-RXR heterodimers and COUP-TF homodimers for DNA binding sites on one side and the formation of heterodimers between VDR and COUP-TF on the other side (Figure 4). This finding alluded to the idea that nuclear receptors may interfere more promiscuously than initially assumed [77]. In this information context, the closest relatives of VDR, RAR, and T_3R were tested for their ability to interact with VDR. In fact, the formation VDR-RAR heterodimers [62,78,79] and VDR-T_3R heterodimers [80,81] was demonstrated on DR- and IP-type VDREs, but their DNA-binding affinity was found to be lower than that of VDR-RXR heterodimers [80]. Moreover, DNA binding assays using in vitro-translated, purified bacterial- or baculovirus-expressed VDR indicated that at high protein concentrations, VDR homodimerization on DR3-, DR6- and IP12-type VDREs could also be obtained [70,82,83]. Taken together, although there is no doubt that the main partner of VDR is RXR [84], VDR appears to have the potential to also contact other nuclear receptors. This understanding modifies the

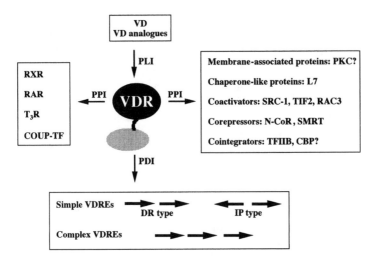

Figure 4   Central role of VDR in VD signaling. VD signaling is based on central involvement of the VDR in protein-ligand (PLI), protein-DNA (PDI), and protein-protein interactions (PPI). The most flexibility appears to be on the level of VDR interaction with other proteins. Protein-protein interactions that have not yet been experimentally proven are indicated by a question mark.

role of RXR from a compulsory partner of VDR to an accessory factor, as described earlier [85], that can be advantageously chosen in the majority of VDR-containing complexes.

IX. THE MODEL OF MULTIPLE VD SIGNALING PATHWAYS

In general, heterodimerization is an elegant way to generate, with a limited number of transcription factors, various functionally different complexes that may explain the multiplicity of nuclear signaling by each of these factors [77,86]. Thus, classification of VDR-containing protein-DNA complexes may show a correlation with a classification of primary VD-responding genes. Taking four types of dimeric VDR complexes (VDR-RXR heterodimers, VDR-RAR heterodimers, VDR-T$_3$R heterodimers, and VDR homodimers) and the two principal VDRE structures (DR- and IP-type) into consideration, eight different complexes can be discriminated. As the polarity of a heterodimeric complex was found to have an influence on its ligand responsiveness [40,81], the number of potentially important VDR-DNA complexes increases to 14. The existence of 7 out of the 14 complexes has been demonstrated on natural VDREs [87], which indicates a relevance for such a classification. However, it is not yet clear if this model implicates all possible VDR-containing complexes or to what extent their relative physiological importance is. In this way, the model of multiple VD signaling pathways [87] should be understood as a suggestion for consideration of alternatives to VDR-RXR heterodimers bound to a DR3-type VDRE. According to the proposed model, the VDR should ideally assume a different conformation in each of the different dimeric receptor complexes, which may then be selectively recognized by VDR ligands. Therefore, such VD analogs should show a sharper biological profile than those for which selectivity for VDR complexes cannot be detected [87].

X. PROMOTER SELECTIVITY OF VD ANALOGUES

The broad variety of physiological actions of VD suggest a potential for therapeutic use in several types of clinical disorders, including cancer, psoriasis, and metabolic bone diseases [88]. However, such pleiotropic actions imply a parallel risk of undesired side effects. Hypercalcemia is the main side effect of the natural hormone, therefore limiting its application range [89]. This prompted chemists to synthesize several hundred structurally divergent VD analogs [90]. Most of them have been tested in animal models and cell culture for their calcemic potential, antiproliferative effect, and ability to compete with radiolabeled VD for binding to the VDR. Unfortunately, most of these compounds have either low receptor affinity (and therefore weak biological effects) or strong calcemic effects. However, a few VD analogs have been identified that demonstrate a desired, selective biological profile—i.e., a high anti-proliferative effect combined with a low calcemic response [91,92]. Studies on VD analog metabolism may already explain a lot of the functional properties of VD analogs; however, a more complete, detailed understanding of their gene regulatory functions is necessary. Cell regulatory properties, VDR, and serum vitamin D binding protein (DBP) binding and calcemic effects of VD analogues have already been summarized [90,93,94]. A selection of VD analogues have been chosen for clinical trials and promising preliminary results give hope that these potent drugs will soon be approved for routine clinical treatment. The multiple VD signaling pathway model predicts that some VD analogues may exhibit selective activation of certain VDRE types. This concept was initially tested with VD, and the analogues KH1060, MC903 (calcipotriol), and EB1089 on DR3- and DR6-type VDREs [95]. Promoter selectivity could not be observed in this system; i.e., there was no significant variation of the ratio between the half-maximal activation levels (EC_{50}-values) for the two types of VDREs for the above-mentioned compounds. In contrast, data obtained from thirteen VD analogs that were tested on DR3- and IP9-type VDREs demonstrated that some analogs show a clear response element selectivity [96–100]. Compared with VD,

EB1089, ZK161422, and MC1288 are 20.3-, 5.9-, and 4.8-times more potent on IP9-type VDREs than on DR3-type VDREs, respectively, whereas CB1093, KH1230, MC1627, and KH1060 demonstrate 22.3-, 17.5-, 8.2-, and 5.5-times higher preference for DR3-type VDREs, respectively [96,97,99].

XI. FUNCTIONAL VDR CONFORMATIONS

Ligand binding to the LBD enables a nuclear receptor to undergo specific protein-protein contacts with other nuclear proteins (Figure 2). It is assumed that in the apo-receptor, the respective contact points are hidden, so that ligand-induced conformational changes are required to activate the receptor. Crystal structures of RXRα [101], RARγ [102], and T$_3$Rβ [103] supported a model by which ligand binding changes the presentation of a small amphiphatic α-helix, called the activation function 2 (AF-2) domain [104,105]. This domain is highly conserved within the nuclear receptor superfamily and is located in close proximity to the carboxy-terminus of the receptor (Figure 2). A crystal structure for the VDR has not yet been resolved, but the crucial role of its AF-2 domain has been demonstrated [106,107]. Therefore, it can be assumed that the mechanisms of ligand-induced conformation described for RARs and T$_3$Rs may also theoretically apply for the VDR. This would suggest that ligand-bound VDR mediates transactivation via a conformational change that also affects the presentation of its AF-2 domain. Ligand binding is usually studied by competition assays using radiolabeled ligand, but this method does not allow for visualization of any conformational changes of the receptor. An attractive alternative is the limited protease digestion assay, which is based on the principle that the binding of ligand to the LBD masks one or more protease cutting sites and creates, under limited reaction conditions, protease-resistant receptor fragments [108,109]. This method has been applied for demonstrating ligand-induced conformational changes of a variety of nuclear receptors, including RXR [110], RAR [111], PPAR [112], and LXR [113]. In the case of ligand-bound VDR, the trypsin endoprotease displays a characteristic digestion pattern: VD and most VD analogs provide two fragments of 33 and 29 kDa in size, respectively, whereas a few analogs also cause stabilization of an additional band 31 kDa in size [96,114]. These VDR fragments have been interpreted as different functional conformations of the VDR. The extent to which the three functional VDR conformations at a given concentration are charged with ligand, is characteristic for each ligand. Briefly, analogs that bind VDR weakly are characterized by preferential stabilization of conformation 3, whereas potent analogs tend to stabilize the high ligand binding conformation 1. It appears that VDR molecules that are in conformation 1 mediate the actions of VD and its analogs, at low concentrations in the physiological range. At present, the function of conformations 2 and 3 are not clear; they may have importance only at high pharmaco-

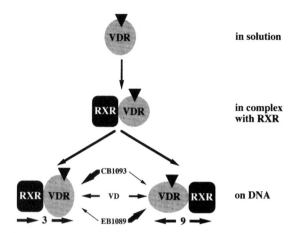

Figure 5 Current model of functional selectivity of VD analogs. The high-affinity conformation of monomeric VDR is stabilized by ligand (small black triangle) in solution. It is assumed that complex formation with RXR influences this conformation. Binding to different VDRE types should theoretically split the conformation into subconformations that are selectively recognized by certain VD analogs.

logical analog concentrations. Amino acids located in the AF-2 domain—e.g., phenylalanine 422 and lysine 417—have recently been demonstrated to have a central role in contacting the ligand [107,115,116]. Until now, the limited protease digestion technique has only been applied to one receptor at a time; i.e. the present results describe the ligand interaction of VDR homodimers, or more likely VDR monomers, in solution. The model shown in Figure 5 illustrates a possible explanation of response element selectivity of VD analogues. According to the model, in the heterodimeric complex of VDR and RXR on DNA the high affinity VDR conformation splits into different subconformations that are selectively recognized by analogs like EB1089 and CB1093. Such DNA- or partner receptor–driven splitting into subconformations has already been reported for T_3R-RXR heterodimers [117], suggesting that similar results may be extrapolated for VDR-RXR heterodimers. Moreover, biochemical evidences have suggested that the exact sequence of the core binding sites induces different conformations within the VDR [118].

XII. NEGATIVE REGULATION BY VD

VDR can mediate downregulation of gene transcription through direct protein-protein contacts. Transactivation of the growth hormone gene by T_3 and all-*trans*

RA is inhibited by VDR, where VDR acts as a competitor by displacing T_3R and RAR from a perfect palindromic T_3 and RA response element [119]. Moreover, unliganded VDR can act in a dominant-negative fashion to repress T_3R-mediated transcription from a DR4-type response element [120]. The repression of inter-leukin-2 gene regulation by VDR-RXR appears to be by direct interaction with and blocking of the $NFAT_p$/AP-1 transcription factor complex [121]. Finally, VDR has been shown to repress retinoid signaling from a RA response element of the tumor necrosis factor–α receptor I [122]. In contrast to these various transre-pressive effects, VD appears not to have an anti-AP-1 effect that is comparable to that described for retinoids and glucocorticoids [96]. Moreover, downregulation of gene transcription by VDR and its ligands appears not only to be mediated through transrepressive effects. A few primary VD-responding genes, such as PTH and ANF, are negatively regulated by VD, but their VDREs act in a heterol-ogous promoter context as positive elements. This indicates that currently un-known proteins mediate the negative regulatory effect on the natural promoters.

XIII. INTERACTION OF VDR WITH THE TRANSCRIPTIONAL MACHINERY

Transcriptional activation through transcription factors, commonly referred to as transactivation, has been shown to be mediated by protein-protein contacts. Many studies now focus on identification of proteins that "relay" transcriptional signals from nuclear receptors to the basal transcriptional machinery. Hence, these cofac-tor activities on gene expression should be considered in the context of DNA, pro-tein, and chromatin contacts [123–126]. Similarly, identification and characteri-zation of novel VDR-interacting proteins that affect VD signaling should also be considered in this way. Cofactors have been categorized into coactivators or core-pressors, which are capable of mediating either "positive" or "negative" transac-tivation, respectively. Additionally, cointegrator proteins such as CREB-binding protein (CBP)/p300 also form a category, functioning as mediator proteins that can integrate incoming and outgoing signals from nuclear receptors, coactivators or corepressors to the basal transcriptional machinery [127–130]. Coactivators function essentially by enhancing ligand-dependent transcriptional activation of nuclear receptors which are bound to DNA responsive elements. These effects have been demonstrated to occur via contacts with nuclear receptor LBDs. The proteins steroid receptor coactivator 1 (SRC-1) [131], transcriptional intermediary factor 2 (TIF2) [132], and receptor associated coactivator 3 (RAC3) [133] repre-sent three main members of the nuclear receptor co-activator gene family (Figure 4). These coactivators typically contain leucine cluster domains of the signature LXXLL sequence motif, that are apparently the interaction interfaces with nuclear receptors [129]. The contact point of the nuclear receptors appears to be their AF-

2 domain [134–136] (Figure 2) and a specific, conserved lysine residue in helix 3 of the LBD [137]. Interestingly, the coactivators identified thus far, appear to be interacting with many nuclear receptors, suggesting an indiscriminate role for interaction. With this is mind, it is theoretically possible that VDR can also interact with a variety of the known cofactors. However, these interaction experiments remain to be further tested and proven specifically for the VDR. This in turn, may largely depend on cellular receptor stoichiometry and DNA- or ligand-induced nuclear conformation, which would provide available cofactor contact sites and possible ligand-signaling variation [138–140]. Yeast two-hybrid studies have demonstrated that the cofactors SRC-1 and RAC3 are able to interact with VDR in a ligand-dependent manner [133,141]. As no major difference between the three coactivator families has been reported thus far, it is quite likely that the VDR, similar to most other nuclear receptors, also interacts with TIF2 [142]. Moreover, the expression pattern of the three cofactor family members in normal tissues as well as in malignant cell lines appears to be rather similar [143]. Furthermore, studies with SRC-1 null mutant mice showed that the different coactivators seem to compensate each other's function [144]. Therefore, it is unlikely that the presently known cofactors are the key for tissue-specific actions of the VDR. However, it is possible that proteins expressed in low abundance, but have preference for the VDR will be identified as the desired cell-specific VDR cofactors. Furthermore, a yeast two-hybrid screen approach identified the ribosomal L7 protein as a modulator of VDR-RXR mediated transcription [145] (Figure 4). However, as L7 is primarily a cytosolic protein, it may primarily function in a chaperone-like fashion. Thus, the yeast two-hybrid system appears to be an extremely powerful method for identifying protein-protein interactions, but it remains to be seen how these interactions take place in the true mammalian cellular context.

XIV. CONCLUSION

VD signaling appears to be more complex than VDR-RXR heterodimers binding to DR3-type VDREs. However, this complexity bears the potential to address only a desired subset of the pleiotropic actions of the nuclear hormone VD. The selective activation of one VDR-containing protein-DNA complex within the variety of other VDR complexes may be the key for a sharp functional profile of a VD analogue. Presently, the most effective, commercially available antipsoriatic VD analog, MC903 (calcipotriol), is applied topically. The apparently most important property of MC903 is its low metabolic stability, so that the analogue acts in a pulse-type fashion only in the skin and not in the rest of the body. However, the future generation of potent VD analogs, such as EB1089 and CB1093, will be applied systemically; they are metabolically much more stable and will have long-lasting effects. Their biological profile is sharp, since they have a high cell-regulatory potential combined with a low calcemic effect. The molecular basis of the sharp profile of these VD analogues is apparently their promoter selectivity. Thus, promoter selectivity may be the key parameter for the selection of even more potent VD analog. However, much less understood is how tissue selectivity of VD analog can be obtained. Initially, there was hope that tissue-specifically expressed cofactors may be the key factors in this process, but the currently known cofactors are widely expressed and show promiscuous interaction with nearly all nuclear receptors, so that presently the expectations are not fulfilled. However, central to all VD signaling pathways is the VDR; i.e., VDR is thus far the single molecular integrator of endocrine signaling of the nuclear hormone VD. Within the last decade, since the cloning of the human VDR cDNA, a lot was learned about the protein VDR. Unfortunately, its crystal structure is not yet known, so that a reasonable part of the understanding of the VDR was still obtained by extrapolation of models of the more intensively studied RARs and T_3Rs. The VDR is composed of a DBD and a LBD, therefore still making protein DNA and protein-ligand interactions involving the VDR the core mechanisms of VD signaling. However, in addition to the specialized interfaces for DNA and ligand contacts, the whole surface of the globular VDR protein may serve as a collection of interfaces with other proteins (Figure 4). These protein partners are other nuclear receptors and cofactors that are, like VDR, mainly located in the nucleus. Some of these interactions are presently only hypothesized by extrapolation of what is known for other nuclear receptors. Thus, future research will in part concentrate on also proving these interactions in the VDR system. However, cytosolic localization of the VDR has convincingly been shown, and this opens up a new field of investigations defining the possible functional role of the VDR outside the nucleus [11].

REFERENCES

1. Walters MR. Newly identified actions of the vitamin D endocrine system. Endocr Rev 1992; 13:719–764.
2. Welsh J, Simboli-Campbell M, Narvaez CJ, Tenniswood M. Role of apoptosis in the growth inhibitory effects of vitamin D in MCF-7 cells. Adv Exp Med Biol 1995; 375:45–52.
3. Manolagas SC, Hustmyer FG, Yu X-P. Immunomodulating properties of 1,25-dihydroxyvitamin D_3. Kidney Int 1990; 38:S9–S16.
4. Stumpf WE, Sar M, Reid FA, Tanaka Y, DeLuca HF. Target cells for 1,25-dihydroxyvitamin D_3 in intestinal tract, stomach, kidney skin, pituitary and parathyroid. Science 1979; 206:1188–1191.
5. Feldman D, Chen T, Hirst M, Colston K, Karasek M, Cone C. Demonstration of 1,25-dihydroxyvitamin D_3 receptor in human skin biopsies. J Clin Endocrinol Metab 1980; 51:1463–1465.

6. Bikle DD, Nemanic MK, Whitney JO, Ellas PW. Neonatal human foreskin keratinocytes produce 1,25-dihydroxyvitamin D_3. Biochemistry 1986; 25:1545–1548.
7. Wright C. Vitamin D therapy in dermatology. Arch Dermatol Syph 1941; 43:145–154.
8. Mangelsdorf DJ, Thummel C, Beato M, Herrlich P, Schütz G, Umesono K, Blumberg B, Kastner P, Mark M, Chambon P, Evans RM. The nuclear receptor superfamily: the second decade. Cell 1995; 83:835–839.
9. Nemere I, Dormanen MC, Hammond MW, Okamura WH, Norman AW. Identification of a specific binding protein for 1α,25-dihydroxyvitamin D_3 in basal-lateral membranes of chick intestinal epithelium and relationship to transcaltachia. J Biol Chem 1994; 269:23750–23756.
10. Baker AR, McDonnell DP, Hughes M, Crisp TM, Mangelsdorf DJ, Haussler MR, Pike JW, Shine J, O'Malley B. Cloning and expression of full-length cDNA encoding human vitamin D receptor. Proc Natl Acad Sci USA 1988; 85:3294–3298.
11. Barsony J, Renyi I, McKoy W. Subcellular distribution of normal and mutant vitamin D receptors in living cells. J Biol Chem 1997; 272:5774–5782.
12. Boyan BD, Posner GH, Greising DM, White MC, Sylvia VL, Dean DD, Schwartz Z. Hybrid structural analogues of 1,25-$(OH)_2D_3$ regulate chondrocyte proliferation and proteoglycan production as well as protein kinase C through a nongenomic pathway. J Cell Biochem 1997; 66:457–470.
13. Marcinkowska E, Wiedlocha A, Radzikowski C. 1,25-dihydroxyvitamin D_3 induced activation and subsequent nuclear translocation of MAPK is upstream regulated by PKC in HL-60 cells. Biochem Biophys Res Commun 1997; 241:419–426.
14. van de Kerkhof PCM. Biological activity of vitamin D analogues in the skin, with special reference to antipsoriatic mechanisms. Br J Dermatol 1995; 132:675–682.
15. Evans RM. The steroid and thyroid hormone receptor superfamily. Science 1988; 240:889–895.
16. Green S, Chambon P. Nuclear receptors enhance our understanding of transcriptional regulation. Trends Genet 1988; 4:309–314.
17. O'Malley BW. The steroid receptor superfamily: more excitement predicted for the future. Mol Endocrinol 1990; 4:363–369.
18. O'Malley BW, Conneely OM. Orphan receptors: in search of a unifying hypothesis for activation. Mol Endocrinol 1992; 6:1359–1361.
19. Laudet V, Adelmant G. Lonesome orphans. Curr Biol 1995; 5:124–127.
20. Levin AA, Sturzenbecker LJ, Kazmer S, Bosakowski T, Huselton C, Allenby G, Speck J, Kratzeisen C, Rosenberger M, Lovey A, Grippo JF. 9-Cis retinoic acid stereoisomer binds and activates the nuclear receptor $RXR\alpha$. Nature 1992; 355:359–361.
21. Heyman RA, Mangelsdorf DJ, Dyck JA, Stein RB, Eichele G, Evans RM, Thaller C. 9-cis retinoic acid is a high affinity ligand for the retinoid X receptor. Cell 1992; 68:397–406.
22. Keller H, Givel F, Perroud M, Wahli W. Signaling cross-talk between peroxisome proliferator-activated receptor/retinoid X receptor estrogen receptor through estrogen response elements. Mol Endocrinol 1995; 5:794–804.
23. Guise TA, Mundy GR. Breast cancer and bone. Curr Opin Endocrinol 1995; 2:548–555.

24. Vink-van-Wijngaarden T, Birkenhäger JC, Kleinekoort WMC, van der Bemd G-J, C.M., Pols HAP, van Leeuwen JPTM. Antiestrogens inhibit in vitro bone resorption stimulated by 1,25-dihydroxyvitamin D_3 and the vitamin D_3 analogues EB1089 and KH1060. Endocrinology 1995; 136:812–815.

25. Kliewer SA, Moore JT, Wade L, Staudinger JL, Watson MA, Jones SA, McKee DD, Oliver SA, Willson TM, Zetterström RH, Perlmann T, Lehmann JM. An orphan nuclear receptor activated by pregnanes defines a novel steroid signaling pathway. Cell 1998; 92:73–82.

26. Smith DP, Mason CS, Jones EA, Old RW. A novel nuclear receptor superfamily member in *Xenopus* that associates with RXR, and shares extensive sequence similarity to the mammalian vitamin D_3 receptor. Nucleic Acids Res 1994; 22:66–71.

27. Szpirer S, Szpirer C, Riviere M, Levan G, Maryen P, Cassiman JJ, Wiese R, DeLuca HF. The SP1 transcription factor gene (SP1) and the 1,25-dihydroxyvitamin D receptor gene (VDR) are colocalized on human chromosomal arm 12q and rat chromosome 7. Genomics 1991; 11:168–173.

28. Lazar MA. Thyroid hormone receptors: multiple forms, multiple possibilities. Endocrinol Rev 1993; 14:184–193.

29. Giguère V. Retinoic acid receptors and cellular retinoid binding proteins: complex interplay in retinoid signaling. Endocrinol Rev 1994; 15:61–79.

30. Nagpal S, Friant S, Nakshatri H, Chambon P. RARs and RXRs: evidence for two autonomous transactivation functions (AF-1 and AF-2) and heterodimerization *in vivo*. EMBO J 1993; 12:2349–2360.

31. Giguère V, Tini M, Flock G, Ong E, Evans RM, Otulakowski G. Isoform-specific amino-terminal domains dictate DNA-binding properties of RORα, a novel family of orphan hormone nuclear receptors. Genes Dev 1994; 8:538–553.

32. Glass CK. Differential recognition of target genes by nuclear receptor monomers, dimers, and heterodimers. Endocrinol Rev 1994; 15:391–407.

33. Umesono K, Murakami KK, Thompson CC, Evans RM. Direct repeats as selective response elements for the thyroid hormone, retinoic acid, and vitamin D_3 receptors. Cell 1991; 65:1255–1266.

34. Yu VC, Delsert C, Andersen B, Holloway JM, Devary OV, Näär AM, Kim SY, Boutin J-M, Glass CK, Rosenfeld MG. RXRβ: a coregulator that enhances binding of retinoic acid, thyroid hormone, and vitamin D receptors to their cognate response elements. Cell 1991; 67:1251–1266.

35. Leid M, Kastner P, Lyons R, Nakshatri H, Saunders M, Zacharewski T, Chen J-Y, Staub A, Garnier J-M, Mader S, Chambon P. Purification, cloning, and RXR identity of the HeLa cell factor with which RAR or TR heterodimerizes to bind target sequences efficiently. Cell 1992; 68:377–395.

36. Perlmann T, Rangarajan PN, Umesono K, Evans RM. Determinants for selective RAR and TR recognition of direct repeat HREs. Genes Dev 1993; 7:1411–1422.

37. Kurokawa R, Yu VC, Näär A, Kyakumoto S, Han Z, Silverman S, Rosenfeld MG, Glass CK. Differential orientations of the DNA-binding domain and carboxy-terminal dimerization interface regulate binding site selection by nuclear receptor heterodimers. Genes Dev 1993; 7:1423–1435.

38. Rastinejad F, Perlmann T, Evans RM, Sigler PB. Structural determinants of nuclear receptor assembly on DNA direct repeats. Nature 1995; 375:203–211.

39. Quélo I, Kahlen J-P, Rascle A, Jurdic P, Carlberg C. Identification and characterization of a vitamin D_3 response element of chicken carbonic anhydrase-II. DNA Cell Biol 1994; 13:118–1187.

40. Schräder M, Nayeri S, Kahlen J-P, Müller KM, Carlberg C. Natural vitamin D_3 response elements formed by inverted palindromes: polarity-directed ligand sensitivity of VDR-RXR heterodimer-mediated transactivation. Mol Cell Biol 1995; 15:1154–1161.

41. Kerner SA, Scott RA, Pike JW. Sequence elements in the human osteocalcin gene confer basal activation and inducible response to hormonal vitamin D_3. Proc Natl Acad Sci USA 1989; 36:4455–4459.

42. Morrison NA, Shine J, Fragonas J-C, Verkest V, McMenemey ML, Eisman JA, 1,25-dihydroxyvitamin D-responsive element and glucocorticoid repression in the osteocalcin gene. Science 1989; 246:1158–1161.

43. Schüle R, Umesono K, Mangelsdorf DJ, Bolado J, Pike JW, Evans RM, Jun-Fos and receptors for vitamins A and D recognize a common response element in the human osteocalcin gene. Cell 1990; 61:497–504.

44. Ozono K, Liao J, Kerner SA, Scott RA, Pike JW. The vitamin D-responsive element in the human osteocalcin gene. Association with a nuclear proto-oncogene enhancer. J Biol Chem 1990; 265:21881–21888.

45. Demay MB, Gerardi JM, DeLuca HF, Kronenberg HM. DNA sequences in the rat osteocalcin gene that bind the 1,25-dihydroxyvitamin D_3 receptor and confer responsiveness to 1,25-dihydroxyvitamin D_3. Proc Natl Acad Sci USA 1990; 87:369–373.

46. Polly P, Carlberg C, Eisman JA, Morrison NA. Identification of a vitamin D_3 response element in the fibronectin gene that is bound by vitamin D_3 receptor homodimers. J Cell Biochem 1996; 60:322–333.

47. Chen K-S, DeLuca HF. Cloning of the human 1α,25-dihydroxyvitamin D_3 24-hydroxylase gene promoter and identification of two vitamin D-responsive elements. Biochim Biophys Acta 1995; 1263:1–9.

48. Zierold C, Darwish HM, DeLuca HF. Two vitamin D response elements function in the rat 1,25-dihydroxyvitamin D 24-hydroxylase promoter. J Biol Chem 1995; 270:1675–1678.

49. Candeliere GA, Jurutka PW, Haussler MR, St-Arnaud R. A composite element binding the vitamin D receptor, retinoid X receptor α, and a member of the CTF/NF-1 family of transcription factors mediates the vitamin responsiveness of the c-*fos* promoter. Mol Cell Biol 1996; 16:584–592.

50. Noda M, Vogel RL, Craig AM, Prahl J, DeLuca HF, Denhardt DT. Identification of a DNA sequence responsible for binding of the 1,25-dihydroxyvitamin D_3 receptor and 1,25-dihydroxyvitamin D_3 enhancement of mouse secreted phosphoprotein 1 (*Spp-1* or osteopontin) gene expression. Proc Natl Acad Sci USA 1990; 87:9995–9999.

51. Zhang Q, Wrana JL, Sodek J. Characterization of the promoter region of the porcine opn (osteopontin, secreted phosphoprotein 1) gene. Eur J Biochem 1992; 207:649–659.

52. Kahlen J-P, Carlberg C. Functional characterization of a 1,25 dihydroxyvitamin D_3 receptor binding site found in the rat atrial natriuretic factor promoter. Biochem. Biophys Res Commun 1996; 218:882–886.

53. Liu SM, Koszewski N, Lupez M, Malluche HH, Olivera A, Russell J. Characterization of a response element in the 5′-flanking region of the avian (chicken) PTH gene that mediates negative regulation of gene transcription by 1,25-dihydroxyvitamin D_3 and binds the vitamin D_3 receptor. Mol Endocrinol 1996; 10:206–215.

54. Liu M, Lee M-H, Cohen M, Bommakanti M, Freedman LP. Transcriptional activation of the Cdk inhibitor p21 by vitamin D_3 leads to the induced differentiation of the myelomonocytic cell line U937. Genes Dev 1996; 10:142–153.

55. Demay MB, Kieran MS, DeLuca HF, Kronenberg HM. Sequences in the human parathyroid hormone gene that bind the 1,25-dihydroxyvitamin D_3 receptor and mediate transcriptional repression in response to 1,25-dihydroxyvitamin D_3. Proc Natl Acad Sci USA 1992; 89:8097–8101.

56. Darwish HM, DeLuca HF. Identification of a 1,25-dihydroxyvitamin D_3-response element in the 5′-flanking region of the rat calbindin D-9k gene. Proc Natl Acad Sci USA 1992; 89:603–607.

57. Zierold C, Darwish HM, DeLuca HF. Identification of a vitamin D-response element in the rat calcidiol (25-hydroxyvitamin D_3) 24-hydroxylase gene. Proc Natl Acad Sci USA 1994; 91:900–902.

58. Kremer R, Sebag M, Champigny C, Meerovitch K, Hendy GN, White J, Goltzman D. Identification and characterization of 1,25-dihydroxyvitamin D_3-responsive repressor sequences in the rat parathyroid hormone-related peptide gene. J Biol Chem 1996; 271:16310–16316.

59. Cao X, Ross FP, Zhang L, MacDonald PN, Chappel J, Teitelbaum SL. Cloning of the promoter for the avian integrin β_3 subunit gene and its regulation by 1,25-dihydroxyvitamin D_3. J Biol Chem 1993; 268:27371–27380.

60. Rhodes SJ, Chen R, DiMattia GE, Scully KM, Kalla KA, Lin S-C, Yu VC, Rosenfeld MG. A tissue-specific enhancer confers Pit-1-dependent morphogen inducibility and autoregulation on the *pit-1* gene. Genes Dev 1993; 7:913–932.

61. Gill RK, Christakos S. Identification of sequence elements in mouse calbindin-D28k gene that confer 1,25-dihydroxyvitamin D_3- and butyrate-inducible responses. Proc Natl Acad Sci USA 1993; 90:2984–2988.

62. Xie Z, Bikle DD. Cloning of the human phospholipase C-γ1 promoter and identification of a DR6-type vitamin D-responsive element. J Biol Chem 1997; 272:6573–6577.

63. Schräder M, Kahlen J-P, Carlberg C. Functional characterization of a novel type of 1α,25-dihydroxyvitamin D_3 response element identified in the mouse c-*fos* promoter. Biochem Biophys Res Commun 1997; 230:646–651.

64. Elder JT, Aström A, Pettersson U, Tavakkol A, Krust A, Kastner P, Chambon P, Voorhees JJ. Retinoic acid receptors and binding proteins in human skin. J Invest Dermatol 1992; 98:36S–41S.

65. Mangelsdorf DJ, Evans RM. The RXR heterodimers and orphan receptors. Cell 1995; 83:841–850.

66. Kliewer SA, Umesono K, Noonan DJ, Heyman RA, Evans RM. Convergence of 9-*cis* retinoic acid and peroxisome proliferator signalling pathways through heterodimer formation of their receptors. Nature 1992; 358:771–774.

67. Perlmann T, Jansson L. A novel pathway for vitamin A signaling mediated by RXR heterodimerization with NGFI-B and NURR1. Genes Dev 1995; 9:769–782.

68. Kahlen J-P, Carlberg C. Allosteric interaction of the 1α,25-dihydroxyvitamin D_3 receptor and the retinoid X receptor on DNA. Nucleic Acids Res 1997; 25:4307–4313.

69. Macdonald PN, Dowd DR, Nakajima S, Galligan MA, Reeder MC, Haussler CA, Ozato K, Haussler MR. Retinoid X receptors stimulate and 9-*cis* retinoic acid inhibits 1,25-dihydroxyvitamin D_3-activated expression of the rat osteocalcin gene. Mol Cell Biol 1993; 13:5907–5917.

70. Cheskis B, Freedman LP. Ligand modulates the conversion of DNA-bound vitamin D_3 receptor (VDR) homodimers into VDR-retinoid X receptor heterodimers. Mol Cell Biol 1994; 14:3329–3338.

71. Lemon BD, Freedman LP. Selective effects of ligands on vitamin D_3 receptor- and retinoid X receptor-mediated gene activation in vivo. Mol Cell Biol 1996; 16:1006–1016.

72. Jensen TJ, Hendriksen LO, Solvesten H, Kragballe K. Inhibition of the 1,25-dihydroxyvitamin D_3-induced increase in vitamin D receptor (VDR) levels and binding of VDR-retinoid X receptor (RXR) to a direct repeat (DR)-3 type response element by an RXR-specific ligand in human keratinocyte cultures. Biochem Pharmacol 1998; 55:767–773.

73. Allegretto EA, Shevde N, Zou A, Howell SR, Boehm MF, Hollis BW, Pike JW. Retinoid X receptor acts as a hormone receptor in vivo to induce a key metabolic enzyme for 1,25-dihydroxyvitamin D_3. J Biol Chem 1995; 270:23906–23909.

74. Zou A, Elgort MG, Allegretto EA. Retinoid X receptor (RXR) ligands activate the human 25-hydroxyvitamin D_3-24-hydroxylase promoter via RXR heterodimer binding to two vitamin D-responsive elements and elict additive effects with 1,25-dihydroxyvitamin D_3. J Biol Chem 1997; 272:19027–19034.

75. Cooney AJ, Leng XL, Tsai SY, O'Malley BW, Tsai MJ. Multiple mechanisms of chicken ovalbumin upstream promoter transcription factor-dependent repression of transactivation by the vitamin D, thyroid hormone, and retinoic acid receptors. J Biol Chem 1993; 268:4152–4160.

76. Cooney AJ, Tsai SY, O'Malley BW, Tsai M-J. Chicken ovalbumin upstream promoter transcription factor (COUP-TF) dimers bind to different GGTCA response elements, allowing COUP-TF to repress hormonal induction of the vitamin D_3, thyroid hormone, and retinoic acid receptors. Mol Cell Biol 1992; 12:4153–4163.

77. Green S. Promiscuous liaisons. Nature 1993; 361:590–591.

78. Schräder M, Bendik I, Becker-André M, Carlberg C. Interaction between retinoic acid and vitamin D signaling pathways. J Biol Chem 1993; 268:17830–17836.

79. Schräder M, Müller KM, Becker-André M, Carlberg C. Response element selectivity for heterodimerization of vitamin D receptors with retinoic acid and retinoid X receptors. J Mol Endocrinol 1994; 12:327–339.

80. Schräder M, Müller KM, Carlberg C. Specificity and flexibility of vitamin D signalling: modulation of the activation of natural vitamin D response elements by thyroid hormone. J Biol Chem 1994; 269:5501–5504.

81. Schräder M, Müller KM, Nayeri S, Kahlen J-P, Carlberg C. VDR-T_3R heterodimer polarity directs ligand sensitivity of transactivation. Nature 1994; 370:382–386.

82. MacDonald PN, Haussler CA, Terpening CM, Galligan MA, Reeder MC, Whitfield GK, Haussler MR. Baculovirus-mediated expression of the human vitamin D receptor. J Biol Chem 1991; 266:18808–18813.

83. Carlberg C, Bendik I, Wyss A, Meier E, Sturzenbecker LJ, Grippo JF, Hunziker W. Two nuclear signalling pathways for vitamin D. Nature 1993; 361:657–660.

84. Carlberg C. The vitamin D_3 receptor in the context of the nuclear receptor superfamily: the central role of retinoid X receptor. Endocrine 1996; 4:91–105.

85. Sone T, Ozono K, Pike JW. A 55-kilodalton accessory factor facilitates vitamin D receptor DNA binding. Mol Endocrinol 1991; 5:1578–1586.

86. Laudet V, Stehelin D. Flexible friends. Curr Biol 1992; 2:293–295.

87. Carlberg C. The concept of multiple vitamin D pathways. J Invest Dermatol Symp Proc 1996; 1:10–14.

88. Ettinger RA, DeLuca HF. The vitamin D endocrine system and its therapeutic potential. Adv Drug Res 1996; 28:269–312.

89. Vieth R. The mechanisms of vitamin D toxicity. Bone Min 1990; 11:267–272.

90. Bouillon R, Okamura WH, Norman AW. Structure-function relationships in the vitamin D endocrine system. Endocr Rev 1995; 16:200–257.

91. Jones G, Calverley MJ. A dialogue on analogues. Trends Endocrinol Metabol 1993; 4:297–303.

92. Pols HAP, Birkenhäger JC, van Leeuven JPTM. Vitamin D analogues: from molecule to clinical application. Clin. Endocrinol 1994; 40:285–291.

93. Bouillon R, Verstuyf A, Verlinden L, Allewaert K, Branisteanu D, Mathieu C, van Baelen H. Non-hypercalcemic pharmacological aspects of vitamin D analogs. Biochem Pharmacol 1995; 50:577–583.

94. Bikle DD. Vitamin D: New actions, new analogs, new therapeutic potential. Endocr Rev 1992; 13:765–784.

95. Carlberg C, Mathiasen I, Saurat J-H, Binderup L. The 1,25-dihydroxyvitamin D_3 analogues MC903, EB1089 and KH1060 function as transcriptional activators: vitamin D receptor homodimers show higher ligand sensitivity than heterodimers with retinoid X receptors. J Ster Biochem Mol Biol 1994; 51:137–142.

96. Nayeri S, Danielsson C, Kahlen J-P, Schräder M, Mathiasen IS, Binderup L, Carlberg C. The anti-proliferative effect of vitamin D_3 analogues is not related to the AP-1 pathway, but related to promoter selectivity. Oncogene 1995; 11: 1853–1858.

97. Nayeri S, Mathiasen IS, Binderup L, Carlberg C. High affinity nuclear receptor binding of 20-epi analogues of 1,25 dihydroxyvitamin D_3 correlates well with gene activation. J Cell Biochem 1996; 62:325–333.

98. Mørk Hansen C, Danielsson C, Carlberg C. The potent anti-proliferative effect of 20-epi analogues of 1,25 dihydroxyvitamin D_3 in human breast cancer MCF-7 cells is related to promoter selectivity. Int J Cancer 1996; 67:739–742.

99. Danielsson C, Nayeri S, Wiesinger H, Thieroff-Ekerdt R, Carlberg C. Potent gene regulatory and antiproliferative activities of 20-methyl analoges of 1,25 dihydroxyvitamin D_3. J Cell Biochem 1996; 63:199–206.

100. Danielsson C, Mathiasen IS, James SY, Nayeri S, Bretting C, Mørk Hansen C, Colston KW, Carlberg C. Sensitive induction of apoptosis in breast cancer cells by a novel 1,25-dihydroxyvitamin D_3 analogue is related to promoter selectivity. J Cell Biochem 1997; 66:552–562.

101. Bourguet W, Ruff M, Chambon P, Gronemeyer H, Moras D. Crystal structure of the ligand binding domain of the human nuclear receptor RXR-α. Nature 1995; 375:377–382.

102. Renaud J-P, Rochel N, Ruff M, Vivat V, Chambon P, Gronemeyer H, Moras D. Crystal structure of the RAR-γ ligand-binding domain bound to all-*trans* retinoic acid. Nature 1995; 378:681–689.

103. Wagner RL, Apriletti JW, McGrath ME, West BL, Baxter JD, Fletterick RJ. A structural role for hormone in the thyroid hormone receptor. Nature 1995; 378:690–697.

104. Danielian PS, White R, Lees JA, Parker MG. Identification of a conserved region required for hormone dependent transcriptional activation by steroid hormone receptors. EMBO J 1992; 11:1025–1033.

105. Durand B, Saunders M, Gaudon C, Roy B, Losson R, Chambon P. Activation function 2 (AF-2) of retinoic acid receptor and 9-*cis* retinoid acid receptor: presence of a conserved autonomous constitutive activating domain and influence of the nature of the response element. EMBO J 1994; 13:5370–5382.

106. Jurutka PW, Hsieh J-C, Remus LS, Whitfield GK, Thompson PD, Haussler CA, Blanco JCG, Ozato K, Haussler MR. Mutations in the 1,25-dihydroxyvitamin D_3 receptor identifying C-terminal amino acids required for transcriptional activation that are functionally dissociated from hormone binding, heterodimeric DNA binding, and interaction with transcription factor IIB, *in vitro*. J Biol Chem 1997; 272:14592–14599.

107. Nayeri S, Kahlen J-P, Carlberg C. The high affinity ligand binding conformation of the nuclear 1,25-dihydroxyvitamin D_3 receptor is functionally linked to the transactivation domain 2 (AF-2). Nucleic Acids Res 1996; 24:4513–4519.

108. Allan GF, Leng X, Tsai SY, Weigel NL, Edwards DP, Tsai M-J, O'Malley BW. Hormone and antihormone induce distinct conformational changes which are central to steroid receptor activation. J Biol Chem 1992; 267:19513–19520.

109. Leng X, Tsai S, O'Malley BW, Tsai M-J. Ligand-dependent conformational changes in thyroid hormone and retinoic acid receptors are potentially enhanced by heterodimerization with retinoid X receptor. J Steroid Biochem Mol Biol 1993; 46:643–661.

110. Leid M. Ligand-induced alteration of the protease sensitivity of retinoid X receptor α. J Biol Chem 1994; 269:14175–14181.

111. Keidel S, Lamour FPY, Apfel CM. Mutational analysis reveals that all-*trans*-retinoic acid, 9-*cis*-retinoic acid, and antagonist interact with distinct binding determinants of RARα. J Biol Chem 1997; 272:18267–18272.

112. Dowell P, Peterson VJ, Zabriskie TM, Leid M. Ligand-induced peroxisome proliferator-activated receptor α conformational change. J Biol Chem 1997; 272:2013–2020.

113. Janowski BA, Willy PJ, Devi TR, Falck JR, Mangelsdorf DJ. An oxysterol signalling pathway mediated by the nuclear receptor LXRα. Nature 1996; 383:728–731.

114. Peleg S, Sastry M, Collins ED, Bishop JE, Norman AW. Distinct conformational changes induced by 20-epi analogues of 1α,25-dihydroxyvitamin D_3 are associated with enhanced activation of the vitamin D receptor. J Biol Chem 1995; 270:10551–10558.

115. Nayeri S, Carlberg C. Functional conformations of the nuclear 1α,25-dihydroxyvitamin D_3 receptor. Biochem J 1997; 235:561–568.

116. Liu Y-Y, Collins ED, Norman AW, Peleg S. Differential interaction of 1α,25-dihydroxyvitamin D_3 analogues and their 20-epi homologues with the vitamin D receptor. J Biol Chem 1997; 272:3336–3345.

117. Ikeda M, Wilcox EC, Chin WW. Different DNA elements can modulate the conformation of thyroid hormone receptor heterodimer and its transcriptional activity. J Biol Chem 1996; 271:23096–23104.

118. Staal A, van Wijnen AJ, Birkenhäger JC, Pols HAP, Prahl J, DeLuca HF, Gaub M-P, Lian JB, Stein GS, van Leeuwen JPTM, Stein JL. Distinct conformations of vitamin D receptor/retinoid X receptor-a heterodimers are specified by dinucleotide differences in the vitamin D-responsive elements of the osteocalcin and osteopontin genes. Mol Endocrinol 1996; 10:1444–1456.

119. Garcia-Villalba P, Jimenez-Lara AM, Aranda A. Vitamin D interferes with transactivation of the growth hormone gene by thyroid hormone and retinoid acid. Mol Cell Biol 1996; 16:318–327.

120. Yen PM, Liu Y, Sugawara A, Chin WW. Vitamin D receptors repress basal transcription and exert dominant negative activity on triiodothyronine-mediated transcriptional activity. J Biol Chem 1996; 271:10910–10916.

121. Alroy I, Towers TL, Freedman LP. Transcriptional repression of the interleukin-2 gene by vitamin D_3: direct inhibition of NFATp/AP-1 complex formation by a nuclear hormone receptor. Mol Cell Biol 1995; 15:5789–5799.

122. Polly P, Carlberg C, Eisman JA, Morrison NA. 1α,25-dihydroxyvitamin D_3 receptor as a mediator of transrepression of retinoid signalling. J Cell Biochem 1997; 67:287–296.

123. Korzus E, Torchia J, Rose DW, Xu L, Kurokawa R, McInerney EM, Mullen T-M, Glass CK, Rosenfeld MG. Transcription factor-specific requirements for coactivators and their acetyltransferase function. Science 1998; 279:703–706.

124. Wu C. Chromatin remodeling and control of gene expression. J Biol Chem 1997; 272:28171–28174.

125. Eckner R. p300 and CBP as transcriptional regulators and targets of oncogenic events. Biol Chem 1996; 377:685–688.

126. Pazin MJ, Kadonaga JT. What's up and down with histone deacetylation and transcription? Cell 1997; 89:325–328.

127. Chakravarti D, LaMorte VJ, Nelson MC, Nakajima T, Schulman IG, Juguilon H, Montminy M, Evans RM. Role of CBP/p300 in nuclear receptor signalling. Nature 1996; 383:99–103.

128. Hanstein B, Eckner R, DiRenzo J, Halachmi S, Liu H, Searcy B, Kurokawa R, Brown M. p300 is a component of an estrogen receptor coactivator complex. Proc Natl Acad Sci USA 1996; 93:11540–11545.

129. Torchia J, Rose DW, Inostroza J, Kamei Y, Westin S, Glass CK, Rosenfeld MG. The transcriptional coactivator p/CIP binds and mediates nuclear-receptor function. Nature 1997; 387:677–684.

130. Dowell P, Ishmael JE, Avram D, Peterson VJ, Nevrivy DJ, Leid M. p300 functions as a coactivator for the peroxisome proliferator-activated receptor. J Biol Chem 1997; 272:22435–33443.

131. Onate SA, Tsai SY, Tsai MJ, O'Malley BW. Sequence and characterization of a coactivator for the steroid hormone receptor superfamily. Science 1995; 270:1354–1357.

132. Voegel JJ, Heine MJS, Zechel C, Chambon P, Gronemeyer H. TIF2, a 160 kDa transcriptional mediator for the ligand-dependent activation function AF-2 of nuclear receptors. EMBO J 1996; 15:3667–3675.

133. Li H, Gomes PJ, Chen JD. RAC3, a steroid/nuclear receptor-associated coactivator that is related to SRC-1 and TIF2. Proc Natl Acad Sci USA 1997; 94:8479–8484.

134. Cavaillès V, Dauvois S, L`Horset F, Lopez G, Hoare S, Kushner PJ, Parker MG. Nuclear factor RIP140 modulates transcriptional activation by the estrogen receptor. EMBO J 1995; 14:3741–3751.

135. Le Dourain B, Zechel C, Garnier J-M, Lutz Y, Tora L, Pierrat B, Heery D, Gronemeyer H, Chambon H, Chambon P, Losson R. The N-terminal part of TIF1, a putative mediator of the ligand-dependent activation function (AF-2) of nuclear receptors, is fused to B-raf in the oncogenic protein T18. EMBO J 1995; 14:2020–2033.

136. vom Baur E, Zechel C, Heery D, Heine MJS, Garnier JM, Vivat V, Le Dourain B, Gronemeyer H, Chambon P, Losson R. Differential ligand-dependent interactions between the AF-2 activating domain of nuclear receptors and the putative transcriptional intermediary factors mSUG1 and TIF1. EMBO J 1996; 15:110–124.

137. Henttu PMA, Kalkhoven E, Parker MG. AF-2 activity and recruitment of steroid receptor coactivator 1 to the estrogen receptor depend on a lysine residue conserved in nuclear receptors. Mol Cell Biol 1997; 17:1832–1839.

138. Zamir I, Zhang J, Lazar MA. Stoichiometrie and steric principles governing repression by nuclear hormone receptors. Genes Dev 1997; 11:835–846.

139. Lin BC, Hong S-H, Krig S, Yoh SM, Privalsky ML. A conformational switch in nuclear hormone receptors is involved in coupling hormone binding to corepressor release. Mol Cell Biol 1997; 17:6131–6138.

140. Wagner BL, Norris JD, Knotts TA, Weigel NL, McDonnell DP. The nuclear coreceptor NCoR and SMRT are key regulators of both ligand- and 8-bromo-cyclic AMP-dependent transcriptional activity of the human progesterone receptor. Mol Cell Biol 1998; 18:1369–1378.

141. Gill RK, Atkins LM, Hollis BW, Bell NH. Mapping the domains of the interaction of the vitamin D receptor and steroid receptor coactivator-1. Mol Endocrinol 1998; 12:57–65.

142. Hong H, Kohli K, Garabedian MJ, Stallcup MR. GRIP1, a transcriptional coactivator for the AF-2 transactivation domain of steroid, thyroid, retinoid, and vitamin D receptors. Mol Cell Biol 1997; 17:2735–2744.

143. Li H, Chen JD. The receptor-associated coactivator 3 activates transcription through CREB-binding protein recruitment and autoregulation. J Biol Chem 1998; 273:5948–5954.

144. Xu J, Qiu Y, DeMayo FJ, Tsai SY, Tsai M-J, O'Malley BW. Partial hormone resistance in mice with disruption of the steroid receptor coactivator-1 (SRC-1) gene. Science 1998; 279:1922–1925.

145. Berghöfer-Hochheimer Y, Zurek C, Wölfl S, Hemmerich P, Munder T. L7 is a coregulator of vitamin D receptor-retinoid X receptor-mediated transactivation. J Cell Biochem 1998; 69:1–12.

2

The Vitamin D Receptor and Its Regulation in the Skin

Henrik Sølvsten
Marselisborg Hospital, University of Aarhus, Aarhus, Denmark

I. THE VITAMIN D RECEPTOR

Vitamin D carries out its physiological functions on calcium and bone metabolism in amphibians, reptiles, birds, mammals, and humans through the active metabolite 1,25-dihydroxyvitamin D_3 [1,25$(OH)_2D_3$]. These effects are mediated through the intracellular located vitamin D receptor (VDR), which functions as a transcription factor and is represented by approximately 0.001% of the total amount of protein in the cell [1]. Through evolution, the VDR has been highly conserved with a strong homology between species, and in the N-terminal portion of the receptor containing the DNA binding domain there is 95% identity between avian and human VDR. The VDR is a member of the nuclear receptor superfamily. Receptors belonging to this family appear to arise from a single ancestral gene and they are all constructed in a similar manner, with a DNA binding domain close to the N-terminal and a ligand-binding domain at the carboxy terminal (Figure 1). The first experimental evidence of a human receptor for vitamin D came with the discovery of a soluble factor of 50.000–70.000 Da able to bind the intestinal metabolite of vitamin D in a saturable fashion [2]. The VDR is a phosphoprotein containing 427 amino acids and has a calculated molecular mass of approximately 48.000 Da (Figure 1).

Like other members of the superfamily, the VDR is made up of several functional domains. The VDR-DNA interactions reside between amino acid residues 22–113, as shown by limited proteolysis [3], site directed mutagenesis [4], and C-terminal deletion mutants [5]. The first eight of nine cysteine residues are important for the tetrahedrally folding and the binding of two zinc ions to form

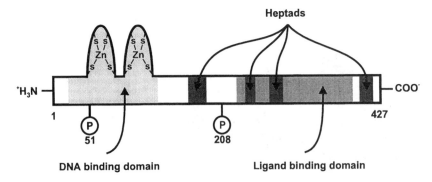

Figure 1   Schematic depiction of the VDR, including the different functional domains and the sites for phosphorylation. See text for further description.

the two zinc fingers [4] (Figure 1). Although not finally established for the VDR, the zinc ions are believed to be important for the DNA binding for all the receptors of the superfamily. The specificity of the VDR binding to specific DNA sequences (vitamin D response elements) seems to rely on the carboxy-terminal portion of the zinc fingers [6]. Substitution of few specific amino acids can change the ability of the DNA binding domain from high affinity for a vitamin D response element (VDRE) to affinity for another type of response element (e.g., thyroid hormone response element).

The ligand-binding domain is less defined than the DNA-binding domain. Using limited proteolysis from the C-terminal region of the chicken VDR, it has been described that deletion of only few amino acids results in a decreased binding of $1,25(OH)_2D_3$. The three-dimensional structure has not been fully described for VDR, but ligand-binding studies have described the ligand-binding domain to be very sensitive to the structure of the ligand. The natural active form of vitamin D $1,25(OH)_2D_3$ binds with highest affinity to the receptor with an equilibrium dissociation constant, Kd, in cultured human keratinocytes of approximately 200 pM (7,8). This binding is clearly lower for other natural forms of vitamin D–like 25-hydroxyvitamin D_3, 1,24,25-trihydroxyvitamin D_3, and 24,25-dihydroxyvitamin D_3. This indicates that the hydroxylation both the C-1 and C-25 are important for the binding to the receptor, while the hydroxylation at C-24, the first metabolic step in the degradation of $1,25(OH)_2D_3$, diminishes the binding to the receptor.

The domain for the protein-protein interactions with VDR and its heterodimeric partner has not finally been established. The "domain" might be have several locations on the protein and then probably connected by folding of the protein to its biologically active three-dimensional structure. Furthermore, the protein-protein contact with the heterodimeric partner might be located at different sites depending on which heterodimeric partner is connected to VDR. Forman and Samuels have described how nine highly conserved heptads (Figure 1) in the ligand binding domain of VDR, RARα, β, and γ, $T_3R\alpha$ and β [9] might participate in protein-protein interactions. By making a hydrophobic surface along one side of a helix, they may act as an dimerization interface. At least two of these heptads have been described to be important for the heterodimerization of VDR with a nuclear accessory factor and the subsequent binding to a VDRE [10]. The nuclear accessory factor was later found to be RXR, the best-described heterodimeric partner for VDR.

The human VDR is a phosphoprotein. The phosphorylation is a ligand-dependent event and occurs shortly (1–2 hr) after stimulation with $1,25(OH)_2D_3$ [11,12]. It has indirectly been described to occur at serine-51 because mutation of this amino acid diminishes the phosphorylation of the receptor [13,14]. These results have, however, not been confirmed by other groups, and phosphorylation has also been described at serine-208 [15–17]. There is no final evidence for the functional effect of the phosphorylation of the VDR. Many transcription factors and all members of the steroid receptor superfamily are phosphoproteins, and phosphorylation has been implicated in DNA binding capacity, transcriptional activation, and cytoplasma to nuclear trafficking [18].

The effects of $1,25(OH)_2D_3$ are closely related to the levels of VDR, but a functionally active and highly expressed VDR is not always sufficient for the growth-inhibitory response of $1,25(OH)_2D_3$. Keratinocytes from a squamous carcinoma cell line have failed to regulate differentiation despite VDR levels equivalent to normal keratinocytes and appropriate regulation of endogenous $25(OH)D_3$ metabolism [19]. This is, however, not constantly demonstrated in squamous carcinoma cell lines, and another study has shown calcipotriol to have the ability to considerably control complex defects in the regulation of proliferation and differentiation [20]. These observations demonstrate that an alteration of the growth inhibitory response to $1,25(OH)_2D_3$ might occur when keratinocytes acquire the malignant phenotype and that the alteration lies beyond the interaction of the ligand with the receptor.

II. LOCALIZATION OF THE VDR IN THE SKIN

The distribution of the vitamin D receptor has not only been restricted to the cells and organs involved in calcium homeostasis and bone metabolism. The VDR is widely distributed in few or all cell types in almost all organs (for review, see Ref. 21), indicating that $1,25(OH)_2D_3$ exerts effects not only on calcium homeostasis. The observation that $1,25(OH)_2D_3$ induces keratinocyte differentiation was first made by Hosomi et al. [22] and provided a rationale for the previous and unexpected finding of the VDR in the skin [23]. In the skin, strong experimental evidence exists that skin diseases other than psoriasis may be responsive to the effects of vitamin D_3 or its analogues (see Chapters 25 to 27). Thus the VDR has been detected by ligand binding or immunoblotting in most cell types in the skin (Table 1), including keratinocytes [23], Langerhans cells [24], melanocytes [25], fibroblasts [26], and endothelial cells [27]. Furthermore, cells involved in inflammatory skin reactions like monocytes and activated T lymphocytes also express the VDR [28].

The subcellular distribution of the unoccupied VDR is a matter of controversy. The unoccupied VDR has both been described to be located mainly in the cytoplasma and in the nucleus. The distribution in human skin has been described by immunohistochemistry [29] and, in mouse skin, by protein extraction of a tissue-homogenate by different ionic strength buffers [30]. However, both methods have their limitation and the description of the VDR always has to be with the reservation that receptor instability might be of concern [31,32] and that VDR only represents approximately 0.001% of the total amount of protein in the cell [1]. In conclusion, previous results indicate that the VDR is located in both the cytoplasm and the nucleus and that VDR is translocated from the cytoplasm to the nucleus in the presence of its ligand.

The in vivo distribution of the VDR in the different layers and appendages of the epidermis in normal human skin is best visualized by immunohistochemistry [29]. However, previously presented data should be interpreted with the precaution that the anti-VDR antibody used is known to have non-VDR cross-reacting proteins as determined by immunoblotting [32]. In general, the staining intensity of VDR was stronger in the basal layers than in upper layers. However, single scattered cells in the upper stratum spinosum and stratum granulosum were found to be heavily stained as well [29]. These in vivo data has been confirmed in vitro in cultured keratinocytes, demonstrating increased VDR levels in undifferentiated compared with differentiated keratinocytes from the same donor [7,33]. Furthermore, by immunohistochemistry, VDR was demonstrated in melanocytes,

Table 1 Target Cells for Vitamin D in the Skin with Detectable VDR

Keratinocytes [21]
Langerhans cells [22]
Melanocytes [23]
Fibroblasts [24]
Endothelial cells [25]
Dermal dendrocytes/monocytes [26]
B and T lymphocytes [27]

Langerhans cells, and the cells of the pilosebaceous apparatus. The cells of the pilosebaceous apparatus contained the most heavily stained nuclei found in the normal skin section. The undifferentiated cells in the outer layer of the sebaceous glands stained more intensively than more differentiated, centrally located cells.

III. HETEROLOGOUS REGULATION OF THE VDR IN THE SKIN

The VDR is fundamental for $1,25(OH)_2D_3$ to exerts its genomic actions. Accordingly the cellular response to $1,25(OH)_2D_3$ has been described to correlate in several tissues with the receptor number. In the skin, similar results have been demonstrated in vitro by the fact that overexpression of VDR in cultured keratinocytes results in increased $1,25(OH)_2D_3$-induced transcriptional activity [34].

Several factors have been described to influence the level of the VDR in different tissues. However, only few studies have been described in cellular systems derived from the skin. As a general rule, VDR levels are correlated to the rate of cell division, as illustrated in T lymphocytes, with resting T lymphocytes having no detectable VDR or VDR mRNA while activated, proliferating T lymphocytes expresses high levels of the VDR [28]. In the skin, similar results are described in vivo and in vitro with increased levels of VDR in proliferating keratinocytes from the basal layers in the epidermis [7,29,33] with mitogenic factors such as serum, epidermal growth factor, insulin-like growth factor I, and insulin causing an increase of the VDR levels in the mouse fibroblasts 3T3 cell line [35]. Furthermore, although not described in the skin, it is of interest that glucocorticoids influence the level of VDR and the sensitivity of $1,25(OH)_2D_3$. In rat calvarial osteoblast-like cells, dexamethasone doubled the VDR level and potentiated the bioresponse of $1,25(OH)_2D_3$ (36). In contrast, when human osteosarcoma cells were stimulated with dexamethasone, the VDR level as well as the VDR mRNA level were decreased [37]. In conclusion, glucocorticoids seems to influence the vitamin D system at the receptor level, but the direction of the involvement at the molecular level is still controversial. However, in the skin combined therapy of psoriasis with twice-daily application of either calcipotriene ointment or a glucocorticoid indicates either additive or a superadditive effect of the combination (see Chapter 13).

IV. HOMOLOGOUS REGULATION OF THE VDR IN THE SKIN

In addition to the classical viewed role of $1,25(OH)_2D_3$-activation of the receptor, other studies have demonstrated that $1,25(OH)_2D_3$ may serve to amplify signal response via homologous upregulation of its own receptor [38,39]. In the literature, no final answer has been given about the mechanism behind the homologous upregulation of the VDR protein.

It has been suggested in studies of mouse fibroblasts 3T6 cells [1,40], human osteosarcoma cells [41], and the breast cancer cell MCF-7 (35) that the upregulation of the VDR is a result of increased transcriptional activity with increased transcriptional level of VDR mRNA. However, the results in the mouse fibroblast 3T6 cell line are in contrast to a study describing the upregulation in the same cell line to be mediated as a result of a ligand-induced stabilization [39].

Cultured keratinocytes are also target cells for homologous upregulation of the VDR after stimulation with $1,25(OH)_2D_3$. As demonstrated by immunoblotting [33] in a time-course study in cultured keratinocytes, VDR was upregulated after 2 hr, having maximum after 8 hr and still having VDR levels above basic level in unstimulated preconfluent cultured human keratinocytes after 24 hr, as demonstrated in Figure 2. However, despite continuous stimulation with $1,25(OH)_2D_3$, VDR decreases below starting level after 2–4 days, probably as a result of increased differentiation of the cells [42]. The VDR increase was preceded by an increase of VDR mRNA after 1/2–2 hr and a later increase after 16–24 hr, indicating that the increase of the receptor level was dependent on mRNA synthesis (Figure 2). The increase of VDR mRNA was statistically insignificant, and another study of VDR mRNA could not confirm the regulation after few hours. However, it also demonstrated an upregulation of the message after 24 hr [43]. The importance of the late upregulation of the VDR mRNA is doubtful and not followed by a regulation at the protein level. The regulation of VDR mRNA after more than 24 hr of stimulation has not been described, but the level is expected to decrease below starting level in a similar way as the VDR protein.

Figure 2 The time-dependent intracellular cascade of events in cultured human keratinocytes after stimulation with $1,25(OH)_2D_3$. (1) VDR mRNA levels with a peak 1–2 hr a lower peak with maximum approximately 24 hr after start of stimulation. VDR mRNA levels are expected to decrease below starting level after 2–3 days of stimulation. The "?" refers to data have not been statistically significant in the cited article (see text). (2) The VDR increases after 2 hr and reaches a maximum after 8 hr. It remain increased above starting level after more than 24 hr but decreases below starting level after 2–3 days of stimulation with $1,25(OH)_2D_3$. The binding of VDR-RXR to the VDRE follow the increase of VDR levels. (3) The transcriptional activity of vitamin D–sensitive genes begins shortly after VDR levels are increased and has a peak activity after 16 hr of stimulation with $1,25(OH)_2D_3$. (4) The biological effects of $1,25(OH)_2D_3$ with increased differentiation and decreased proliferation in cultured keratinocytes begins after day of stimulation and slowly reach maximum after 3–4 days of stimulation with $1,25(OH)_2D_3$. The dotted line in all graphs indicates the level prior to stimulation with $1,25(OH)_2D_3$.

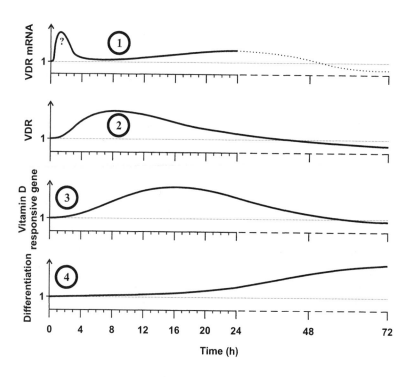

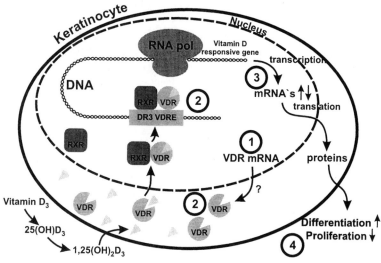

The biological relevance of the homologous upregulation of the VDR have been demonstrated by the concurrent increase of the transcriptional activity of a vitamin D–sensitive gene. The 1,25-dihydroxyvitamin D_3-24-hydroxylase (24-OHase), a vitamin D–sensitive gene with two DR-3 vitamin D response elements (VDRE) in its promotor region [44], was upregulated in a time-dependent manner with a maximum after 16–24 hr in the same keratinocytes where the ligand-induced receptor-upregulation was demonstrated after 8 hr (Figure 2) (45). Furthermore, although not demonstrated in the same cells, these intracellular events in the keratinocyte correspond well with the biological response of $1,25(OH)_2D_3$, with increased differentiation and decreased proliferation after 2–4 days [42].

A similar cascade of intracellular events has been demonstrated after topical application of $1,25(OH)_2D_3$ or the vitamin D analogue calcipotriene in vivo in normal human skin. After topical application of calcipotriene under occlusion for 4 days, the VDR levels were increased approximately 50% from 56 pg/µg protein to 82 pg/µg protein in normal human skin [46]. The ligand-induced VDR increase was accompanied by increased binding to a DR-3 vitamin D response element, indicating that the receptor upregulation is biological relevant and an important mechanism whereby calcipotriene mediates its effects in human skin. However, the underlying mechanism behind the upregulation of the VDR increase in vivo in normal human skin has not finally been described with concurrent measurement of VDR and VDR mRNA in a time study.

In psoriatic skin, VDR has been detected both by immunoblotting and immunohistochemistry [29,32]. In protein extracts from keratomed biopsies similar levels (approximately 50 pg/µg protein) of VDR were found in lesional psoriatic skin, nonlesional psoriatic skin, and normal human skin as determined by immunoblotting. Furthermore, no differences of VDR mRNA were observed either [32]. By immunohistochemistry a small increase of VDR was found in basal as well as suprabasal layers of keratinocytes in lesional compared with nonlesional psoriatic skin [32]. These two studies seems to contradicts each other. However, studies were carried out with different methods and small differences of VDR levels in psoriatic skin, including inflammatory cells and hyperproliferative dedifferentiated keratinocytes compared with nonlesional skin, seem not to be of major importance. Furthermore, the biological function of the receptor are also preserved in psoriatic skin as demonstrated by its ability to bind to vitamin D response elements, and also in psoriatic skin the receptor level are strictly correlated to the receptor level [47]. In conclusion, VDR and its message are detectable and biologically active in psoriatic skin.

The homologous regulation of the VDR after topical application of $1,25(OH)_2D_3$ or its analogs has not been intensively described in psoriatic skin. A study has demonstrated that VDR mRNA levels were increased after topical application of $1,25(OH)_2D_3$ in patients with clinical improvement in contrast to patients with no clinical improvement [48]. The upregulation might, however, be explained by a heterologous regulation and secondary to the clinical improvement of $1,25(OH)_2D_3$ with differentiation of the keratinocytes and effects on epidermal immunoregulatory cells.

A full description of the VDR and its influence at the vitamin D system should also include the interaction with the heterodimeric partner RXR and its natural and synthetic ligands. The molecular cross-talk between $1,25(OH)_2D_3$, retinoids and their cognate receptors in vivo is important and may provide information about an eventual synergistic effect, - an interesting topic from a clinical point of view. This description is beyond the scope of this chapter and is discussed in Chapter 10.

In conclusion, the ability of $1,25(OH)_2D_3$ and its analog to regulate growth and differentiation in human skin is closely linked to the level and regulation of the VDR, and homologous VDR upregulation is one of the first steps of the intracellular cascade of events responsible for the biological effects of $1,25(OH)_2D_3$.

REFERENCES

1. McDonnell DP, Mangelsdorf DJ, Pike JW, Haussler MR, O'Malley BW. Molecular cloning of complementary DNA encoding the avian receptor for vitamin D. Science 1987; 235:1214–1217.
2. Haussler MR, Norman AW. Chromosomal receptor for a vitamin D metabolite. Proc Natl Acad Sci USA 1969; 62:155–162.
3. Allegretto EA, Pike JW, Haussler MR. Immunochemical detection of unique proteolytic fragments of the chick 1,25-dihydroxyvitamin D_3 receptor: distinct 20-kDa DNA-binding and 45-kDa hormone-binding species. J Biol Chem 1987; 262:1312–1319.
4. Sone T, Kerner S, Pike JW. Vitamin D receptor interaction with specific DNA: association as a 1,25-dihydroxyvitamin D_3-modulated heterodimer. J Biol Chem 1991; 266:23296–23305.
5. McDonnell DP, Scott RA, Kerner SA, O'Malley BW, Pike JW. Functional domains of the human vitamin D_3 receptor regulate osteocalcin gene expression. Mol Endocrinol 1989; 3:635–644.
6. Ing NH, O'Malley BW. The steroid hormone receptor superfamily: molecular mechanisms of action. In: Molecular Endocrinology: Basic Concepts and Clinical Correlations. New York: Raven Press, 1995, pp. 195–215.
7. Pillai S, Bikle DD, Elias PM. 1,25-Dihydroxyvitamin D production and receptor binding in human keratinocytes varies with differentiation. J Biol Chem 1988; 263:5390–5395.
8. Fogh K, Sølvsten H, Jønhke H, Kragballe K. All-trans retinoic acid inhibits binding of 1,25-dihydroxyvitamin D_3 to the vitamin D receptor in cultured human keratinocytes. Exp Dermatol 1996; 5:24–27.
9. Forman BM, Samuels HH. Interactions among a subfamily of nuclear hormone receptors: the regulatory zipper model. Mol Endocrinol 1990; 4:1293–1301.

10. Nakajima S, Hsieh JC, MacDonald PN, Galligan MA, Haussler CA, Whitfield GK, Haussler MR. The C-terminal region of the vitamin D receptor is essential to form a complex with a receptor auxiliary factor required for high affinity binding to the vitamin D-responsive element. Mol Endocrinol 1994; 8:159–172.

11. Brown TA, DeLuca HF. Phosphorylation of the 1,25-dihydroxyvitamin D_3 receptor. A primary event in 1,25-dihydroxyvitamin D_3 action. J Biol Chem 1990; 265:10025–10029.

12. Pike JW, Sleator NM. Hormone-dependent phosphorylation of the 1,25-dihydroxyvitamin D_3 receptor in mouse fibroblasts. Biochem Biophys Res Commun 1985; 131:378–385.

13. Hsieh JC, Jurutka PW, Galligan MA, Terpening CM, Haussler CA, Samuels DS, Shimizu Y, Shimizu N, Haussler MR. Human vitamin D receptor is selectively phosphorylated by protein kinase C on serine 51, a residue crucial to its trans-activation function. Proc Natl Acad Sci USA 1991; 88:9315–9319.

14. Hsieh JC, Jurutka PW, Nakajima S, Galligan MA, Haussler CA, Shimizu Y, Shimizu N, Whitfield GK, Haussler MR. Phosphorylation of the human vitamin D receptor by protein kinase C: biochemical and functional evaluation of the serine 51 recognition site. J Biol Chem 1993; 268:15118–15126.

15. Hilliard GM, Cook RG, Weigel NL, Pike JW. 1,25-dihydroxyvitamin D_3 modulates phosphorylation of serine 205 in the human vitamin D receptor: site-directed mutagenesis of this residue promotes alternative phosphorylation. Biochemistry. 1994; 33:4300–4311.

16. Brown TA, DeLuca HF. Sites of phosphorylation and photoaffinity labeling of the 1,25-dihydroxyvitamin D_3 receptor. Arch Biochem Biophys. 1991; 286:466–472.

17. Jurutka PW, Hsieh J-C, MacDonald PN, Terpening CM, Hausler CA, Haussler MR. Phosphorylation of serine 208 in the human vitamin D receptor. J Biol Chem 1993; 268:6791–6799.

18. Kuiper GG, Brinkmann AO. Steroid hormone receptor phosphorylation: is there a physiological role? Mol Cell Endocrinol 1994; 100:103–107.

19. Ratnam AV, Bikle DD, Su MJ, Pillai S. Squamous carcinoma cell lines fail to respond to 1,25-dihydroxyvitamin D despite normal levels of the vitamin D receptor. J Invest Dermatol 1996; 106:522–525.

20. Cho KO, Son YS, Lee DY, Chung EK, Hur KC, Hong SI, Fuchs E. Calcipotriol (MC 903), a synthetic derivative of vitamin D_3 stimulates differentiation of squamous carcinoma cell line in the raft culture. Anticancer Cancer Res 1996; 16:337–347.

21. Hannah SS, Norman AW. 1a,25(OH)$_2$ Vitamin D_3-regulated expression of the eukaryotic genome. Nutr Rev 1994; 52:376–382.

22. Hosomi J, Hosoi J, Abe E, Suda T, Kuroki T. Regulation of terminal differentiation of cultured mouse epidermal cells by 1 alpha,25-dihydroxyvitamin D_3. Endocrinology 1983; 113:1950–1957.

23. Feldman D, Chen T, Hirst M, Colston K, Karasek M, Cone C. Demonstration of 1,25-dihydroxyvitamin D_3 receptors in human skin biopsies. J Clin Endocrinol Metab 1980; 51:1463–1465.

24. Dam TN, Møller B, Hindkjaer J, Kragballe K. The vitamin D analog calcipotriol suppresses the number and antigen-presenting function of Langerhans cells in normal human skin. J Invest Dermatol 1996; 1:S72–S77.

25. Ranson M, Posen S, Manson R. Human melanocytes as a target tissue for hormones: in vitro studies with 1,25-dihydroxyvitamin D_3, apha-melanocyte stimulating hormone, beta-estradiol. J Invest Dermatol 1988; 91:593–598.

26. Eil C, Marx S. Nuclear uptake of 1,25-dihydroxy cholecalciferol in dispersed fibroblasts cultured from normal human skin. Proc Natl Acad Sci USA 1981; 78:2562–2566.

27. Merke J, Milde P, Lewicka S, Hugel U, Klaus G, Mangelsdorf DJ, Haussler MR, Rauterberg EW, Ritz E. Identification and regulation of 1,25-dihydroxyvitamin D_3 receptor activity and biosynthesis of 1,25-dihydroxyvitamin D_3: studies in cultured bovine aortic endothelial cells and human dermal capillaries. J Clin Invest 1989; 83:1903–1915.

28. Bhalla AK, Amento EP, Clemens TL, Holick MF, Krane SM. Specific high-affinity receptors for 1,25-dihydroxyvitamin D_3 in human peripheral blood mononuclear cells: presence in monocytes and induction in T lymphocytes following activation. J Clin Endocrinol Metab 1983; 57:1308–1310.

29. Milde P, Hauser U, Simon T, Mall G, Ernst V, Haussler MR, Frosch P, Rauterberg EW. Expression of 1,25-dihydroxyvitamin D_3 receptors in normal and psoriatic skin. J Invest Dermatol 1991; 97:230–239.

30. Clemens TL, Horiuchi N, Nguyen M, Holick MF. Binding of 1,25-dihydroxy-[3H]vitamin D_3 in nuclear and cytosol fractions of whole mouse skin in vivo and in vitro. FEBS Lett 1981; 134:203–206.

31. Norman AW, Hunziker W, Walters MR, Bishop JE. Differential effects of protease inhibitors on 1,25-dihydroxyvitamin D_3 receptors. J Biol Chem 1983; 258:12876–12880.

32. Sølvsten H, Fogh K, Svendsen ML, Kristensen P, Kumar R, Kragballe K. Normal levels of the vitamin D receptor and its message in psoriatic skin. J Invest Dermatol 1996; 1:S28–S32.

33. Sølvsten H, Svendsen ML, Fogh K, Kragballe K. Upregulation of vitamin D receptor levels by 1,25(OH)$_2$-vitamin D_3 in cultures of normal human keratinocytes. Arch Dermatol Res 1997; 289:367–372.

34. Henriksen LØ, Kragballe K, Jensen TG, Fogh K. Transcriptional activation by 1,25-dihydroxyvitamin D_3 and synthetic analogues in transfected cultures of human keratinocytes. Skin Pharmacol 1997; 10:12–20.

35. Krishnan AV, Feldman D. Stimulation of 1,25-dihydroxyvitamin D_3 receptor gene expression in cultured cells by serum and growth factors. J Bone Min Res 1991; 6:1099–1107.

36. Chen TL, Hauschka PV, Feldman D. Dexamethasone increases 1,25-dihydroxyvitamin D_3 receptor levels and augments bioresponses in rat osteoblast-like cells. Endocrinology 1986; 118:1119–1126.

37. Godschalk M, Levy JR, Downs RW Jr. Glucocorticoids decrease vitamin D receptor number and gene expression in human osteosarcoma cells. J Bone Min Res 1992; 7:21–27.

38. Santiso-Mere D, Sone T, Hilliard GM 4th, Pike JW, McDonnell DP. Positive regulation of the vitamin D receptor by its cognate ligand in heterologous expression systems. Mol Endocrinol 1993; 7:833–839.

39. Wiese RJ, Uhland Smith A, Ross TK, Prahl JM, DeLuca HF. Up-regulation of the vitamin D receptor in response to 1,25-dihydroxyvitamin D_3 results from ligand-induced stabilization. J Biol Chem 1992; 267:20082–20086.

40. Mangelsdorf DJ, Pike JW, Haussler MR. Avian and mammalian receptors for 1,25-dihydroxyvitamin D_3: in vitro translation to characterize size and hormone-dependent regulation. Proc Natl Acad Sci USA 1987; 84:354–358.

41. Dokoh S, Donaldson CA, Haussler MR. Influence of 1,25-dihydroxyvitamin D_3 on cultured osteogenic sarcoma cells: correlation with the 1,25-dihydroxyvitamin D_3 receptor. Cancer Res 1984; 44:2103–2109.

42. Svendsen ML, Daneels G, Geysen J, Binderup L, Kragballe K. Proliferation and differentiation of cultured human keratinocytes is modulated by 1,25(OH)$_2$D$_3$ and synthetic vitamin D_3 analogues in a cell density-, calcium- and serum-dependent manner. Pharmacol Toxicol 1997; 80:49–56.

43. Hanafin NM, Persons KS, Holick MF. The mRNA expression of the human 1,25-dihydroxyvitamin D_3 receptor and the c-*myc* protooncogene in cultured human keratinocytes. In Vitro Cell Dev Biol 1994; 30A:187–191.

44. Chen KS, DeLuca HF. Cloning of the human 1a,25-dihydroxy-vitamin D_3 24-hydroxylase gene promoter and identification of two vitamin D-responsive elements. Biochem Biophys Acta 1995; 1263:1–9.

45. Jensen TJ. Regulation of the vitamin D receptor in human skin and its DNA binding ability. Master's thesis, University of Aarhus, Aarhus, Denmark, 1997.

46. Sølvsten H, Jensen TJ, Sørensen S, Kragballe K. Calcipotriol increases the vitamin D receptor (VDR) levels and the binding of the VDR-retinoid X receptor heterodimer to DNA in normal human skin. Submitted.

47. Jensen TJ, Sørensen S, Sølvsten H, Kragballe K. The vitamin D receptor and retinoid X receptors in psoriatic skin: the receptor levels correlate with the receptor binding to DNA. Br J Dermatol 1998; 138:225–228.

48. Chen ML, Perez A, Sanan DK, Heinrich G, Chen TC, Holick MF. Induction of vitamin D receptor mRNA expression in psoriatic plaques correlates with clinical response to 1,25-dihydroxyvitamin D_3. J Invest Dermatol 1996; 106:637–641.

3
Photobiology of Vitamin D$_3$

Michael F. Holick
Boston University School of Medicine,
Boston, Massachusetts

I. EVOLUTIONARY PERSPECTIVE

Vitamin D is a very ancient photochemical, the origin of which dates back at least 800 million years, when it was first produced in ocean-dwelling phytoplankton while they were being exposed to sunlight [1]. Today, most plants and animals exposed to sunlight have the capacity to produce vitamin D [1]. Although it is well known that vitamin D is critically important for calcium and bone metabolism in land vertebrates, it remains unclear what the function of vitamin D was in earlier life forms. What is most intriguing is that the precursor of vitamin D, known as provitamin D, is found in very high concentrations in phytoplankton [1]. Therefore, when phytoplankton are exposed to sunlight and conduct photosynthetic activity, they also produce vitamin D from its precursor. It has been speculated that provitamin D may have either acted as a natural sunscreen, since provitamin D's ultraviolet (UV) absorption spectrum is similar to the UV absorption spectrum of DNA and protein [1]. The UV absorption characteristics of provitamin D demonstrate that it has a high absorbability (extinction coefficient) and, when absorbing ultraviolet radiation, it does not result in free radical formation but rather the energy is used to open the steroid ring system (Figure 1). A second possible use of the provitamin D was to alter membrane permeability. Once the B ring of provitamin D was opened, the resulting vitamin D had increased flexibility, which, ultimately, could either increase membrane fluidity or exit the membrane perturbing it in some fashion. A third possible explanation is that every photon of ultraviolet radiation that provitamin D absorbs results in the production of photoproducts (Figure 1). Thus, the provitamin D system may have acted as a photon counter and could have provided the photochemical signal for early life forms that

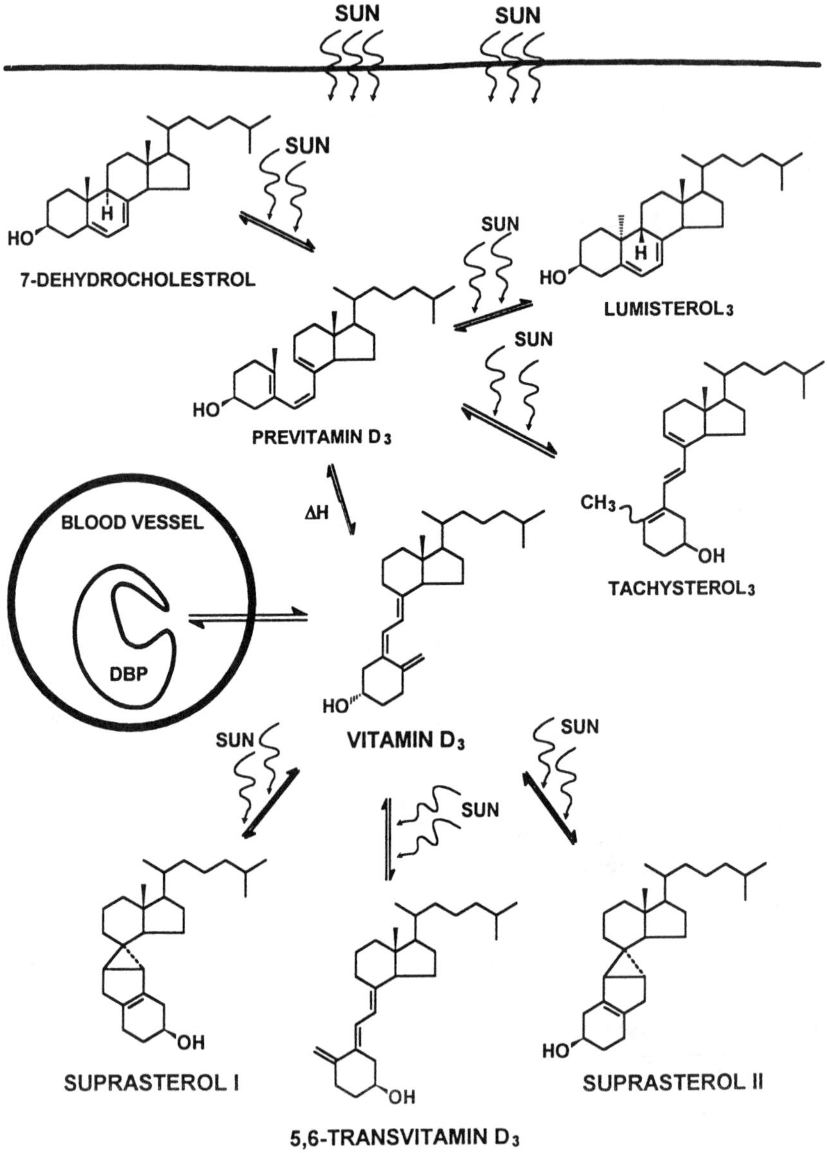

Figure 1 Photochemical events that lead to the production of vitamin D_3 and the regulation of vitamin D_3 in the skin. (From Ref. 2.)

were dependent on sunlight for their energy source but needed to determine photochemically when enough exposure occurred to induce it to return to deeper waters, thereby avoiding potential damage to its UV-sensitive macromolecules, including DNA, RNA, and proteins. For whatever reason vitamin D first evolved, there is no doubt that as our aquatic ancestors left their ocean environment (which had a plentiful supply of calcium) and ventured onto land (a calcium-deficient environment), they depended on vitamin D for their calcium needs. Their only calcium came from their diets. In order to utilize dietary calcium efficiently, vitamin D became critically important for the regulation of intestinal absorption of dietary calcium. How and why exposure of sunlight on the surface of the skin, resulting in the production of vitamin D, is so intimately involved in calcium and bone metabolism remains an enigma.

II. HISTORICAL PERSPECTIVE

Although there is some evidence from early Greek and Roman times to suggest that rickets was a health problem, this was most likely due to secondary effects of other chronic diseases. In the seventeenth century, as the industrial revolution began to take hold in northern Europe, people came to congregate in cities that were heavily polluted by the pall due to the burning of coal [2] (Figure 2). In the mid-1600s, Glissen, Whistler, and DeBoot called attention to a bone disease identified by deformities of the skeleton, including enlargement of the joints of the long bones and rib cage, curvature of the spine, enlargement of the head, short stature, and bowed legs or knock knees (Figure 3) [2,3]. The disease was seen within the first 2 years of childhood and the deformities persisted throughout the afflicted's life. This disease was insidious in nature and not only stunted the growth of both boys and girls but also resulted in a flattened the pelvis in young women, causing high incidence of maternal and infant morbidity and mortality. Indeed, it was this problem that gave rise to cesarean sectioning as a means of mitigating a difficult childbirth. The incidence of this crippling bone disease, commonly known as rickets or English disease, continued to increase during the industrial revolution; by the turn of the twentieth century, it was epidemic in the industrialized cities of northern Europe and the northeastern United States. One study conducted in Leiden, The Netherlands, reported that more than 80% of young children dying of various causes had clinical manifestations of this bone-deforming disease [2,3].

Sniadecki, in 1822 [4], recognized that his young patients who lived in Warsaw had a high incidence of rickets, while his young patients that lived in the outskirts of Warsaw did not. He concluded that the major difference between the two groups was that the children who lived in the rural areas outside Warsaw were exposed to sunlight while children living in the densely populated inner city were not. He suggested that it was the lack of exposure to sunlight that was responsible

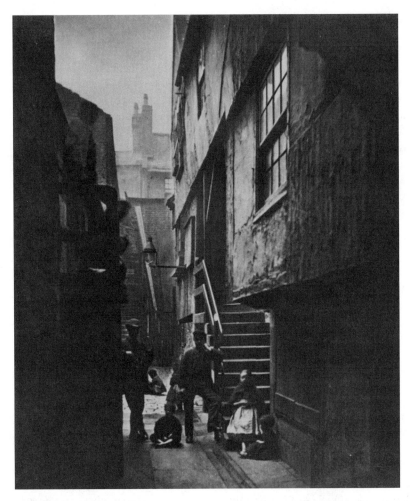

Figure 2   Photograph of a street in Glasgow between 1877 and 1898. (From Ref. 2.)

for this severe bone disease. His insightful observation went unheeded, and 70 years later Palm [5] also recognized that the lack of sunlight was a common denominator that could be associated with the high incidence of rickets in children living in the inner cities of Great Britain as compared with children living in underdeveloped countries. He encouraged systematic sunbathing as a means of preventing and curing rickets, much as Sniadecki had proposed 70 years before.

In the early 1800s, it was a common practice, supported by folklore, to give children cod liver oil to prevent and cure rickets. However, it was not until 1918,

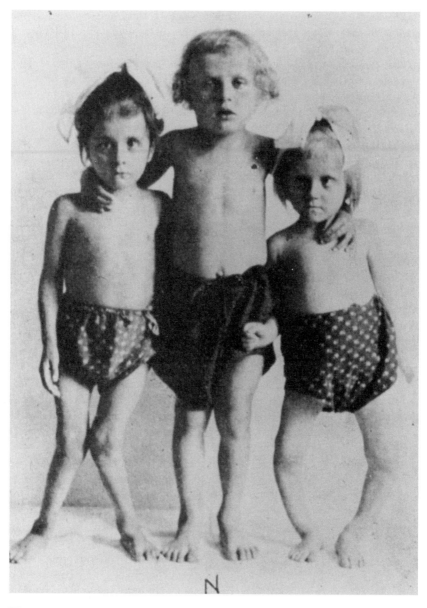

Figure 3 Typical presentation of two children with rickets. The child in the middle is normal; the children on either side have severe muscle weakness and bone deformities including bowed legs (right) and knock knees (left). (From Ref. 32.)

when Mellanby reported that he could make beagles rachitic and reverse the bone disease with cod liver oil, that the concept of a nutritional antirachitic factor arose. At the same time, Finsen [6] made the dramatic report that phototherapy was effective in treating a wide variety of skin disorders, including lupus vulgaris. This prompted several scientists to evaluate various light sources as a means of curing rickets. The first demonstration was by Huldchinsky [7], who exposed rachitic children to radiation from a mercury arc lamp. He was successful in curing the disease within 4 months. In 1921, Hess and Unger [8] exposed rachitic children in New York City to sunlight and reported by x-ray examination that there was marked improvement in the rickets of each child. The appreciation that exposure to sunlight or artificial ultraviolet radiation could cure rickets led to the concept of treating food with ultraviolet radiation. This ultimately led to the fortification of milk in the 1930s, which eradicated rickets as a significant health problem in countries using this practice [2,3]. Today milk, a few cereals, and bread are the major fortified foods containing vitamin D in the United States, Canada, and Mexico. Europe and Japan do no fortify their milk with vitamin D; instead, margarine, some cereals, and bread are so fortified. These simple practices have eradicated rickets as a significant health problem among most children worldwide.

III. PHOTOSYNTHESIS OF VITAMIN D

During exposure to sunlight, one does not directly photosynthesize vitamin D_3. Instead, the high-energy ultraviolet B radiation (photons with energies between 290 and 315 nm) penetrate into the skin, where they are absorbed by epidermal and dermal stores of 7-dehydrocholesterol (provitamin D_3, the immediate precursor in the cholesterol biosynthetic pathway). Once provitamin D_3 absorbs the ultraviolet radiation, it undergoes bond cleavage between carbons 9 and 10 to form a 9,10-secosteroid known as previtamin D_3 (Figure 1). Previtamin D_3 is biologically inert and is thermodynamically unstable. As a result, its double bonds rearrange spontaneously to form vitamin D_3 (Figure 1). At a physiological temperature of 37°, this process would take approximately 24 to 48 hr to reach completion. However, it is now recognized that previtamin D_3 is rapidly converted to vitamin D_3 in human skin and that almost 100% is converted to vitamin D_3 within 4 hr [9]. The explanation for this is that previtamin D_3 exists in two conformeric forms known as the cis,cis and cis,trans forms. Only the cis,cis conformer can be converted to vitamin D_3. The cis,trans form is thermodynamically more stable but cannot be converted to vitamin D_3, thus accounting for the prolonged isomerization time. It takes time for the cis,trans form to isomerize to the cis,cis conformer before it can be converted to vitamin D_3. However, a unique mechanism is apparently operative that permits the efficient conversion of previtamin D_3 to vitamin D_3 within hours after it is made in the skin. It has been suggested that the provitamin D_3 is

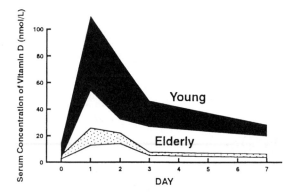

Figure 4 Circulating concentrations of vitamin D in response to a whole-body exposure to one minimal erythemal dose in healthy young and elderly subjects. (From Ref. 13.)

sandwiched in between the fatty acids within the bilipid membrane [10]. Once exposed to ultraviolet radiation, the B ring opens up, but only the cis,cis conformer can exist. Thus, it is efficiently converted to vitamin D_3. Once vitamin D_3 is made, it undergoes a conformational change, which likely helps it exit the membrane into the extracellular space to eventually find its way into the dermal capillary bed. Since most of the ultraviolet B radiation is absorbed in the epidermis, greater than 70% of previtamin D_3 synthesis occurs in the epidermis [11]. Aging decreases the thickness of both the dermis and epidermis; therefore, it is not surprising that there is an age-dependent decline in provitamin D_3 [11,12]. This results in a decrease at a capacity of elderly to produce vitamin D_3 in the skin [13,14] (Figure 4).

IV. REGULATION OF VITAMIN D SYNTHESIS IN THE SKIN

A. Photoisomerization

During exposure to sunlight, provitamin D_3 is converted to previtamin D_3 (Figure 1), which has the capacity to absorb ultraviolet radiation. This absorption results in its isomerization to two photoproducts known as lumisterol and tachysterol [15]. Both of these photoisomers are inert in calcium metabolism. Once formed in the skin, vitamin D_3 is also able to absorb ultraviolet radiation. As a result, when it is exposed to ultraviolet radiation, vitamin D_3 undergoes an isomerization to form at least three photoproducts, known as 5,6-trans vitamin D_3, supersterol I, and supersterol II (Figure 1) [16]. None of these vitamin D_3 photoproducts has any effect on calcium metabolism at physiological concentrations.

B. Melanin, Sunscreens, Clothing, and Glass

Any process that decreases or prevents ultraviolet B photons from reaching the viable epidermis to be absorbed by provitamin D_3 results in a diminution in the photosynthesis of previtamin D_3. Melanin and sunscreens are effective in absorbing ultraviolet B radiation. Thus, an increase in skin pigmentation can markedly diminish the cutaneous production of vitamin D_3 [17]. The application of a sunscreen with a sun protection factor (SPF) of 8 will reduce, by more than 95%, the cutaneous production of previtamin D_3 (Figure 5) [18]. Most clothing completely absorbs ultraviolet B radiation; therefore, clothing completely prevents the cutaneous production of vitamin D_3 on the areas it covers (Figure 6) [19].

It is well known that exposure of sunlight through glass will not result in any significant vitamin D_3 production. The reason for this is that there are substances in the glass, including lead, that absorb the ultraviolet B radiation [2].

C. Latitude

The zenith angle of the sun has a dramatic effect on the total number of ultraviolet B photons reaching the earth's surface. During the winter, at latitudes above 40° north and below 40° south of the equator, the ultraviolet B photons are efficiently absorbed by the ozone layer, thereby essentially eliminating the ability of the skin to produce vitamin D_3 [20,21]. At latitudes above and below 34° south and north, respectively, there is cutaneous production of vitamin D_3 the year round [20]. In far northern and southern latitudes, cutaneous production of vitamin D is essentially eliminated for almost 6 months of each year (Figure 6).

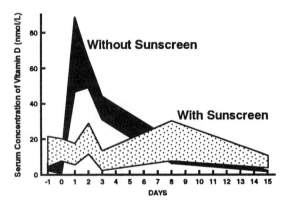

Figure 5 Circulating concentrations of vitamin D after a single exposure to one minimal erythemal dose of simulated sunlight either with a sunscreen, with a sun protection factor of 8, or a topical placebo cream. (From Ref. 18.)

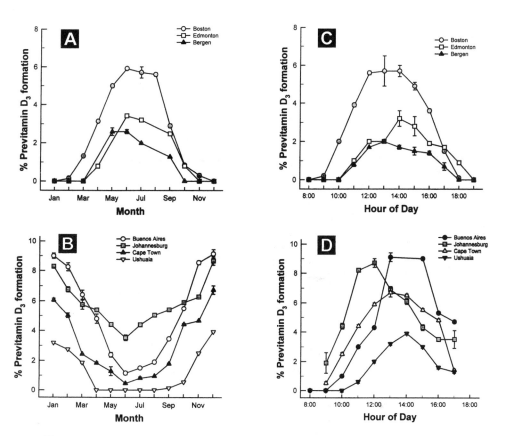

Figure 6 Influence of season, time of day, and latitude on the synthesis of previtamin D_3 in northern (A and C) and southern hemispheres (B and D). The hour indicated in C and D is the end of the 1-hr exposure time. (From Ref. 21.)

The zenith angle of the sun changes not only with changing season but also with time of day. Thus, in the early and late afternoons, there is a marked diminution in the cutaneous production of vitamin D_3.

V. VITAMIN D AND HUMAN HEALTH

A. Metabolism

It has been estimated that between 90 and 95% of most people obtain their vitamin D (D represents vitamin D_2 or D_3) requirement from casual exposure to sunlight

[2]. For people who live in climates where they can make vitamin D_3 only in the spring, summer, and fall, this is often adequate, because the vitamin D_3 that is made in the skin or ingested from the diet can be stored in the body fat to be released into the circulation later, during times when there is an inadequate cutaneous production of vitamin D_3. Vitamin D's principal function is to maintain serum calcium levels in the normal range to support most metabolic activities. Thus, it is critically important for neuromuscular function and bone mineralization.

However, vitamin D is biologically inert and must be metabolized in the liver on carbon 25 to form the major circulating form of vitamin D, 25-hydroxyvitamin D [25(OH)D] (Figure 7). 25(OH)D is used clinically to measure vitamin D status for vitamin D deficiency, sufficiency, and intoxication [2,22].

Because 25(OH)D is biologically inert at physiologic concentrations, it must be converted in the kidney to its activated form, 1,25-dihydrovitamin D [1,25(OH)$_2$D] (Figure 7). 1,25(OH)$_2$D travels to the small intestine, where it interacts with a specific receptor, the vitamin D receptor (VDR), resulting in an increase in the efficiency of intestinal calcium absorption. Normally, without vitamin D, the small intestine absorbs about 10–15% of dietary calcium. However, in a vitamin D sufficiency state, approximately 30% of the calcium is absorbed from the diet. During periods of growth, the increased calcium demand by the skeleton results in an increased production of 1,25(OH)$_2$D, thereby increasing the efficiency of intestinal calcium transport to between 60–80% [22].

However, if there is an inadequate amount of dietary calcium to satisfy the body's requirement, then 1,25(OH)$_2$D mobilizes stem cells and interacts with osteoblasts to signal an increase in osteoclastic activity, resulting in a mobilization of precious calcium stores from the skeleton [22]. Thus, contrary to what may be intuitive—i.e., that vitamin D plays an important, active role in bone mineralization—in fact, the function of vitamin D is to maintain the blood calcium in the normal range to keep most metabolic functions active. Only when there is adequate dietary calcium and phosphorus, so that the calcium phosphate product is in a supersaturating state, will the collagen matrix laid down by osteoblasts be mineralized. This has been confirmed in animal models whereby vitamin D–deficient rats either receiving a diet high in calcium and phosphorus [23] or being infused with calcium and phosphorus [24] were able to mineralize their skeletons. In addition, children with the rare disease vitamin D–dependent rickets type II [22,25], whereby they have a resistance to 1,25(OH)$_2$D because of a defective VDR, can mineralize their skeletons by receiving calcium and phosphorus intravenously [26].

B. Vitamin D Deficiency

Vitamin D deficiency causes a transient decrease in ionized calcium, which leads to an increase in parathyroid hormone synthesis and secretion [2,22,23]. Parathyroid hormone increases tubular reabsorption of calcium in the kidney, stimulates osteoclastic calcium mobilization from the skeleton, and causes increased loss of

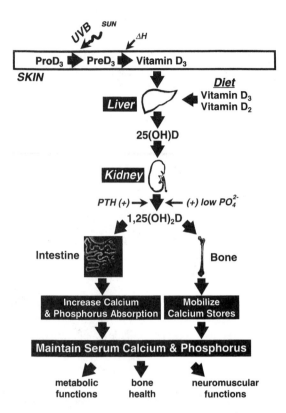

Figure 7 Schematic representation of the synthesis of vitamin D and its metabolism and biological functions on calcium and phosphorus homeostasis. 7-Dehydrocholesterol (provitamin D_3; ProD$_3$) in the skin is photolyzed to previtamin D_3 (PreD$_3$) during its exposure to ultraviolet B (UVB) radiation from sunlight. Once formed, previtamin D_3 undergoes a thermally induced (ΔH) transformation to vitamin D_3. Vitamin D_3 from the skin and vitamin D_3 and vitamin D_2 from the diet enter the blood and are metabolized to their 25-hydroxy counterparts: 25-hydroxyvitamin D [25(OH)D]. Once formed, 25(OH)D is metabolized in the kidney to 1,25(OH)$_2$D. Parathyroid hormone (PTH) and low serum phosphorus both enhance (+) the production of 1,25(OH)$_2$D. Once formed, 1,25(OH)$_2$D regulates serum calcium and phosphorus levels by increasing the efficiency of intestinal calcium and phosphorus absorption and by mobilizing calcium stores from bone. The ultimate role of vitamin D is to maintain the serum within the normal range in order to sustain a wide variety of metabolic and physiological functions as well as to optimize bone health. (From Ref. 28.)

phosphorus in the urine [22,23]. Thus, in vitamin D deficiency, the serum calcium is usually normal, accompanied by a low normal serum phosphorus. This results in an inadequate product of calcium × phosphorus, thereby resulting in defective mineralization. A defect in the mineralization of a young, growing skeleton results in rickets. However, in adults, whose epiphyseal plates are fused, the effect of vitamin D deficiency is more subtle. Vitamin D deficiency in adults causes a mineralization defect of the newly laid out osteoid, resulting in the bone disease osteomalacia. In addition, the secondary hyperparathyroidism associated with vitamin D deficiency results in a mobilization of skeletal calcium stores, causing and exacerbating osteoporosis and increased risk of fracture [23].

VI. RECOMMENDATIONS FOR ADEQUATE INTAKE

The Institute of Medicine of the National Academy of Sciences reviewed the literature on vitamin D requirements for all age groups [27] and concluded that although most humans can obtain the majority of their vitamin D from exposure to sunlight, all humans need dietary supplemental vitamin D in the absence of adequate sunlight exposure. For infants and neonates, it was recommended that 200 IU (5 μg) was adequate. However, twice that recommendation would not be inappropriate [27,28]. For children as well as young and middle-aged adults up the age of 49 years, 200 IU of vitamin D per day was considered to be adequate. However, the committee recognized that vitamin D deficiency is becoming a significant health problem for adults over the age of 50 years. In two recent studies, it has been estimated that between 40 and 60% of outpatient and inpatients were deficient in vitamin D [29,30]. Thus, the adequate intake for adults aged 50–70 is 400 IU (10 μg) per day [27].

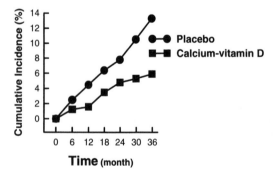

Figure 8 Cumulative percentage of 389 men and women older than 65 years with a first nonvertebral fracture, according to study group. By 36 months, 26 of 202 subjects in the placebo group and 11 of 187 subjects in the calcium–vitamin D group had had a fracture (p = 0.02). (From Ref. 33.)

The elderly are especially prone to developing vitamin D deficiency. This is in part due to their lack of outdoor activities, decreased ability to make vitamin D in the skin, and avoidance of foods containing vitamin D. There is strong evidence that at least 600 IU of vitamin D is necessary to satisfy the vitamin D requirement in this age group. For example, in a French nursing home, residents receiving 800 IU of vitamin D a day along with 800 mg of calcium showed an increase in their bone mineral density and had a marked decrease in vertebral and nonvertebral fractures [31]. Similarly, in a study in Boston, there was a 116% reduction in the risk of nonvertebral fractures among both men and women who were supplemented with 700 IU of vitamin D a day [32] (Figure 8).

VII. CONCLUSION

How much sunlight is necessary to satisfy the body's requirement? This is an especially relevant question in view of concern about the damaging effects of excessive exposure to sunlight. A study was conducted whereby medical students received a whole-body exposure to 1 minimal erythemal dose (MED) of solar simulated sunlight as well as graded doses of vitamin D. The circulating levels of vitamin D were then measured at various intervals. It was found that a whole-body exposure to 1 MED of ultraviolet B radiation resulted in a blood level of vitamin D that was comparable to taking between 10,000 and 25,000 IU of vitamin D orally (Figure 9) [2,31]. Thus, if 6% of the body were exposed to 1 MED, this

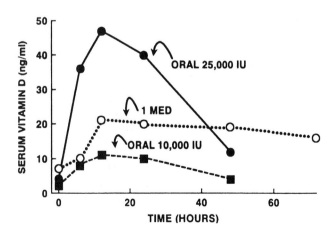

Figure 9   Comparison of serum vitamin D levels after a whole body exposure to 1 MED (minimal erythemal dose) of simulated sunlight compared with a single oral dose of either 10,000 or 25,000 IU of vitamin D₂.

would be equal the production of approximately 600–1000 IU of vitamin D. Thus, it is recommended that suberythemal exposure of hands, face, and arms two to three times a week is more than adequate to satisfy the body's requirement. A sunscreen application after that initial exposure will prevent the damaging effects of excessive exposure to sunlight.

For children, there is no need to be concerned about sunscreen use and lack of vitamin D synthesis. Children and young adults will not always wear a sunscreen before going outdoors, nor will they use the proper amount. Therefore, they are making adequate amounts of vitamin D in the skin to satisfy their requirements during the spring, summer, and fall. The excess vitamin D is stored in the body's fat and released when there is an insufficiency of vitamin D.

ACKNOWLEDGMENT

This work was supported in part by grants from NIH M01 00533 and AR 36963.

REFERENCES

1. Holick MF. Phylogenetic and evolutionary aspects of vitamin D from phytoplankton to humans. In: Pang PKT, Schreibman MP, eds. Vertebrate Endocrinology: Fundamentals and Biomedical Implications, Vol. 3. Orlando, FL: Academic Press (Harcourt Brace Jovanovich) 1989, pp. 7–43.
2. Holick MF. McCollum Award Lecture, 1994. Vitamin D: new horizons for the 21st century. Am J Clin Nutr 60:619–630, 1994.
3. Holick MF. Vitamin D: photobiology, metabolism, mechanism of action, and clinical application. In: Favus MJ, ed. Primer on the Metabolic Bone Diseases and Disorders of Mineral Metabolism, 3d ed. New York: Lippincott-Raven, 1996, pp. 74–81.
4. Sniadecki J. Jerdrzej Sniadecki (1768–1838) on the cure for rickets (1840). Cited by W. Mozolowski. Nature 143:121, 1939.
5. Palm TA. The geographic distribution and etiology of rickets. Practioner 45:270–342, 1890.
6. Finsen NR. In: Phototherapy. London: Edward Arnold Publishing, 1901.
7. Huldschinsky K. Heilung von Rachitis durch kunstliche Honensonne. Dtsch Med Wochenschr 45:712–713, 1919.
8. Hess AF, Unger LF. Cure of infantile rickets by sunlight. JAMA 77:39, 1921.
9. Tian XQ, Chen TC, Matsuoka LY, Wortsman J, Holick MF. Kinetic and thermodynamic studies of the conversion of previtamin D_3 to vitamin D_3 in human skin. J Biol Chem 268:14888–14892, 1993.
10. Holick MF, Tian XQ, Allen M. Evolutionary importance for the membrane enhancement of the production of vitamin D_3 in the skin of poikilothermic animals. Proc Natl Acad Sci USA 92:3124–3126, 1995.
11. Holick M, MacLaughlin J, Clark M, Holick S, Potts J, Anderson R, Blank I, Parrish

J. Photosynthesis of previtamin D_3 in human skin and the physiologic consequences. Science 210:203–205, 1980.

12. MacLaughlin J, Holick MF. Aging decreases the capacity of human skin to produce vitamin D_3. J Clin Invest 76:1536–1538, 1985.

13. Need AG, Morris HA, Horowitz M, Nordin BEC. Effects of skin thickness, age, body fat, and sunlight on serum 25-hydroxyvitamin D. Am J Clin Nutr 58:882–885, 1993.

14. Holick MF, Matsuoka LY, Wortsman J. Age, Vitamin D, and solar ultraviolet radiation. Lancet ii:1104–1105, 1989.

15. Holick MF, MacLaughlin JA, Doppelt SH. Regulation of cutaneous previtamin D_3 photosynthesis in man: skin pigment is not an essential regulator. Science 211: 590–593, 1981.

16. Webb AR, DeCosta BR, Holick MF. Sunlight regulates the cutaneous production of vitamin D_3 by causing its photodegradation. J Clin Endocrinol Metab 68:882–887, 1989.

17. Clemens TL, Henderson SL, Adams JS, Holick MF. Increased skin pigment reduces the capacity of skin to synthesize vitamin D_3. Lancet 74–76, 1982.

18. Matsuoka LY, Ide L, Wortsman J, MacLaughlin J, Holick MF. Sunscreens suppress cutaneous vitamin D_3 synthesis. J Clin Endocrinol Metab 64:1165–1168, 1987.

19. Matsuoka LY, Wortsman J, Dannenberg MJ, Hollis BW, Lu Z, Holick MF. Clothing prevents ultraviolet-B radiation-dependent photosynthesis of vitamin D. J Clin Endocrinol Metab 75:1099–1103, 1992.

20. Webb AR, Kline L, Holick MF. Influence of season and latitude on the cutaneous synthesis of vitamin D_3: exposure to winter sunlight in Boston and Edmonton will not promote vitamin D_3 synthesis in human skin. J Clin Endocrinol Metab 67:373–378, 1988.

21. Chen TC. Photobiology of vitamin D. In: Holick MF, ed. Vitamin D Physiology, Molecular Biology, and Clinical Applications. Totowa, NJ: Human Press, 1998, pp. 39–56.

22. Holick MF. Vitamin D: photobiology, metabolism, and clinical applications. In: DeGroot L, ed. Endocrinology. Philadelphia: Saunders, 1995, pp. 990–1013.

23. Holtrop ME, Cox KA, Carnes DL, Holick MF. Skeletal mineralization in vitamin D-deficient rats. Am J Physiol 251:E20, 1986.

24. Underwood JL, DeLuca HF. Vitamin D is not directly necessary for bone growth and mineralization. Am J Physiol 246:E493–E498, 1984.

25. Holick MF, Krane S, Potts JR Jr. Calcium, phosphorus, and bone metabolism: calcium-regulating hormones. In: KJ Isselbacher KJ, Braunwald E, Wilson JD, et al., eds. Harrison's Principles of Internal Medicine. New York: McGraw-Hill, 1994, pp. 2137–2151.

26. Balsan S, Garabedian M, Larchet M, Gorski AM, Cournot G, Tau C, Bourdeau A, Silve C, Ricour C. Long-term nocturnal calcium infusions can cure rickets and promote normal mineralization in hereditary resistance to 1,25-dihydroxyvitamin D. J Clin Invest 77:1661–1667, 1986.

27. Standing Committee on the Scientific Evaluation of Dietary Reference Intakes. Dietary reference intakes for calcium, phosphorus, magnesium, vitamin D, and fluoride. In: Dietary Reference Intakes. Washington, DC: Institute of Medicine, National Academy Press, 1997, pp. 1–30.

28. Holick MF. Vitamin D requirements for humans of all ages: new increased requirements for women and men 50 years and older. Osteoporos Int (Suppl) 8:S24–S29, 1998.

29. Malabanan A, Veronikis IE, Holick MF. Redefining vitamin D insufficiency. Lancet 351:805–806, 1998.

30. Thomas MK, Lloyd-Jones DM, Thadhani RI, Shaw AC, Deraska DJ, Kitch BT, Vamvakas EC, Dick IM, Prince RL, Finkelstein JS. Hypovitaminosis D in medical inpatients. N Engl J Med 338:777–783, 1998.

31. Holick MF. Sunlight, vitamin D, and human health. In: Jung EG, Holick MF, eds. Biologic Effects of Light (proceedings of symposium, Basel, Switzerland). Berlin: Walter de Gruyter, 1994, pp. 3–15.

32. Bicknell F, Prescott F. Vitamin D. In: Heineman W, ed. The Vitamins in Medicine, 2d ed. London: Random House, 1948, pp. 630–708.

33. Holick MF. Evolution, biologic functions, and recommended dietary allowances for vitamin D. In: Holick MF, ed. Vitamin D: Physiology, Molecular Biology, and Clinical Applications. Totowa, NJ: Humana Press, 1998, pp. 1–16.

4

Metabolism of Vitamin D and Its Role in Calcium Metabolism

Henning Glerup and Erik Fink Eriksen
Aarhus Amtssygehus, University Hospital of Aarhus, Aarhus, Denmark

I. INTRODUCTION

The aim of this chapter is to review the calcemic actions of vitamin D on the classic target organs: bone, kidney, and intestine. When vitamin D was discovered approximately 80 years ago [1], it was classified as a vitamin. With the knowledge we now have about vitamin D, it is more correct to classify it as a secosteroid hormone (a secosteroid is a steroid with a disrupted B ring). The most important source of vitamin D is endogenous production of vitamin D in the skin when exposed to ultraviolet B (UV-B) radiation (290–315 nm). Under normal conditions, the skin will be able to supply the body with 80–100% of the requirements of vitamin D [2]. If, however, the exposure to direct sunlight is limited, the vitamin D supply of the body depends on the intake of vitamin D, and vitamin D becomes a true vitamin [3–8]. Most food items contains very limited amounts of vitamin D, the most important being fatty fish (herring, mackerel, sardine, salmon, etc.). But even when one is eating very large amounts of fish, it is difficult to get enough vitamin D without exposure to sunlight. This means that any limitations in exposure to direct sunlight will increase the risk of developing vitamin D deficiency if one is not supplied with a relatively high dose vitamin D (800–1000 IU or 20–25 μg of vitamin D per day) [2,9–13].

II. METABOLISM OF VITAMIN D

Cholecalciferol (vitamin D_3) is the naturally occurring form of vitamin D from animal food. Ergocalciferol (vitamin D_2) is produced in plants, primarily yeast, when exposed to UV-B. The metabolism of the two forms of vitamin D is identical (Figure 1). The first step in the metabolism is 25-hydroxylation in the liver. This process is very fast and not very tightly regulated. The resulting 25-OH-vit-D is transported by vitamin D–binding protein (DBP) and stored in the lipid phase of the body for later use. As a result of this, serum-25-OH-vit-D can be measured as a good marker of the body content of vitamin D. The next step in the metabolism is 1-hydroxylation, which occurs in the proximal tubular cells of the kidney. The formation of 1,25-OH$_2$-vit-D is tightly regulated. The most important regulator is PTH. A lowering of s-Ca^{2+} or a rise in phosphate will immediately result in liberation of PTH from the parathyroid glands. The rise in PTH results in a fast increase in 1,25-OH$_2$-vit-D production (Figure 1). 1,25-OH$_2$-vit-D hydroxylation is suppressed by an increase in s-Ca^{2+} or by 1,25-OH$_2$-vit-D itself.

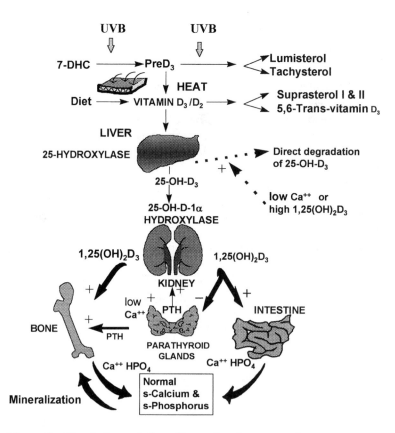

Figure 1   Vitamin D metabolism. (For explanation, see text.)

The biological activity of $1,25$-OH_2-vit-D is 500- to 1000-fold higher than that of 25-OH-vit-D [3,14], but as the serum concentration of 25-OH-vit-D normally is about 100 times higher than $1,25$-OH_2-vit-D, the biological activity of 25-OH-vit-D cannot be ruled out. This issue is still poorly investigated. Recent research in the field of osteomalacic myopathy [9], however, strongly supports that 25-OH-vit-D may exert biological actions of its own.

The first step in the degradation of vitamin D is 24-hydroxylation with formation of $24,25$-OH_2-vit-D and $1,24,25$-OH_3-vit-D. These compounds may have some biological activity, albeit this issue is still controversial [4]. After several further hydroxylations and oxidations, the final degradation product, calcitroic acid, is excreted in the urine [2]. Vitamin D metabolites also undergo enterohepatic circulation, and part of the vitamin D pool may be lost with the bile.

III.   CALCEMIC ACTIONS OF VITAMIN D

For many years vitamin D has been known to regulate calcium homeostasis—the so-called "calcemic actions" on the "classical target organs": bone, intestine, and kidney. The effects of vitamin D are (1) calcification of bone and mobilization of Ca^{2+} from bone, (2) increased absorption of Ca^{2+} from the intestine, and (3) increased reabsorption of Ca^{2+} in the kidney.

In addition to these vital calcemic actions, the discovery of the nuclear receptor of $1,25$-OH_2-vit-D opened the possibility that vitamin D might exert many noncalcemic actions as well [6,15–19]. The Vitamin D receptor has now been demonstrated in most "nonclassical target" tissues of the body (cells of the immune system, heart, skeletal muscle, smooth muscle, gonads, prostate, uterus, mammary gland, placenta, brain, pancreas, thyroid and parathyroid glands, liver, lung, colon, bladder, stomach, skin, hair follicle, melanocytes) [6,15]. In agreement with these findings, vitamin D has been found to be important in the differentiation of most cells, which gives vitamin D potential as an antiproliferative drug, as reviewed elsewhere in this volume.

The mechanisms of action of vitamin D are discussed in details in Chapter 1. The calcaemic actions of vitamin D are mediated through both genomic and nongenomic actions. The genomic actions are mediated through binding of $1,25$-OH_2-vit-D to a nuclear receptor, resulting in de novo synthesis of RNA and protein. The nongenomic actions are mediated through binding of vitamin D to a membrane receptor. The binding to the receptor initiates a cascade, which results in intracellular formation of a second messengers (cAMP, DAG, IP_3, AA) or phosphorylation of intracellular proteins (Figure 2). Typically these reactions results in activation of an intracellular enzyme or ion channel.

The relative importance of these nongenomic action is still open for discussion. The best-documented effect is the transcaltachia of the kidney [5,20,21], but nongenomic actions have also been well documented in muscle [22].

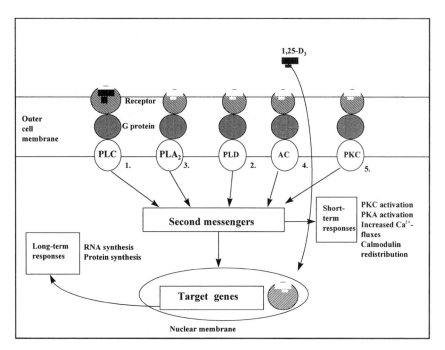

Figure 2 Genomic and nongenomic pathways of vitamin D. Binding to putative membrane receptors may affect several different intracellular signaling pathways and elicit a wide array of short-term responses. PLC, phospholipase C; PLA₂, phospholipase A₂; PLD, phospholipase D; AC, adenylate cyclase; PKC, phosphokinase C.

A. Calcemic Actions of Vitamin D in the Intestine

In vitamin D–deficient individuals, the intestinal absorption of calcium is very low. When vitamin D is given to a vitamin D–depleted individual, calcium increases within 30 min, with a further increase seen after approximately 5 hr. The intracellular levels of calcium are very low (10^{-7} mol/L) compared with millimolar concentrations in the intestinal lumen [23]. The concentration gradient allows a passive diffusion over the brush border into the enterocyte. The fast increase in calcium absorption seen after vitamin D administration is thought to be due to the nongenomic action of transcaltachia [21], an absorption process involving formation of calcium-containing endocytotic vesicles, which are exocytosed at the transluminar cell membrane of the enterocyte. Transportation of calcium through the cell and excretion of calcium against the concentration gradient at the transluminal cell membrane are energy-requiring processes, involving genome-mediated synthesis of proteins (calbindin D's, calcium pumps), that proceed more slowly.

This explains the secondary increase in calcium absorption seen 5 hr after administration of vitamin to vitamin D–depleted individuals.

B. Calcemic Actions of Vitamin D in the Kidney

About 8 g of calcium is filtered at the glomerulus per day. Approximately 98% is reabsorbed. The reabsorption process is influenced by several factors, including sodium intake and several hormones (parathyroid hormone [PTH], calcitonin $1,25\text{-OH}_2\text{-vit-D}$). Vitamin D has been shown to be important for the synthesis of a number of proteins involved in the intracellular handling of calcium (calbindin D's, calcium pumps, vitamin D receptor) [24]. The net effect of vitamin D on the kidney is an increased efficiency in the reabsorption of calcium.

C. Calcemic Actions of Vitamin D in Bone

Although the effect of vitamin D on bone cells has been extensively studied, the effector mechanisms of vitamin D in mineralization and resorption of bone are only partly understood. Most of the effects seems to be mediated by $1,25\text{-OH}_2\text{-vit-}$ D via the vitamin D receptor. Vitamin D is important for both mineralization and resorption. In vitamin D deficiency, accumulation of unmineralized osteoid is seen. If the vitamin D deficiency is not corrected, osteomalacia characterized by increased alkaline phosphatase, secondary hyperparathyroidism, increased bone resorption, marrow fibrosis, and tunnelling resorption will develop [25]. When vitamin D is given, bone mineralization will increase. It has been speculated that this effect on bone mineralization could be due to increased intestinal calcium absorption, resulting in an increased amount of calcium available for the mineralization process [3]. Vitamin D also increases calcium liberation from bone. This effect is mediated through an increased osteoclastogenesis and stimulation of osteoclastic resorption. The activation of osteoclasts is probably mediated by cells of the osteoblastic lineage [2].

Vitamin D–dependent intestinal calcium absorption is most likely of great importance for the risk of development of senile osteoporosis. Intestinal calcium absorption is decreased among osteoporotic elderly individuals. This decrease seems to be due to an age-related decline in intestinal sensitivity to vitamin D; however, the calcium balance can be improved be supplementation of higher doses of 25-OH-vit-D_3 [26]. The age-related decline in calcium absorption is possibly related to the genotype of the vitamin D receptor, as it has been shown that the genotype BB has a lower calcium absorption compared to genotype bb [27]. Recently Francis et al. [28] showed that treatment with alfacalcidol in osteoporotic elderly individuals improved calcium absorption despite normal levels of 25-OH-vit-D and $1,25\text{-OH}_2\text{-vit-D}$ prior to initiation of treatment. Moreover, no changes in $1,25\text{-OH}_2\text{-vit-D}$ levels were detectable during treatment. In agreement with their findings, alfacalcidol [29] and calcitriol [30] treatment have been shown to reduce fracture risk.

D. Calcemic Actions on Other Organs

Exact regulation of intracellular levels of calcium is of vital importance for most of the cells of the body. Vitamin D seems to play an important role in the regulation of intracellular calcium levels in most cells. The effects are mediated through both genomic and nongenomic pathways, as, for example, in muscles, where vitamin D plays an important regulatory role in determining the calcium pool available for muscle contraction [9,31,32].

IV. VITAMIN D DEFICIENCY

Measurement of serum levels of 25-OH-vit-D gives us a measure of the body content of vitamin D, But the lower limit for s-25-OH-vit-D has been subject to intensive debate. In 1985 Peacock et al. [33] proposed the following definition of vitamin D deficiency based on s-25-OH-vit-D concentrations:

1. Serum levels ≤10 nmol/L where evident secondary hyperparathyroidism and reduced calcium malabsorption were seen and osteomalacia and osteomalacic myopathy was likely were defined as vitamin D deficiency.
2. Serum levels 10–50 nmol/L where mild hyperparathyroidism, suboptimal calcium absorption [26], and reduced BMD could be seen were defined as vitamin D insufficiency.
3. Serum levels 50–200 nmol/L where no abnormalities in calcium metabolism are seen were defined as vitamin D sufficiency.

A different definition of vitamin D deficiency is based on the demonstration of PTH elevations and s-25-OH-vit-D levels at which further supplementation with vitamin D did not result in an increase of s-1,25-OH$_2$-vit-D. Based on these definitions, the lower limit was defined as 30 nmol/L [34,35], while others have proposed 37 nmol/L [36–38] or 50 nmol/L [39]. Recently it was shown that intestinal calcium absorption is suboptimal if serum levels of 25-OH-vit-D are below 65 nmol/L [14].

In our view the definition of vitamin D deficiency should be based on deficiency at the tissue level—i.e., of bone and/or muscle disease. We have recently shown [9] that osteomalacic myopathy is common with serum levels <20 nmol/L. Based on these observations, we propose that vitamin D deficiency is defined as serum levels of 25-OH-vit-D <20 nmol/L and that serum levels between 20–50 nmol/L are defined as vitamin D insufficiency.

A. Symptoms Related to Vitamin D Deficiency

Severe vitamin D deficiency is accompanied by a number of unspecific muscular and skeletal symptoms, and if the clinician is not aware of the disease, the diagnosis can easily be missed. The first systematic description of the clinical picture of vitamin D deficiency was given by Smith and Stern [40] and Chalmers [41] in 1967. In the following decades little interest was paid to the myopathic symptoms, but in the nineties they were rediscovered [42,43]. Lately we reviewed the clinical symptoms [9]:

1. Bone pain. Often described by the patient as deep pain, typically located in the long bones, ribs, pelvis, and shoulder with the same localization of the pain every day.
2. Muscle pain. Often more diffuse, located in the muscles in femur, crura, neck, shoulders, and upper arms. Typically the pain can move from day to day.
3. Muscle weakness. The patient often complains of a change in gait, difficulties in climbing a staircase and difficulties in rising from a kneeling position or from a chair.
4. Fatigue. Often a prominent symptom.
5. Muscle cramps. Mostly in the extremities.
6. Paresthesia. Very much like the symptoms seen in hyperventilation syndrome.

The most important differential diagnoses are rheumatic diseases, polymyalgia rheumatica, fibromyalgia, hyperventilation syndrome, hysteriform cramps, and malignant disease.

The final confirmation of the diagnosis is dependent on blood tests. Serum 25-OH-vit-D below 20 nmol/L and intact PTH above normal levels will strongly support the diagnosis. Alkaline phosphatase can be increased in osteomalacic bone disease but not in isolated myopathy. The diagnosis osteomalacic bone disease is dependent on histomorphometric evaluation of a bone biopsy (osteoid thickness $> 12,5$ μm and mineralization lag time > 100 days [44–46]).

V. RISK FACTORS FOR THE DEVELOPMENT OF VITAMIN D DEFICIENCY

A. Sunlight Exposure

Direct exposure of the skin to sunlight is by far the most important source of vitamin D. It is therefore understandable that any limitation in the exposure to direct sunlight is critical. The latitude, the season, and the time of day of the exposure are very important. In studies performed in Boston (42°N) Holick et al. [12,37,47] demonstrated that the maximal production of vitamin D was seen around noon in July, with decreasing production in spring and autumn and no production between November 1 and March 15. In countries nearer the equator, the production is constant throughout the year. With the skin production of vitamin D shut down for several month in winter, it could be expected that there would be a seasonal variation in s-25-OH-vit-D, and this is indeed what is seen [48–51]. The most pronounced seasonal variations are seen in nonobese elderly persons. Oral supplementation of vitamin D can exclude these seasonal variations [52,53].

The skin production of vitamin D is dependent on UV-B radiation. Glass and plastic exclude 100% of the UV-B waves [12] and the use of sunscreen factor 8 excludes 95% [54–56]. Clothing style is important as well. Black wool excludes 100% of UV-B radiation. The habit of being veiled and wearing long sleeves when outside is a risk factor for the development of vitamin D deficiency. In agreement with these findings, we found extremely low values of 25-OH-vit-D (mean $\pm$ SEM 7.1 $\pm$ 1.1 nmol/L) among veiled Arab women living in Denmark [9]. Low values of 25-OH-vit-D among Asians exposed to limited amounts of sunlight have also been reported from the United Kingdom [57–60] and Norway [61,62]. Even in sunny countries like Saudi Arabia and Kuwait, where it is the custom to wear long sleeves and veils, low values of 25-OH-vit-D are common [63–67]. The skin type is also important [68] as melanin acts as a natural UV-B filter. The vitamin D production capacity of the skin is, however, the same in persons with dark skin, but a longer exposure of UV-B is needed.

B. Age

S-25-OH-vit-D declines with advancing age [69,70], thus secondary hyperparathyroidism [36,51,52,71–79] is prevalent in the elderly.

1.   Synthesis of Vitamin D in the Skin

The most important factor determining impaired vitamin D status among the elderly is reduced vitamin D synthesis in the skin. The elderly tend to protect their skin more from the sun with long sleeves and sunscreen than younger adults do. In addition, many elderly are relatively immobile and have greater difficulty in getting outside. Furthermore, the vitamin D production capacity of the skin is reduced with age. The reason for this seems to be a combination of the skin getting thinner and a reduction of the 7-dehydrochlesterol content of the skin. It has been estimated that, above age 70, the vitamin D production capacity of the skin is reduced to one-third that of 20-year-olds [12,80,81].

2.   Vitamin D Intake

When the vitamin D synthesis of the skin is reduced, the elderly become very dependent on an intake of vitamin D with their food. The vitamin D intake in this age group is, however, very low (approximately 100 IU/day) [51,76,82,83].

3. Intestinal Absorption of Vitamin D

The intestinal absorption has been found to be reduced by 40% in the elderly [84], whereas others have reported no reduction [85].

4. Liver Function

The 25-hydroxylation takes place in the liver. There is no data suggesting an age related reduction in the 25-hydroxylation capacity. Liver insufficiency must be very severe (reduced by 90%) before the 25-hydroxylation is affected [2,86,87].

5. 1α-Hydroxylation in the Kidney

The data on the levels of s-1,25-OH$_2$-vit-D in the elderly are very divergent. Some have found them reduced, while others have reported their being normal or even increased [88,89].

With increasing age, a reduction in renal function is often seen, and when GFRs are reduced below 60–70 mL/min [90,91], a reduction in the 1α-hydroxylation is seen [92,93]. The decline in renal function, however, varies a lot, and many elderly exhibit normal renal function until they reach the age of 80 or 90. In a recent French study [51] of 444 women in the age range of 75–90 years, renal function was found to be of lesser importance for the vitamin D status of the elderly.

C. Malabsorption

It is well known that malabsorption states with steatorrhea result in malabsorption of the fat soluble vitamin D [44]. In addition, steatorrhea and other malabsorption diseases result in malabsorption of calcium, leading to secondary hyperparathyroidism and finally to increased 1,25-OH$_2$-vit-D synthesis. Recently Clemens and others [94,95] investigated vitamin D metabolism in calcium-deprived rats. They documented that increased s-1,25-OH$_2$-vit-D leads to increased hepatic degradation of 25-OH-vit-D to inactive metabolites (see Figure 1). It is now well documented that the same inactivation process is taking place in humans with increased s-1,25-OH$_2$-vit-D [96,97], and this seems to be the most likely explanation for the high frequency of hypovitaminosis D seen in patients with gastrectomy [98–100], intestinal bypass [46], Crohn's disease [101–103], and pancreatic insufficiency [44]. In untreated celiac disease, osteomalacia is extremely common (50–70%) [44,104]. As mentioned above, vitamin D deficiency is uncommon in liver insufficiency, but in cholestatic liver disease, a state of fat malabsorption can be seen, and vitamin D deficiency may evolve [44,86,87].

D. Renal Insufficiency

As mentioned above, declining renal function will lead to reduced production of 1,25-OH$_2$-vit-D. This results in reduced calcium absorption and subsequent secondary hyperparathyroidism. Many similarities exist between uremic and osteomalacic myopathy and bone disease [105–108], but the picture is somewhat more complicated in renal failure, where electrolyte perturbations and phosphate retention are seen. In addition, renal production of erythropoitin is reduced [109]. Improvement in muscle function after treatment with 1α-hydroxylated vitamin D preparations has been reported [110,111].

VI. RECOMMENDATIONS FOR PROPHYLAXIS AND TREATMENT OF VITAMIN D DEFICIENCY

The Recommended daily allowance (RDA) for vitamin D is 200 IU (5 μg) per day for adults and 400 IU (10 μg) per day for children and the elderly. The RDA for healthy active adults seems to be sufficient, but many studies [11,26,36,42,77,79,112] have shown that the RDA for elderly and other risk groups is too low. In a study on ethnic Danish veiled Moslems [9], we have recently shown that a daily intake of 17,5 μg of vitamin D was not sufficient to maintain a normal serum level of 25-OH-vit-D. In agreement with our findings, Holick et al. [12] reported that a dosage of 600 IU ergocalciferol was insufficient to maintain normal serum levels of 25-OH-vit-D in a group of submariners deprived of direct sunlight for 3 months. These findings indicate that individuals exposed to limited amounts of direct sunlight should have a prophylactic dosage of 800–1000 IU (20–25 μg) of vitamin D daily. This recommendation is further supported by the findings of Chapuy et al. [51,113–115] and Lips et al. [116]. Both groups studied the effects of vitamin D prophylaxis in the elderly. Chapuy et al. used a daily dose of 800 IU cholecalciferol and demonstrated a 42% decrease in the number of hip fractures after 1 1/2 years treatment. Further, they demonstrated that the regimen effectively suppressed secondary hyperparathyroidism. Lips et al. used a daily dose of 400 IU. They found no significant reduction in the number of fractures and the secondary hyperparathyroidism was only partly suppressed. We conclude that there is an increasing amount of evidence [10] that the RDA for the elderly should be a daily dose of at least 800–1000 IU cholecalciferol/ergocalciferol.

If the patient has developed clinical signs of vitamin D deficiency and has both a low 25-OH-vit-D (<20 nmol/L) and an increased intact PTH, higher doses of vitamin D are required. The vitamin D supplementation can be given either by mouth or by intramuscular injection. In our department we have found that a regimen consisting of intramuscular injections of 100.000 IU weekly for a month followed by a monthly injection for another 5 months constitute a safe and effective treatment. The treatment should always be followed by supplementation of 1000–1500 mg elemental calcium per day.

VII. TOXICOLOGY

The toxic effects of vitamin D compounds are mainly if not exclusively mediated through its hypercalcemic and hypercalciuric actions. The clinical presentation of vitamin D intoxication is the same no matter which kind of vitamin D compound is causing the intoxication. The classical symptoms of vitamin D intoxication are anorexia, nausea, vomiting, polyuria, polydipsia, constipation, weakness, muscle pain, changes in mental status with fatigue, confusion, difficulty in concentration, drowsiness, apathy, and eventually coma. Metastatic calcification of the soft tissues may develop. The clinically most important ectopic calcinosis is nephrocalcinosis, causing a gradual decline in kidney function.

The likelihood of the different formulations of vitamin D to cause a full-blown vitamin D intoxication is dependent on the hypercalcemic potency, the systemic half-life like the storage capacity of the body, and the systemic availability of the compound. The best-known vitamin D intoxications were caused by over-fortification of milk with 70–600 times the legal limit for vitamin D fortification (400 IU per quart or 423 IU/L) [117]. The body has a large storage capacity for the unhydroxylated vitamin D's, cholecalciferol (vitamin D_3) and ergocalciferol (vitamin D_2). Furthermore, these compounds have long half-lives (20–60 days). The result is a high risk for accumulation in the body, with prolonged vitamin D intoxication. Vitamin D_2 seems to be a little less toxic than vitamin D_3. If administered properly, the therapeutic windows of both compounds seems to be quite broad. Recent American guidelines [118] have prescribed 2400 IU as the maximal daily dose of vitamin D. These recommendations were, however, based on the observation of hypercalcemia in a single Indian study. Others have described treatment with much larger doses of vitamin D without any side effects. A single dose of 400,000 IU of cholecalciferol has been given to elderly people with unknown pretreatment vitamin D status without any negative effects [119]. If a daily dose of 40,000–60,000 IU of cholecalciferol is given for a long period, the risk of vitamin D intoxication increases; if the daily dose of cholecalciferol exceeds 100,000–500,000 IU, metastatic calcifications and nephrocalcinosis may develop [120,121]. In children, more caution is advisable, as intoxication has been demonstrated at daily doses of 2,000–4,000 IU cholecalciferol [122].

The hydroxylated compounds (calcitriol, alfacalcidol) have a much higher calcemic potency than the unhydroxylated forms. Their half-lives, on the other hand, are very short (15–35 hr). These characteristics indicate a high risk for the development of hypercalcemia if treatment is not very carefully monitored and titrated with small increases in doses (0.5 μg/day is usually well tolerated). If hypercalcemia develops during treatment, however, discontinuation of the treatment will very quickly normalize serum calcium levels.

New vitamin D analogs with less hypercalcemic action have been developed. Calcipotriol, a new analog developed as an antiproliferative drug, has

100–200 times less calcemic potency than calcitriol. Topical administration of the compound minimizes its systemic availability (<5%), although administration of excessive amounts can cause hypercalcemia (See Chapter 18).

The diagnosis of vitamin D intoxication is based partly on a typical clinical picture combined with knowledge of the intake of vitamin D preparations. An obligatory laboratory finding is increased values of serum calcium and/or increased urine calcium. If the patient has been treated with either ergocalciferol, cholecalciferol, or 25-hydroxyvitamin D, the diagnosis can often be confirmed by measuring serum values of 25-hydroxyvitamin D, where the typical findings are values above 110 nmol/L. Measurement of serum 1,25-dihydroxyvitamin D is often less informative, as both normal and increased values can be seen in vitamin D intoxication. The obligatory safety control parameters for patients taking high-dose or high-potency vitamin D preparations are serum calcium and serum creatinine.

The maximum tolerated dose of vitamin D preparations varies from one individual to another. Special caution should be observed with certain groups of patients. Individuals with reduced kidney function and patients in treatment with pharmacological doses of vitamin A preparations are more likely to develop hypercalcemia. Patients suffering from granulomatous diseases have a high capacity for extrarenal 1,25-dihydroxyvitamin D synthesis, making them hypersensitive to vitamin D treatment. The granulomatous diseases best known for causing vitamin D intoxication are sarcoidosis, tuberculosis, and lymphoma, but cases have also been reported in leprosy, coccidioidomycosis, histoplasmosis, candidiasis, eosinophilic granuloma, berylliosis and silicone-induced granuloma [117].

When vitamin D intoxication has been diagnosed or suspected, discontinuation of the vitamin D treatment is the most important step. Furthermore fluid intake should be increased (to 3–4 L/day) and calcium intake restricted (to <400 mg/day). This regimen will cure most cases. In more severe cases of hypercalcemia, forced diuresis with the use of loop diuretics (e.g., furosemide) can be considered. Hypercalcemia and hypercalciuria in vitamin D intoxication are mediated through stimulation of intestinal calcium absorption and of osteoclastic bone resorption. In more prolonged cases of vitamin D intoxication, treatment with either glucocorticoids or bisphosphonates has been shown to effective. Glucocorticoids decrease vitamin D–stimulated intestinal calcium uptake and bisphosphonates decrease osteoclastic bone resorption.

REFERENCES

1. McCollum EF, Simmonds N, Becker JE, Shipley PG. Studies on experimental rickets; and experimental demonstration of the existence of a vitamin which promotes calcium deposition. J Biol Chem 1922; 53:293–312.

2. Holick MF. Vitamin D: Photobiology, metabolism, mechanism of action, and clinical applications. In: Favus MD, ed. Primer on Metabolic Bone Diseases and Disorders of Mineral Metabolism, 3d ed. New York: Lippincott-Raven, 1996:74–81.

3. Reichel H, Koeffler HP, Norman AW. The role of the vitamin D endocrine system in health and disease. N Engl J Med 1989; 320:980–991.

4. Hurwitz S. Homeostatic control of plasma calcium concentration. Crit Rev Biochem Mol Biol 1996; 31:41–100.

5. Norman AW, Nemere I, Zhou LX, Bishop JE, Lowe KE, Maiyar AC, et al. 1,25(OH)2-vitamin D3, a steroid hormone that produces biologic effects via both genomic and nongenomic pathways. J Steroid Biochem Mol Biol 1992; 41: 231–240.

6. Holick MF. Noncalcemic actions of 1,25-dihydroxyvitamin D3 and clinical applications. Bone 1995; 17:107S–111S.

7. Ljunghall S, Charles P, Falch J, Haug E, Melhus H, Mellstrom D, et al. Vitamin D and osteoporosis. Nord Med 1995; 110:253–257.

8. Fraser DR. Vitamin D. Lancet 1995; 345:104–107.

9. Glerup H. Investigations on the role of vitamin D in muscle function—A study of muscle function in vitamin D deficient humans and the effect of treatment with vitamin D. PhD-thesis. University of Aarhus, Denmark, 1998.

10. Utiger RD. The need for more vitamin D. N Engl J Med 1998; 338:828–829.

11. Thomas MK, Lloyd-Jones DM, Thadhani RI, Shaw AC, Deraska DJ, Kitch BT, et al. Hypovitaminosis D in medical inpatients. N Engl J Med 1998; 338:777–783.

12. Holick MF. McCollum Award Lecture, 1994: vitamin D—new horizons for the 21st century. Am J Clin Nutr 1994; 60:619–630.

13. Holick MF. Photobiology of vitamin D. In: Feldman D, Glorieux FH, Pike JW, eds. Vitamin D. San Diego, CA: Academic Press, 1997:33–39.

14. Barger-Lux MJ, Heaney RP, Lanspa SJ, Healy JC, DeLuca HF. An investigation of sources of variation in calcium absorption efficiency. J Clin Endocrinol Metab 1995; 80:406–411.

15. Walters MR. Newly identified actions of the vitamin D endocrine system. Endocrinol Rev 1992; 13:719–764.

16. Bouillon R, Okamura WH, Norman AW. Structure-function relationships in the vitamin D endocrine system. Endocrinol Rev 1995; 16:200–257.

17. Lowe KE, Maiyar AC, Norman AW. Vitamin D-mediated gene expression. Crit Rev Eukaryot Gene Exp 1992; 2:65–109.

18. Minghetti PP, Norman AW. 1,25(OH)2-vitamin D3 receptors: Gene regulation and genetic circuitry. FASEB J 1988; 2:3043–3053.

19. Pike JW. Vitamin D3 receptors: Structure and function in transcription. Annu Rev Nutr 1991; 11:189–216.

20. Nemere I, Dormanen MC, Hammond MW, Okamura WH, Norman AW. Identification of a specific binding protein for 1 alpha,25-dihydroxyvitamin D3 in basal-lateral membranes of chick intestinal epithelium and relationship to transcaltachia. J Biol Chem 1994; 269:23750–23756.

21. Zhou LX, Nemere I, Norman AW. 1,25-Dihydroxyvitamin D3 analog structure-function assessment of the rapid stimulation of intestinal calcium absorption (transcaltachia). J Bone Min Res 1992; 7:457–463.

22. de Boland AR, Boland RL. Non-genomic signal transduction pathway of vitamin D in muscle. Cell Signal 1994; 6:717–724.

23. Wasserman RH. Vitamin D and the intestinal absorption of calcium and phosphorus. In: Feldman D, Glorieux FH, Pike JW, eds. Vitamin D. San Diego, CA: Academic Press, 1997:259–273.

24. Kumar R. Vitamin D and the kidney. In: Feldman D, Glorieux FH, Pike JW, eds. Vitamin D. San Diego, CA: Academic Press, 1997:275–292.

25. Parfitt AM. Osteomalacia and related disorders. In: Avioli LV, Krane SM, eds. Metabolic Bone Diseases and Clinically Related Disorders, 2d ed. Philadelphia: Saunders, 1990:329–396.

26. Francis RM, Peacock M, Storer JH, Davies AE, Brown WB, Nordin BE. Calcium malabsorption in the elderly: The effect of treatment with oral 25-hydroxyvitamin D3. Eur J Clin Invest 1983; 13:391–396.

27. Dawson Hughes B, Harris S, Finneran S. Calcium absorption on high and low calcium intakes in relation to vitamin D receptor genotypes. J Clin Endocrinol Metab 1995; 80:3657–3661.

28. Francis RM, Boyle IT, Moniz C, Sutcliffe AM, Davis BS, Beastall GH, et al. A comparison of the effects of alfacalcidol treatment and vitamin D2 supplementation on calcium absorption in elderly women with vertabral fractures. Osteoporos Int 1996; 6:284–290.

29. Orimo H, Shiraki M, Hayashi T, Nakamura T. Reduced occurrence of vertebral crush fractures in senile osteoporosis treated with 1 alpha (OH)-vitamin D3. Bone Min 1987; 3:47–52.

30. Tilyard MW, Spears GF, Thomson J, Dovey S. Treatment of postmenopausal osteoporosis with calcitriol or calcium. N Engl J Med 1992; 326:357–362.

31. de Boland AR, Boland RL. Rapid changes in skeletal muscle calcium uptake induced in vitro by 1,25-dihydroxyvitamin D3 are suppressed by calcium channel blockers. Endocrinology 1987; 120:1858–1864.

32. Toury R, Stelly N, Boisonneau E, Convert M, Dupuis Y. Relationship between vitamin D status and deposition of bound calcium in skeletal muscle of the rat. Biol Cell 1990; 69:179–189.

33. Peacock M, Selby PL, Francis RM, Brown WB, Hordon L. Vitamin D deficiency, insufficiency, sufficiency and intoxication: What do they mean? In: Norman A, Schaefer K, Grigoletti MG, Herrath DV, eds. Sixth Workshop on Vitamin D. Berlin and New York: de Gruyter, 1985:569–570.

34. Chapuy MC, Chapuy P, Meunier PJ. Calcium and vitamin D supplements: Effects on calcium metabolism in elderly people. Am J Clin Nutr 1987; 46:324–328.

35. Lips P, Wierzinga A, van Ginkel FC, Jongen MJM, Netelenbos JC. The effect of vitamin D supplementation on vitamin D status and parathyroid function in the elderly. J Clin Endocrinol Metab 1988; 67:324–328.

36. Gloth FM, Gundberg CM, Hollis BW, Haddad JG Jr, Tobin JD. Vitamin D deficiency in homebound elderly persons. JAMA 1995; 274:1683–1686.

37. Webb AR, Pilbeam C, Hanafin N, Holick MF. An evaluation of the relative contributions of exposure to sunlight and of diet to the circulating concentrations of 25-hydroxyvitamin D in an elderly nursing home population in Boston. Am J Clin Nutr 1990; 51:1075–1081.

38. O'Dowd KJ, Clemens TL, Kelsey JL, Lindsay R. Exogenous calciferol (vitamin D) and vitamin D endocrine status among elderly nursing home residents in the New York City area. J Am Geriatr Soc 1993; 41:414–421.

39. Malabanan A, Veronikis IE, Holick MF. Redefining vitamin D insufficiency. Lancet 1998; 351:805–806.

40. Smith R, Stern G. Myopathy, osteomalacia and hyperparathyroidism. Brain 1967; 90:593–602.

41. Chalmers J, Conacher WDH, Gardner DL, Scott PJ. Osteomalacia—A common disease in elderly women. J Bone Joint Surg 1967; 49B:403–423.

42. Gloth FM, Lindsay JM, Zelesnick LB, Greenough WB. Can vitamin D deficiency produce an unusual pain syndrome? Arch Intern Med 1991; 151:1662–1664.

43. Rimaniol JM, Authier FJ, Chariot P. Muscle weakness in intensive care patients: initial manifestation of vitamin D deficiency. Intensive Care Med 1994; 20:591–592.

44. Rao DS, Honasoge M. Metabolic bone disease in gastrointestinal, hepatobiliary and pancreatic disorders. In: Favus MJ, ed. Primer on the Metabolic Bone Diseases and Disorders of Mineral Metabolism, 3d ed. New York: Lippincott-Raven, 1997: 306–310.

45. Melsen F, Mosekilde L. The role of bone biopsy in metabolic bone disease. Orthop Clin North Am 1981; 12:571–600.

46. Parfitt AM, Podenphant J, Villanueva AR, Frame B. Metabolic bone disease with and without osteomalacia after intestinal bypass surgery: a bone histomorphometric study. Bone 1985; 6:211–220.

47. Webb AR, Kline L, Holick MF. Influence of season and latitude on the cutaneous synthesis of vitamin D3: exposure to winter sunlight in Boston and Edmonton will not promote vitamin D3 synthesis in human skin. J Clin Endocrinol Metab 1988; 67:373–378.

48. Poskitt EME, Cole TJ, Lawson DEM. Diet, sunlight, and 25-hydroxy vitamin D in healthy children and adults. BMJ 1979; 1:221–223.

49. Need AG, Morris HA, Horowitz M, Nordin C. Effects of skin thickness, age, body fat, and sunlight on serum 25-hydroxyvitamin D. Am J Clin Nutr 1993; 58:882–885.

50. Bouillon RA, Auwerx JH, Lissens WD, Pelemans WK. Vitamin D status in the elderly: Seasonal substrate deficiency causes 1,25-dihydroxycholecalciferol deficiency. Am J Clin Nutr 1987; 45:755–763.

51. Chapuy MC, Schott AM, Garnero P, Hans D, Delmas PD, Meunier PJ. Healthy elderly French women living at home have secondary hyperparathyroidism and high bone turnover in winter. EPIDOS Study Group. J Clin Endocrinol Metab 1996; 81: 1129–1133.

52. Khaw KT, Scragg R, Murphy S. Single-dose cholecalciferol suppresses the winter increase in parathyroid hormone concentrations in healthy older men and women: A randomized trial. Am J Clin Nutr 1994; 59:1040–1044.

53. Krall EA, Sahyoun N, Tannenbaum S, Dallal GE, Dawson Hughes B. Effect of vitamin D intake on seasonal variations in parathyroid hormone secretion in postmenopausal women. N Engl J Med 1989; 321:1777–1783.

54. Matsuoka LY, Ide L, Wortsman J, MacLaughlin JA, Holick MF. Sunscreens suppress cutaneous vitamin D3 synthesis. J Clin Endocrinol Metab 1987; 64: 1165–1168.

55. Fine RM. Sunscreens and cutaneous vitamin D synthesis. Int J Dermatol 1988; 27: 300–301.
56. Devgun MS, Johnson BE, Paterson CR. Tanning, protection against sunburn and vitamin D formation with a UV-A "sun-bed." Br J Dermatol 1982; 107:275–284.
57. Finch PJ, Ang L, Colston KW, Nisbet J, Maxwell JD. Blunted seasonal variation in serum 25-hydroxy vitamin D and increased risk of osteomalacia in vegetarian London Asians. Eur J Clin Nutr 1992; 46:509–515.
58. Nisbet JA, Eastwood JB, Colston KW, Ang L, Flanagan AM, Chambers TJ, et al. Detection of osteomalacia in British Asians: A comparison of clinical score with biochemical measurements. Clin Sci Colch 1990; 78:383–389.
59. Solanki T, Hyatt RH, Kemm JR, Hughes EA, Cowan RA. Are elderly Asians in Britain at a high risk of vitamin D deficiency and osteomalacia? Age Ageing 1995; 24:103–107.
60. Smith R. Asian rickets and osteomalacia. Q J Med 1990; 76:899–901.
61. Henriksen C, Brunvand L, Stoltenberg C, Trygg K, Haug E, Pedersen JI. Diet and vitamin D status among pregnant Pakistani women in Oslo. Eur J Clin Nutr 1995; 49:211–218.
62. Brunvand L, Haug E. Vitamin D deficiency amongst Pakistani women in Oslo. Acta Obstet Gynecol Scand 1993; 72:264–268.
63. Woodhouse NJY, Norton WL. Low vitamin D levels in Saudi Arabians. King Faisal Spec Hosp Med J 1982; 2:127–131.
64. Fonseca V, Tongia R, el Hazmi M, Abu Aisha H. Exposure to sunlight and vitamin D deficiency in Saudi Arabian women. Postgrad Med J 1984; 60:589–591.
65. el Sonbaty MR, Abdul Ghaffar NU. Vitamin D deficiency in veiled Kuwaiti women. Eur J Clin Nutr 1996; 50:315–318.
66. Sedrani SH, Elidrissy AWTH, El Arabi KM. Sunlight and vitamin D status in normal Saudi subjects. Am J Clin Nutr 1983; 38:129–132.
67. Al Arabi KM, Elidrissy AW, Sedrani SH. Is avoidance of sunlight a cause of fractures of the femoral neck in elderly Saudis? Trop Geogr Med 1984; 36:273–279.
68. Lo CW, Paris PW, Holick MF. Indian and Pakistani immigrants have the same capacity as Caucasians to produce vitamin D in response to ultraviolet irradiation. Am J Clin Nutr 1986; 44:683–685.
69. van der Wielen RP, Lowik MR, van den Berg H, de Groot LC, Haller J, Moreiras O, et al. Serum vitamin D concentrations among elderly people in Europe. Lancet 1995; 346:207–210.
70. McKenna MJ. Differences in vitamin D status between countries in young adults and the elderly. Am J Med 1992; 93:69–77.
71. Chapuy MC, Durr F, Chapuy P. Age-related changes in parathyroid hormone and 25 hydroxycholecalciferol levels. J Gerontol 1983; 38:19–22.
72. McMurtry CT, Young SE, Downs RW, Adler RA. Mild vitamin D deficiency and secondary hyperparathyroidism in nursing home patients receiving adequate dietary vitamin D. J Am Geriatr Soc 1992; 40:343–347.
73. Compston JE, Silver AC, Croucher PI, Brown RC, Woodhead JS. Elevated serum intact parathyroid hormone levels in elderly patients with hip fracture. Clin Endocrinol Oxf 1989; 31:667–672.

74. Falch JA, Mowe M, Bohmer T, Haug E. Serum levels of intact parathyroid hormone in elderly patients with hip fracture living at home. Acta Endocrinol Copenh 1992; 126: 10–12.
75. Ooms ME, Roos JC, Bezemer PD, van der Vijgh WJ, Bouter LM, Lips P. Prevention of bone loss by vitamin D supplementation in elderly women: A randomized double-blind trial. J Clin Endocrinol Metab 1995; 80:1052–1058.
76. Omdahl JL, Garry PJ, Hunsaker LA, Hunt WC, Goodwin JS. Nutritional status in a healthy elderly population: Vitamin D. Am J Clin Nutr 1982; 36:1225–1233.
77. Gloth FM, Tobin JD, Sherman SS, Hollis BW. Is the recommended daily allowance for vitamin D too low for the homebound elderly? J Am Geriatr Soc 1991; 39: 137–141.
78. Benhamou CL, Tourliere D, Gauvain JB, Picaper G, Audran M, Jallet P. Calciotropic hormones in elderly people with and without hip fracture. Osteoporos Int 1995; 5:103–107.
79. Gloth FM, Tobin JD. Vitamin D deficiency in older people. J Am Geriatr Soc 1995; 43:822–828.
80. Holick MF, Matsuoka LY, Wortsman J. Age, vitamin D, and solar ultraviolet. Lancet 1989; 2:1104–1105.
81. MacLaughlin J, Holick MF. Aging decreases the capacity of human skin to produce vitamin D3. J Clin Invest 1985; 76:1536–1538.
82. Klein GL, Simmons DJ. Nutritional rickets: thoughts about pathogenesis. Ann Med 1993; 25:379–384.
83. Osler M, Schroll M. A dietary study of the elderly in the City of Roskilde 1988/1989: II. A nutritional risk assessment. Dan Med Bull 1991; 38:410–413.
84. Barragry JM, France MW, Corless D, Gupta SP, Switala S, Boucher BJ, et al. Intestinal cholecalciferol absorption in the elderly and in the younger adults. Clin Sci Mol Med 1978; 55:213–220.
85. Clemens TL, Zhou XY, Myles M, Endres D, Lindsay R. Serum vitamin D2 and vitamin D3 metabolite concentrations and absorption of vitamin D2 in elderly subjects. J Clin Endocrinol Metab 1986; 63:656–660.
86. Dibble JB, Sheridan P, Losowsky MS. A survey of vitamin D deficiency in gastrointestinal and liver disorders. Q J Med 1984; 53:119–134.
87. Hay JE. Bone disease in cholestatic liver disease. Gastroenterology 1995; 108: 276–283.
88. Lips P, Netelenbos JC, Jongen MJ, van Ginkel FC, Althuis AL, van Schaik CL, et al. Histomorphometric profile and vitamin D status in patients with femoral neck fracture. Metab Bone Dis Rel Res 1982; 4:85–93.
89. Epstein S, Bryce G, Hinman JW. The influence of age on bone mineral regulating hormones. Bone 1986; 7:421–425.
90. Tsai KS, Heath H, Kumar R, Riggs BL. Impaired vitamin D metabolism with aging in women: Possible role in pathogenesis of senile osteoporosis. J Clin Invest 1984; 73:1668–1672.
91. Llach F, Massry SG. On the mechanism of secondary hyperparathyroidism in moderate renal insufficiency. J Clin Endocrinol Metab 1985; 61:601–606.

92. Freaney R, McBrinn Y, McKenna MJ. Secondary hyperparathyroidism in elderly people: Combined effect of renal insufficiency and vitamin D deficiency. Am J Clin Nutr 1993; 58:187–191.

93. Lund B, Sorensen OH, Agner E. Serum 1,25(OH)2D in normal subjects and in patients with postmenopausal osteopenia. Horm Metab Res 1982; 14:271–274.

94. Clements MR, Johnson L, Fraser DR. A new mechanism for induced vitamin D deficiency in calcium deprivation. Nature 1987; 325:62–65.

95. Halloran BP, Bikle DD, Levens MJ, Castro ME, Globus RK, Holton E. Chronic 1,25-dihydroxyvitamin D3 administration in the rat reduces the serum concentration of 25-hydroxyvitamin D by increasing metabolic clearance rate. J Clin Invest 1986; 78:622–628.

96. Clements MR, Davies M, Hayes ME, Hickey CD, Lumb GA, Mawer EB, et al. The role of 1,25-dihydroxyvitamin D in the mechanism of acquired vitamin D deficiency. Clin Endocrinol Oxf 1992; 37:17–27.

97. Davies M, Heys SE, Selby PL, Berry JL, Mawer EB. Increased catabolism of 25-hydroxyvitamin D in patients with partial gastrectomy and elevated 1,25-dihydroxyvitamin D levels: Implications for metabolic bone disease. J Clin Endocrinol Metab 1997; 82:209–212.

98. Bisballe S, Eriksen EF, Melsen F, Mosekilde L, Sorensen OH, Hessov I. Osteopenia and osteomalacia after gastrectomy: Interrelations between biochemical markers of bone remodelling, vitamin D metabolites, and bone histomorphometry. Gut 1991; 32:1303–1307.

99. Bisballe S, Buus S, Lund B, Hessov I. Food intake and nutritional status after gastrectomy. Hum Nutr Clin Nutr 1986; 40:301–308.

100. Nilas L, Christiansen C, Christiansen J. Regulation of vitamin D and calcium metabolism after gastrectomy. Gut 1985; 26:252–257.

101. Driscoll RH Jr, Meredith SC, Sitrin M, Rosenberg IH. Vitamin D deficiency and bone disease in patients with Crohn's disease. Gastroenterology 1982; 83: 1252–1258.

102. Harries AD, Brown R, Heatley RV, Williams LA, Woodhead S, Rhodes J. Vitamin D status in Crohn's disease: Association with nutrition and disease activity. Gut 1985; 26:1197–1203.

103. Talabiska DG, Seidner DL, Jensen GL. Acute tetany in the Crohn's patient with osteomalacia. Nutrition 1993; 9:159–162.

104. Russell JA. Osteomalacic myopathy. Muscle Nerve 1994; 17:578–580.

105. Ritz E, Boland R, Kreusser W. Effects of vitamin D and parathyroid hormone on muscle: Potential role in uremic myopathy. Am J Clin Nutr 1980; 33:1522–1529.

106. Matthews C, Heimberg KW, Ritz E, Agostini B, Fritzsche J, Hasselbach W. Effect of 1,25-dihydroxycholecalciferol on impaired calcium transport by the sarcoplasmic reticulum in experimental uremia. Kidney Int 1977; 11:227–235.

107. Clyne N, Esbjornsson M, Jansson E, Jogestrand T, Lins LE, Pehrsson SK. Effects of renal failure on skeletal muscle. Nephron 1993; 63:395–399.

108. Laville M, Fouque D. Muscular function in chronic renal failure. Adv Nephrol Necker Hosp 1995; 24:245–269.

109. Clyne N, Jogestrand T. Effect of erythropoietin treatment on physical exercise capacity and on renal function in predialytic uremic patients. Nephron 1992; 60:390–396.

110. Bertoli M, Luisetto G, Arcuti V, Urso M. Uremic myopathy and calcitriol therapy in CAPD patients. ASAIO Trans 1991; 37:M397–M398

111. Wanic Kossowska M, Grzegorzewska A, Plotast H, Bombicki K. Does calcitriol therapy improve muscle function in uremic patients. Perit Dial Int 1996; 16 (suppl 1): S305–S308.

112. Gloth FM, Smith CE, Hollis BW, Tobin JD. Functional improvement with vitamin D replenishment in a cohort of frail, vitamin D-deficient older people. J Am Geriatr Soc 1995; 43:1269–1271.

113. Chapuy MC, Arlot ME, Delmas PD, Meunier PJ. Effect of calcium and cholecalciferol treatment for three years on hip fractures in elderly women. BMJ 1994; 308:1081–1082.

114. Chapuy MC, Arlot ME, Duboeuf F, Brun J, Crouzet B, Arnaud S, et al. Vitamin D3 and calcium to prevent hip fractures in the elderly women. N Engl J Med 1992; 327:1637–1642.

115. Chapuy MC, Meunier PJ. Prevention of secondary hyperparathyroidism and hip fractures in elderly women with calcium and vitamin D3 supplements. Osteoporos Int 1996; suppl 3:S60–S63.

116. Lips P, Graafmans WC, Ooms ME, Bezemer PD, Bouter LM. Vitamin D supplementation and fracture incidence in elderly persons: a randomized, placebo-controlled clinical trial. Ann Intern Med 1996; 124:400–406.

117. Thys-Jacobs S, Chan FKW, Koberle LMC, Bilezikian JP. Hypercalcemia due to vitamin D toxicity. In: Feldman B, Glorieux FH, Pike JW, eds. Vitamin D. San Diego, CA: Academic Press, 1997:883–901.

118. Standing Committee on the Scientific Evaluation of Dietary Reference Intakes. Dietary Reference Intake for Calcium, Phosphorus, Magnesium, Vitamin D, and Fluoride. Washington DC: National Academy Press, 1997.

119. Heikinheimo RJ, Inkovaara JA, Harju EJ, Haavisto MV, Kaarela RH, Kataja JM, et al. Annual injection of vitamin D and fractures of aged bones. Calcif Tissue Int 1992; 51:105–110.

120. Jacobus CH, Holick MF, Shao Q, Chen TC, Holm IA, Kolodny JM, et al. Hypervitaminosis D associated with drinking milk. N Engl J Med 1992; 326:1173–1177.

121. Allen SH, Shah JH. Calcinosis and metastatic calcification due to vitamin D intoxication: A case report and review. Horm Res 1992; 37:68–77.

122. Mehls O, Wolf H, Wille L. Vitamin D requirements and vitamin D intoxication in infancy. Int J Vitam Nutr Res Suppl 1989; 30:87–94.

5

Effect of Vitamin D on Keratinocyte Proliferation and Differentiation

Daniel D. Bikle
University of California, San Francisco and Veterans Affairs Medical Center, San Francisco, California

I. INTRODUCTION

The epidermis is the sole source of cholecalciferol or vitamin D_3, the precursor for a family of vitamin D metabolites whose best-understood role is the regulation of bone mineral homeostasis. In Chap. 3 Dr. Holick describes this process. Vitamin D may also be ingested in the diet, generally in vitamin D–supplemented dairy products. Both cholecalciferol and ergocalciferol (D_2) are used for such supplementation, and their metabolic pathways with respect to activation and biologic activity are comparable. Accordingly, in this chapter I will use the subscript (2 or 3) only when one or the other form of vitamin D is specifically indicated. Otherwise, lack of subscript includes both. Vitamin D has little biological activity per se but must be metabolized first in the liver to 25OHD and then in the kidney to a number of metabolites, the most important of which is $1,25(OH)_2D$. This is the classic pathway and quantitatively the most important for producing $1,25(OH)_2D$ for the body overall. However, the keratinocyte is fully capable of producing its own $1,25(OH)_2D$ [1]. In fact we [2] used RNA from the keratinocyte to clone and sequence the 25OHD 1α hydroxylase, the enzyme that converts 25OHD to $1,25(OH)_2D$, because the expression of this enzyme was higher in keratinocytes than in any other cell including the renal proximal tubule cell. Furthermore, Lehmann and collaborators [3,4] recently demonstrated that the keratinocyte could also convert vitamin D directly to $1,25(OH)_2D$, indicating that the vitamin D 25 hydroxylase was also present in these cells. These results are consistent with the finding by Ichikawa et al. [5] in mouse skin of the mRNA for the sterol 26(27) hydroxylase, the only clearly identified enzyme with 25 hydroxylase activity [6].

Thus it is conceivable that the keratinocyte makes its own $1,25(OH)_2D$ from endogenously produced vitamin D. Why? This chapter is devoted to answering this question. In brief, $1,25(OH)_2D$ in combination with calcium and protein kinase C plays an important role in keratinocyte differentiation.

II. CUTANEOUS PRODUCTION OF $1,25(OH)_2D$

A. The Epidermal Enzymes Metabolizing Vitamin D_3 to Its Active Products

Keratinocytes are not only capable of producing vitamin D_3 from endogenous sources of 7-dehydrocholesterol (7-DHC) in a regulated fashion (Chap. 3) but are also capable of producing a variety of D metabolites, including $1,25(OH)_2D$; $24,25(OH)_2D$; and $1,24,25(OH)_3D$ [1,7,8] from exogenous and endogenous sources of 25OHD. The latter two metabolites are the products of the 24 hydroxylase acting on 25OHD and $1,25(OH)_2D$, respectively, whereas $1,25(OH)_2D$ is the product of the 1α hydroxylase. The process by which $1,25(OH)_2D$ is produced and catabolized is tightly regulated and coupled to the differentiation of these cells.

Extrarenal production of $1,25(OH)_2D$ has been clearly demonstrated in both anephric humans [9,10] and pigs [11], although the tissue(s) responsible for the circulating levels of $1,25(OH)_2D$ in anephric animals has not been established. The epidermis is likely to contribute, as human keratinocytes rapidly and extensively convert 25OHD to $1,25(OH)_2D$. Peak levels of $1,25(OH)_2D$ are reached in the cell within 1 hr after adding 25OHD. By 1 hr, $1,25(OH)_2D$ is the main metabolite observed; however, other metabolites appear with continued incubation, many of which represent degradation products of $1,25(OH)_2D$ [7]. The apparent Km for the enzyme (25OHD-1α hydroxylase) metabolizing 25OHD to $1,25(OH)_2D$ is estimated to be 5×10^{-8} M, a value lower than that estimated for the kidney. The production of $1,25(OH)_2D$ by isolated keratinocytes in culture has been confirmed using intact pig skins perfused with 25OHD [12]. However, when renal production of $1,25(OH)_2D$ is normal the circulating levels of $1,25(OH)_2D$ are sufficient to limit the contribution from epidermal production.

The 1α hydroxylase and the 24 hydroxylase are cytochrome P-450 enzymes residing in the inner membrane of the mitochondrion, where they function as mixed function oxidases at the end of an electron transport chain that includes ferrodoxin and ferrodoxin reductase. Despite the cloning of the 25 hydroxylase (sterol 26[27] hydroxylase) [13] and the 24 hydroxylase [14] several years ago, the cloning of the 1α hydroxylase has only recently been accomplished [2,15–18]. It is now clear that the epidermal 1α hydroxylase and the renal 1α hydroxylase are the same protein. The 1α hydroxylase is a 56-kDa protein with 506 amino acids. A region containing a putative mitochondrial signal sequence is found near the N-terminus. The heme-binding domain has 73 and 65% homology with the heme-binding domains of the human 25 and 24 hydroxylases, with overall homology of 39 and 30%, respectively. The intron/exon boundaries for the 1α hydroxylase gene occur at the same location (except for intron 1 of the 1α hydroxylase gene and an additional two introns in the 24 hydroxylase gene) as found for the 25 and 24 hydroxylase genes and for the genes encoding the homologous mitochondrial P-450 side chain cleavage enzyme (SCC) and 11β hydroxylase.

B. Hormonal Regulation

Both the formation and catabolism of $1,25(OH)_2D$ are under hormonal control (Figure 1). Parathyroid hormone (PTH) exerts a modest stimulatory effect on

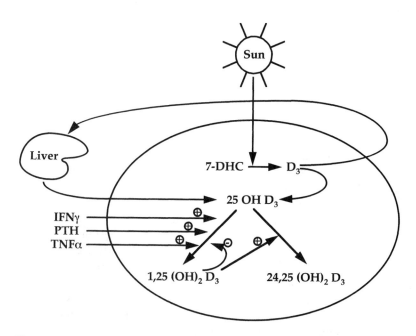

Figure 1   Regulation of $1,25(OH)_2D$ production in the keratinocyte. 7-dehydrocholesterol (7-DHC) is converted to vitamin D_3 under the influence of UV light. The D_3 produced is transported out of the keratinocyte to the liver, where it is converted to $25OHD_3$. Some of the D_3 produced may be converted directly in the epidermis to $25OHD_3$. $25OHD_3$ is then metabolized either to $24,25(OH)_2D_3$ or to $1,25(OH)_2D_3$. Parathyroid hormone (PTH) secreted by the parathyroid gland stimulates the production of $1,25(OH)_2D_3$ as does tumor necrosis factor-alpha (TNF-α) secreted by keratinocytes and interferon-gamma (IFN-γ) secreted by macrophages. $1,25(OH)_2D$ inhibits its own production and stimulates its catabolism by inducing the 24 hydroxylase.

1,25(OH)$_2$D production, whereas the phosphodiesterase inhibitor isobutyl-methylxanthine (IBMX) inhibits its degradation [7]. In combination, PTH and IBMX markedly increase the amount of 1,25(OH)$_2$D that accumulates within the keratinocyte following the addition of 25OHD. These effects are not reproduced by cAMP or its membrane-permeable derivatives, suggesting that the actions of PTH and IBMX may be operating through a mechanism independent of cAMP. The effects of PTH and IBMX are maximal after a 4-hr incubation of cells with these agents before adding 25OHD; i.e., the effects are not immediate. In renal cells, PTH displays a more acute stimulation of 1,25(OH)$_2$D production [19], and cAMP appears to play a second-messenger role [20]. The promoter of the 1α hydroxylase gene contains three potential cAMP response elements, which, in appropriate cells, may allow cAMP to stimulate expression of this gene [21]. But the regulation of 1,25(OH)$_2$D production in keratinocytes by PTH and cAMP differs from their regulation of 1,25(OH)$_2$D production in renal cells. The mechanism by which PTH stimulates 1,25(OH)$_2$D production in keratinocytes is unclear, since PTH receptors have been difficult to detect in normal keratinocytes and PTH fails to stimulate adenyl cyclase activity in these cells.

1,25(OH)$_2$D regulates its own levels negatively within the cell. This negative feedback loop is similar to that observed in the kidney but differs from that seen in the macrophage, where this feedback loop is missing. The mechanism by which 1,25(OH)$_2$D exerts this negative regulation is unclear, since the promoter of the 1α hydroxylase gene is not suppressed by 1,25(OH)$_2$D in its basal activity and is only marginally suppressed by 1,25(OH)$_2$D when stimulated by PTH [21]. Incubation of keratinocytes with exogenous 1,25(OH)$_2$D inhibits 1,25(OH)$_2$D production and stimulates 1,25(OH)$_2$D catabolism in part through induction of the 24 hydroxylase. Unlike the promoter of the 1α hydroxylase gene, the promoter of the 24-hydroxylase gene contains at least one vitamin D response element, which mediates 1,25(OH)$_2$D-stimulated gene expression [22]. Although inhibition of the 1α hydroxylase occurs within 4 hr of the addition of 1,25(OH)$_2$D (IC50 = 10^{-11} M), induction of the 24 hydroxylase requires more time (within 16 hr) and higher concentrations of 1,25(OH)$_2$D (EC50 = 2.3×10^{-11}) [23]. The concentrations required to regulate 25OHD metabolism in keratinocytes are free concentrations and are independent of vitamin D–binding proteins. Addition of serum (which contains DBP) or albumin reduces the free fraction of 1,25(OH)$_2$D and increases the apparent EC50 (IC50) for total 1,25(OH)$_2$D. However, using direct measurements of the free fraction of 1,25(OH)$_2$D, we [24] showed that the EC50 (IC50) for the free concentration was not altered by serum or albumin. An important difference in the regulation of 25OHD metabolism by 1,25(OH)$_2$D between keratinocytes and renal cells is that the concentration of 1,25(OH)$_2$D required to inhibit the 1α hydroxylase and induce the 24 hydroxylase in renal cells appears to be several orders of magnitude greater than that required for comparable effects in keratinocytes [7,23,25,26]. Thus, 1,25(OH)$_2$D production by keratinocytes is exquisitely sensitive to exogenous $1,25(OH)_2D$. This difference in sensitivity to feedback inhibition by $1,25(OH)_2D$ between keratinocytes and renal cells may account for the observation that following acute nephrectomy, extrarenal production of $1,25(OH)_2D$ is very low [27,28]; only with time after renal production has ceased does extrarenal production emerge. A similar observation was made in pig skins perfused with 25OHD: the amount of $1,25(OH)_2D$ produced was initially low but increased after 4–8 hr of perfusion [12].

C. Effects of Differentiation

The role of $1,25(OH)_2D$ in promoting differentiation of the keratinocyte is reviewed below. In this section, the ability of differentiation to regulate $1,25(OH)_2D$ production is considered. In the presence of adequate levels of calcium, keratinocytes progress from rapidly proliferating cells to cells capable of making cornified envelopes, one of the most distinctive features of epidermal terminal differentiation. The cornified envelope is formed by the cross-linking of precursor molecules such as involucrin and loricrin into an insoluble, durable sheet by the membrane-bound enzyme transglutaminase. As the cells differentiate in culture, there is a successive increase in involucrin, transglutaminase, and cornified envelope formation [29,30]. The 25OHD-1α hydroxylase and 24 hydroxylase also change with differentiation [29]. Preceding the rise in transglutaminase and involucrin is a rise in 1α hydroxylase activity; the 1α hydroxylase activity, transglutaminase activity, and involucrin then fall as cornified envelopes appear; the appearance of cornified envelopes and the fall in 1α hydroxylase activity coincide with a rise in 24 hydroxylase activity [29]. Growing the cells in 0.1 mM calcium, which retards differentiation [30], permits the cells to maintain higher 1α hydroxylase activity than when they are grown in 1.2 mM calcium [31], although acute changes in calcium have little effect on $1,25(OH)_2D$ production [7].

D. Regulation by Cytokines

Both tumor necrosis factor-alpha (TNF) and interferon-gamma (IFN-γ) bind to and promote the differentiation of keratinocytes [32–34]. Epidermal growth factor (EGF) and transforming growth factor-alpha (TGF-α) stimulate proliferation of keratinocytes via the EGF receptor [32], although these cytokines may promote the antiproliferative, prodifferentiating actions of $1,25(OH)_2D$ [33,34]. All four cytokines stimulate $1,25(OH)_2D$ production by keratinocytes [31,35,36]. These cytokines require 16–24 hr of incubation with the keratinocytes before their effects on $1,25(OH)_2D$ production are observed, and their effects are blocked by actinomycin D and cycloheximide, implicating an effect on gene expression [31,35,36]. These cells are exquisitely sensitive to IFN, with maximal stimulation of $1,25(OH)_2D$ production at concentrations less than 10 pM. Higher concentrations are inhibitory, but such concentrations also profoundly inhibit the proliferation of these cells and limit their ability to differentiate. Keratinocytes grown in 0.1 mM calcium are more sensitive to IFN than cells grown in 1.2 mM calcium [31]. Serum markedly reduces the potency of IFN in this system for reasons which are obscure. TNF stimulates $1,25(OH)_2D$ production and transglutaminase activity in preconfluent cells [35], and it can reverse the inhibition seen with the higher concentrations of IFN. The effects of TNF and IFN are not additive at the lower and stimulatory concentrations of IFN. When TNF is added after the cells have reached confluence, a time after which $1,25(OH)_2D$ production (and transglutaminase activity) has peaked, TNF inhibits $1,25(OH)_2D$ production (and transglutaminase activity) even as it stimulates cornified envelope formation. Although IFN is not made in keratinocytes, TNF is, and its production is stimulated by ultraviolet light [37] and barrier disruption [38]. Thus, environmental perturbations could enhance $1,25(OH)_2D$ production in the skin, leading to accelerated repair.

E. 1,25(OH)₂D Production by Transformed Keratinocytes

Keratinocytes from squamous cell carcinomas (SCC) do not differentiate normally in response to calcium [39] or $1,25(OH)_2D$ [40] despite having genes for the differentiation markers that can be induced by serum [41]. Nevertheless, these cells produce $1,25(OH)_2D$ [and $24,25(OH)_2D$]; in some cases, these rates of production are comparable to those of normal keratinocytes [40]. Furthermore, the SCC lines respond to exogenous $1,25(OH)_2D$ with a reduction in $1,25(OH)_2D$ production and an increase in $24,25(OH)_2D$ production, although in some cases the sensitivity of the SCC line to $1,25(OH)_2D$ is less than normal [40]. The levels of the VDR mRNA and protein in SCC are comparable to those in normal keratinocytes [41], suggesting that the reason why $1,25(OH)_2D$ can regulate 25OHD metabolism but not differentiation in SCC lies in other transcription factors required for calcium and $1,25(OH)_2D$ regulation of the differentiation pathway.

F. Clinical Implications

The finding of $1,25(OH)_2D$ production by keratinocytes indicates that the skin is at least one source for extrarenal production of this important metabolite. The kidney is the major source, but in anephric individuals the circulating level of $1,25(OH)_2D$ may fall sufficiently low that the cutaneous production of $1,25(OH)_2D$ is no longer inhibited and its degradation is no longer induced. Thus, the epidermis may provide $1,25(OH)_2D$ to the body in patients with decreased or absent renal function, accounting for the normalization of $1,25(OH)_2D$ levels when such individuals are provided with adequate amounts of 25OHD [42]. Although a variety of squamous cell carcinomas are associated with hypercalcemia, this appears to be due to their elaboration of a parathyroid hormone–like protein and not to uncontrolled $1,25(OH)_2D$ production. Most likely the $1,25(OH)_2D$ produced by keratinocytes serves an autocrine or paracrine function, regulating the proliferation and differentiation of these cells. The ability of the epidermis to produce $1,25(OH)_2D$ from 25OHD and to catabolize the D metabolites quickly offers several possibilities for the topical administration of vitamin D compounds in the treatment of skin disorders.

III. REGULATION OF KERATINOCYTE DIFFERENTIATION

A. The Microanatomy of the Epidermis

The epidermis is composed of four layers of cells at different stages of differentiation (Figure 2). The basal layer (stratum basale) rests on the basal lamina separating the dermis and epidermis. These cells proliferate, providing the cells for the upper differentiating layers. They are large, columnar cells forming intercellular

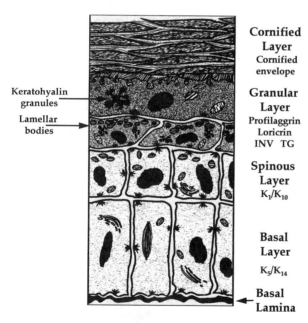

Figure 2 Cartoon of the four principal layers of the epidermis. The basal layer rests on the basal lamina separating the epidermis from the dermis. The cornified layer provides the major barrier to the outside environment. The basal layer provides the cells which differentiate as they pass through the different layers to become corneocytes. Each layer has its distinct appearance, function, and differentiation markers as described in the text.

attachments with adjacent cells through desmosomes. An asymmetrical distribution of integrins on their lateral and basal surfaces may also regulate their attachment to the basal lamina and adjacent cells [43–45]. They contain an extensive keratin network made up principally of keratins K5 (58 kDa) and K14 (50 kDa) [46]. By a process we are only beginning to understand, cells migrate upward from this basal layer, acquiring the characteristics of a fully differentiated corneocyte, which is eventually sloughed off. The layer above the basal cells is the spinous layer (stratum spinosum). These cells initiate the production of the keratins, K1 and K10, which are the keratins characteristic of the more differentiated layers of the epidermis [47]. Cornified envelope precursors such as involucrin [48] also appear in the spinous layer, as does the enzyme transglutaminase, responsible for the ε-(γ-glutamyl) lysine cross-linking of these substrates into the insoluble cornified envelope [49]. The keratinocyte contains both a soluble (tissue, TG-C, or type II) and a membrane bound (particulate, TG-K, or type I) form of transglutaminase. It is the membrane-bound form that correlates with differentiation and is thought to be responsible for the formation of the cornified envelope [49]. The granular layer (stratum granulosum), lying above the spinous layer, is characterized by electron-dense keratohyalin granules. These are of two types [50]. The larger of the two granules contains profilaggrin, the precursor of filaggrin, a protein thought to facilitate the aggregation of keratin filaments [51]. The smaller granule contains loricrin, a major component of the cornified envelope [52]. The granular layer also contains lamellar bodies, lipid-filled structures that fuse with the plasma membrane, divesting their contents into the extracellular space, where the lipid contributes to the permeability barrier of skin [53]. As the cells pass from the granular layer to the cornified layer (stratum corneum), they undergo destruction of their organelles, with further maturation of the cornified envelope into an insoluble, highly resistant structure surrounding the keratin-filaggrin complex and linked to the extracellular lipid milieu [54].

B.   Regulators of Growth and Differentiation—General

The ability to grow keratinocytes in culture in a manner that permits at least partial differentiation has made it possible to study the regulation of this process [55]. Although this chapter emphasizes the interacting roles of calcium, protein kinase C, and 1,25(OH)$_2$D in keratinocyte differentiation, a number of hormones, cytokines, and ions are involved that influence or are influenced by 1,25(OH)$_2$D.

1.   Vitamin A

Vitamin A and its metabolites and analogs have long been known to influence epidermal development. Vitamin A deficiency induces squamous metaplasia, causing even normal keratinizing epithelia (e.g., the epidermis) to become hyperkeratotic [56]. In contrast, pharmacological doses of retinoids can induce a mucous metaplasia in what is otherwise a keratinizing epithelium [57]. In culture, it has long been appreciated that retinoids block the terminal differentiation of keratinocytes [58]. Retinoids block the appearance of the suprabasal keratins (K1 and K10) while enhancing the appearance of keratins characteristic of undifferentiated cells [59–61]. Retinoids decrease cornified envelope formation [62] by decreasing type 1 (or type K) transglutaminase [63,64] and substrate (involucrin, loricrin) [63–65] levels and the expression of filaggrin [65]. These effects are opposite to and antagonize the prodifferentiating actions of $1,25(OH)_2D_3$. Similarly, all-*trans* retinoic acid blocks the ability of $1,25(OH)_2D$ to increase the levels of TGF-β, the cell cycle inhibitor p21[wafl], and hypophosphorylation of the retinoblastoma protein [66], all actions likely to account for the ability of low doses of retinoids to block the antiproliferative actions of $1,25(OH)_2D$ [65,66].

Like the actions of $1,25(OH)_2D_3$, many of the actions of retinoic acid (tRA) are mediated through changes in gene expression. Two members of the retinoic acid receptor family (RAR$\alpha\gamma$), whose structures are homologous to steroid hormone receptors (including the VDR), have been identified in keratinocytes [67–69]. Recently, it was found that epidermal differentiation was blocked in a transgenic mouse with a dominant negative form of RAR in the skin [70]. The RARs are found in transformed as well as normal keratinocytes [71,72], although their expression in SCC may not be normal [71]. Certain retinoic acid metabolites (e.g., 9-*cis* retinoic acid) also bind to another family of receptors, the RXRs. The major member of this family in skin is RXRα [69,73]. It is likely, because of the similarity of the vitamin A and vitamin D response elements in genes [74–76], that tRA and $1,25(OH)_2D_3$ will interact at the genomic level in their control of keratinocyte differentiation. Furthermore, since RARs and VDR each form heterodimers with RXR [76–80], competition between RARs and VDR for RXR heterodimer formation is likely. Thus, the antagonism between retinoic acid and $1,25(OH)_2D$ on keratinocyte proliferation and differentiation has its explanation at the molecular level. However, the interaction between $1,25(OH)_2D$ and retinoic acid is not always competitive. The phospholipase C γ (PLCγ) gene in keratinocytes has a vitamin D response element in its promoter that binds both VDR and RAR [75]. $1,25(OH)_2D$ and all-*trans* retinoic acid synergistically induce the expression of this gene [81]. Similarly, the vitamin D response element in the 24-hydroxylase gene binds both VDR and RXR and is synergistically stimulated by $1,25(OH)_2D$ and 9-*cis* retinoic acid [82]. Therefore, at the level of individual genes regulated by $1,25(OH)_2D$, one cannot predict whether $1,25(OH)_2D$ and the retinoids will be antagonistic or synergistic.

2. Cytokines and Peptide Growth Factors

Keratinocytes produce a large array of cytokines and growth factors, many of which have autocrine activity and respond to still other cytokines and growth factors produced by stromal cells in the dermis [83,84]. Transforming growth factor-alpha (TGF-α) is produced by the keratinocyte and acts through the EGF receptor to stimulate proliferation and migration [85]. Transforming growth factors beta 1 and 2 (TGF-β1, TGF-β2) are also produced by keratinocytes [86,87], but they inhibit proliferation [88]. Part of the antiproliferative action of 1,25(OH)$_2$D may be mediated by its induction of this cytokine [89,90]. TGF-β exerts a number of effects on keratinocytes, including reducing the differentiation markers K1 and filaggrin [91]; increasing fibronectin, laminin β1, and α1 (IV) collagen [61,91] increasing type II transglutaminase without altering type I transglutaminase [92]; and decreasing c-*myc* expression [93]. The c-*myc* gene has been shown to have a response element for TGF-β [93], but whether the other actions of TGF-β are mediated through a similar response element in other genes remains to be demonstrated. Even though TGF-α and TGF-β exert opposite effects on keratinocyte proliferation, neither promotes keratinocyte differentiation, although, as discussed previously, both stimulate 1,25(OH)$_2$D production. Basic fibroblast growth factor (bFGF) is produced by keratinocytes [94] and stimulates their proliferation [95]. A related molecule, keratinocyte growth factor (KGF), is produced by stromal fibroblasts but stimulates the proliferation of keratinocytes [96,97]. The ability of EGF [or TGF-α], bFGF, and KGF to stimulate keratinocyte proliferation is markedly enhanced by the presence of high concentrations of insulin, indicating that insulin-like growth factors 1 and 2 (IGF-1 and IGF-2) are also keratinocyte mitogens [97,98]. Receptors for IGF-1 on keratinocytes have been found [99]. In contrast to its ability to enhance the proliferative actions of EGF, insulin blocks the antiproliferative actions of 1,25(OH)$_2$D. EGF activates phospholipase Cγ, an enzyme induced by 1,25(OH)$_2$D [75]. However, the ability of 1,25(OH)$_2$D to modulate the actions of EGF has not been reported. Tumor necrosis factor-alpha (TNF-α) is produced by keratinocytes [83] and promotes their differentiation with only a modest antiproliferative effect [35]. Interferon-gamma (IFN-γ), on the other hand, is not made by keratinocytes but markedly inhibits their proliferation, with little effect on differentiation (31,100). IFN-γ increases class II antigens (HLA-DR) [32,101] and the intercellular adhesion molecule (ICAM-1) [102] of these cells. Whether any of the actions of TNF-α or IFN-γ involve their ability to stimulate 1,25(OH)$_2$D production is not known. Keratinocytes produce platelet derived growth factors (PDGF) but do not have the PDGF receptor [83]. Parathyroid hormone–related peptide (PTHrP) is also produced by keratinocytes [103], but, like PDGF, receptors for PTHrP on normal keratinocytes, have been difficult to demonstrate [104,105]. Nevertheless, PTHrP and/or its C-terminal fragments have been reported to inhibit or stimulate keratinocyte proliferation [106,107], and a 7-34 PTH antagonist has been claimed to promote hair growth by reversing the antiproliferative effects of PTHrP on the epidermis [106]. 1,25(OH)$_2$D inhibits the production of PTHrP in keratinocytes. PTHrP, like PTH, would be expected to stimulate 1,25(OH)$_2$D production, but this has not been reported. Interleukins 1 (IL-α and β) [108,109], IL-3 [110], IL-6 (111), and IL-8 (112) are all produced by keratinocytes, as are the colony-stimulating factors (CSF) granulocyte/macrophage (GM)-CSF [113], G-CSF, and M-CSF [114]. The roles the interleukins and colony-stimulating factors play in keratinocyte proliferation, migration, and differentiation are uncertain, but, acting in a coordinated fashion, they probably regulate important aspects of wound healing, inflammation, and cell growth [115] in the epidermis. Their roles in $1,25(OH)_2D$ production and/or action have not been tested.

C. Calcium-Regulated Differentiation

Calcium is the best-studied prodifferentiating agent for keratinocytes (Figure 3). In vivo, a calcium gradient exists in the epidermis such that in the basal and spinous layers calcium is found primarily intracellularly and in low amounts, but in the upper granular layers calcium accumulates in large amounts in the intercellular matrix [116]. Dissipation of this calcium gradient by barrier disruption or iontophoresis results in increased proliferation, increased lamellar body secretion, and disarray of the differentiated cell layers [117–121], suggesting that it plays an important role in maintaining the ordered differentiation process of the epidermis. However, most of the information regarding calcium-induced differentiation comes from in vitro studies with cultured keratinocytes. In low-calcium-containing media, keratinocytes proliferate readily but differentiate slowly if at all and remain as a monolayer in culture. Upon switching the cells to higher calcium concentrations (referred to as the *calcium switch*), keratinocytes undergo a coordinated set of responses at both the genomic and nongenomic levels, eventuating in a stratified culture in which the cells contain many of the features of the differentiated epithelium. For reasons that are not apparent, mouse keratinocytes are more sensitive to the antiproliferative effects of calcium and require lower concentrations of calcium for differentiation than do human keratinocytes; but the qualitative effects of calcium on human and murine cells are comparable.

1. Changes Induced by the Calcium Switch

Within minutes to hours of the calcium switch, morphological changes are apparent, with rapid development of cell-to-cell contact [122], desmosome formation [122], and a realignment of actin and keratin bundles near the cell membrane at the point of intercellular contacts [123]. Desmoplakin (a component of desmosomes), fodrin (an actin- and calmodulin-binding spectrin, like protein), and calmodulin are redistributed to the membrane shortly after the calcium switch by a mechanism that is blocked by cytochalasin, an agent which disrupts microfilament reorganization [123–125]. These effects do not appear to be under genomic control, although this has not been tested rigorously. Within hours to days of the calcium switch, the cells begin to make involucrin [63,126,127], loricrin (128),

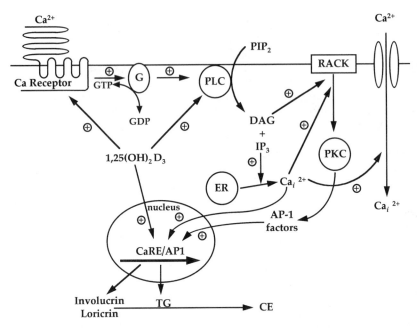

Figure 3 Interactions among calcium, PKC, and 1,25(OH)$_2$D in regulating keratinocyte differentiation. The keratinocyte contains a calcium receptor which increases intracellular calcium by activating phospholipase C (PLC) via a G protein coupled process. 1,25(OH)$_2$D enhances this process by increasing the number of calcium receptors and inducing PLC. PLC hydrolyzes phosphatidyl inositol bisphosphate (PIP$_2$) to inositol tris phosphate (IP$_3$) and diacylglyderol (DAG). IP$_3$ releases calcium (Cai) from intracellular stores such as the endoplasmic reticulum (ER). In combination with DAG, Cai stimulates the translocation (and activation) of the classic isozymes of PKC (primarily PKCα in keratinocytes) to the membrane where they bind to their specific receptors (RACK). Activated PKC then induces or activates AP-1 factors, which serve as transcription factors along with the vitamin D receptor (VDR) to induce the expression of the genes important for differentiation, such as the involucrin, loricrin, and transglutaminase (TG) genes. TG under the stimulation of calcium catalyzes the crosslinking of involucrin, loricrin, and other substrates to form the cornified envelope (CE). Cai and possibly PKC also regulate various cation channels through which calcium can enter the keratinocyte.

transglutaminase [63,126,127], keratins K1 and K10 [128], and filaggrin [128] and start to form cornified envelopes [126,128]. As evidenced by a rise in mRNA levels for these proteins following the calcium switch [65,127,128], these effects of calcium represent genomic actions. Calcium response regions have been identified in the involucrin [129] and K1 [130] genes. As is to be discussed, these calcium response regions contain AP-1 sites and are also under the control of protein kinase C (PKC). The redistribution of integrin isoforms within days following the calcium switch [43,45,131] may participate in the mechanism by which cells begin to stratify. Calcium-induced increases in TGF-β [86,132] may contribute to the decrease in proliferation that accompanies the calcium switch, but as discussed above, TGF-β does not stimulate differentiation.

2. Role of Intracellular Calcium

The mechanisms by which calcium exerts its effects on keratinocyte differentiation are multiple. The intracellular free calcium concentration (Cai) increases as keratinocytes differentiate, correlating closely with their ability to form cornified envelopes [133]. Raising the extracellular calcium concentration (Cao) increases Cai [133–135]. This response is saturable, reaching a maximum at 2mM Cao in human foreskin keratinocytes [133]. The acute response to Cao with respect to an increase in Cai is maximal in undifferentiated cells and is lost as the cells differentiate in response to calcium [136,137]. Transformed keratinocytes, which do not differentiate under the influence of calcium, do not lose this acute response of Cai to Cao [134,138,139]. The plateau phase of the rise in Cai is not lost with differentiation [136,137] and is not seen or is of shorter duration in transformed keratinocytes [139]. Inositol 1,4,5 tris phosphate (IP$_3$) and diacylglycerol (DAG) levels increase within seconds to minutes after the calcium switch, implicating activation of the phospholipase C (PLC) pathway [140,141]. As for the acute Cai response, the acute IP$_3$ response to calcium is blunted with differentiation [142]. Although not firmly established, the rise in IP$_3$ is believed to account for the initial rise in Cai by release of calcium from intracellular stores. As cells differentiate, their basal levels of Cai increase [126] which in other cells reduces the ability of IP$_3$ to stimulate calcium release from the intracellular pools [143]. This may contribute to the loss of the acute Cai response with differentiation. Similar to Cai, the levels of inositol phosphates (IPs) remain elevated for hours after the calcium switch, indicating ongoing activation of the PLC pathway. This prolonged increase in IPs appears to be due to calcium activation of PLCγ [144], not PLCβ as might be expected by continued stimulation via a G protein coupled membrane receptor. ATP, on the other hand, results in only a transient increase in IP$_3$ and other IPs through its effects on the G protein coupled P2 receptor [145]. The prolonged increase in IPs after the calcium switch may contribute to the plateau phase of Cai elevation by participating in the regulation of calcium channel activity, but this has not been established in the keratinocyte.

3. Calcium Channels

The plateau phase of the Cai response to Cao is most likely due to increased calcium influx. Unlike the loss of the acute Cai response to calcium with differentiation, the calcium activated calcium influx [141] increases substantially as the cells differentiate [136]. Nickel [141,146] blocks calcium influx and blocks the rise in Cai after increases in Cao. Similarly, lanthanum blocks calcium influx, the increase in Cai after increases in Cao, and calcium-induced differentiation [147]. Inhibition of the sustained rise in Cai using the intracellular calcium chelator BAPTA prevents calcium induced differentiation despite increasing calcium influx [148]. The mechanism by which calcium stimulates calcium influx is not clear. Several channels have been identified in the keratinocyte membrane that are candidates for mediating calcium induced calcium influx [149–152]. These include calcium-activated chloride channels, which could hyperpolarize the membrane and increase calcium influx [149,150]; nonselective cation channels, in which the open time is increased by calcium [138,151]; nicotinic acetylcholine receptors [152]; and a newly discovered cGMP gated channel [152] nearly identical to such a channel in the retinal rod and olfactory neurons [153] and known to contain a calcium/calmodulin regulatory element. The extent to which any or all of these channels are activated by the initial release of calcium from intracellular stores following calcium stimulation is unclear, although such currents have been described in other cells [154,155]. Of particular interest with respect to the increase in calcium-activated calcium influx with differentiation is the cGMP gated channel, which in the keratinocyte exists in two alternatively spliced forms. Undifferentiated cells have a form lacking the calcium/calmodulin regulatory domain, whereas the full-length sequence appears as the cells differentiate [156].

4. The Calcium Receptor

The response of the keratinocyte to calcium resembles that of the parathyroid cell [157]. The parathyroid cell senses Cao via a seven-transmembrane domain, G protein–coupled receptor (CaR) [158,159]. This receptor is not limited to the parathyroid gland, being found in the kidney, thyroid, brain, lung, and intestine [160], and we have identified the same structure in the keratinocyte [136,142]. The human CaR cDNA predicts a structure with 1078 amino acids with a calculated molecular weight of 120 kDa (Figure 4). The first 612 residues are predicted to be in the extracellular domain, residues 613–862 in the transmembrane and connecting loops domain, and residues 863–1078 in the C-terminal intracellular tail [159]. However, we also observed that the keratinocyte produces an alternatively spliced variant of the CaR as it differentiates, which lacks exon 5 and so would be missing residues 461–537 in the extracellular domain [142]. A mouse model in which the full-length CaR has been deleted but which continues to produce the alternatively spliced form of CaR contains markedly lower levels of the terminal differentiation markers loricrin and profilaggrin, suggesting the requirement for the full-length CaR in terminal differentiation. The alternatively spliced form of CaR is unable to mediate Cao-stimulated IP formation or involucrin gene expression,

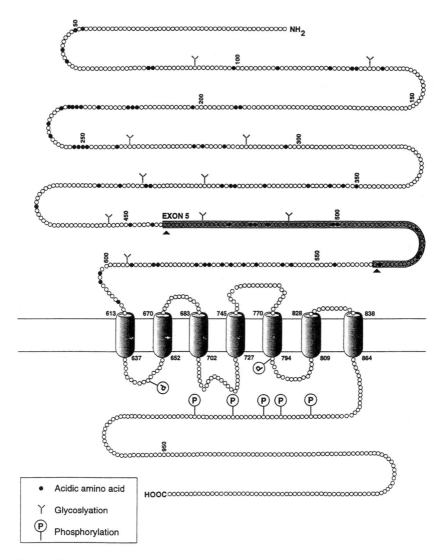

Figure 4 A putative structure of the CaR showing the region encoded by exon 5 (shadowed). The spliced variant lacks exon 5. This region contains 77 amino acids including 10 acidic amino acids (shown by closed circles) and two potential N-linked glycosylation sites (shown by branches). The potential phosphorylation sites (P) are also shown.

unlike the full-length form. As mentioned above, keratinocytes lose their acute response to Cao with respect to increases in Cai and IP. This change in calcium responsiveness is paralleled by the fall in full-length CaR levels. No changes are seen in transformed keratinocytes which do not lose this aspect of calcium responsiveness [136,138]. 1,25(OH)$_2$D increases the CaR mRNA levels and prevents their decrease with time [161]. Furthermore, 1,25(OH)$_2$D potentiates the ability of these cells to respond to Cao with a rise in Cai [161]. Thus, the CaR appears to be important in mediating the Cai response of keratinocytes to Cao and provides a mechanism by which 1,25(OH)$_2$D can regulate calcium induced epidermal differentiation.

D. Protein Kinase C Regulated Differentiation

The rise in diacyl glycerol (DAG) and Cai following the calcium switch provides a means to link the abilities of both calcium and phorbol esters to stimulate keratinocyte differentiation, and that link is protein kinase C (PKC). Phorbol esters, which bind to and activate protein kinase C, are well-known tumor promoters in skin [162–165]. However, the initial effects of phorbol esters in vitro are to promote differentiation in cells grown in low calcium [162,163,166–171], effects potentiated by calcium. Phorbol esters stimulate PKC, and PKC inhibitors block the ability of both calcium and phorbol esters to promote differentiation. Nevertheless, differences between the acute effects of phorbol esters and calcium on differentiation are clear. Phorbol esters block rather than promote calcium induction of K1 and K10 (early differentiation markers) [171], in contrast to their synergistic effects with calcium on the later differentiation markers. Phorbol esters as well as calcium stimulate the expression of involucrin gene constructs containing the calcium response element (CaRE). If the AP-1 site within the CaRE is mutated, neither calcium nor phorbol esters are effective [Ng and Bikle, unpublished data]. A similar situation is seen for the CaRE in the keratin 1 gene [172]. AP-1 sites have also been implicated in the expression of loricrin and transglutaminase [173]. Calcium does not duplicate all the changes in protein phosphorylation caused by phorbol esters [174–176], and phorbol esters, unlike calcium, do not activate the phospholipase C (PLC) pathway [140,144]. Calcium activation of the PLC pathway, by increasing the amount of DAG, is a likely means by which calcium stimulates PKC, whereas phorbol esters tend to reduce hormonal activation of PLC and the increase in Cai at least in other cells [177,178]. Thus, it seems certain that although calcium regulated differentiation involves the PKC pathway, the effects of calcium are not solely due to PKC activation and are not mimicked in their entirety by phorbol esters.

1. PKC Isozymes

The study of PKC in differentiation is complicated by the large number of isozymes of PKC in the epidermis, most of which are separate gene products and under different modes of regulation and distribution within the epidermis. Mouse keratinocytes contain α, δ, ε, ζ and η [179]. Transformed mouse keratinocytes lose their responsiveness to calcium but retain the same complement of isozymes [179,180]. Human keratinocytes and at least one human SCC line (SCC4) contain the same set of isozymes as mouse keratinocytes [181,182], although HaCaT cells (an immortalized human keratinocyte cell line) reportedly contain α, δ, ε, and ζ but not η [183]. PKCα is a classic PKC activated by calcium, phorbol esters and DAG. In contrast, PKCδ, ε, and η are novel PKCs activated by phorbol esters and DAG, like the classic PKCs, but not by calcium. PKCζ is an atypical PKC which does not respond to calcium or phorbol esters. Cholesterol sulfate appears to stimulate ζ, ε, and η more than α and δ, and its ability to stimulate keratinocyte differentiation may utilize a different set of PKCs than that used by calcium [184]. The activation process for most if not all PKCs involves translocation from one site to another—e.g., movement of PKCα from the cytosol to the membrane [185]. A group of proteins termed RACKS (receptors for activated C kinase) bind the activated PKCs in an isozyme-specific manner and have been shown to be important for their function [185–188]. The cDNAs for these isozymes have been sequenced and the structural basis for their differences identified [189]. For example, the classic PKCs contain a region near the N terminus (C2) that confers calcium responsiveness and is missing from the other forms of PKC. The C2 region of the classic PKCs also contains the RACK binding domain, whereas this domain is found in the V1 region of the novel PKCs [186–188]. Peptides of these regions when expressed or incorporated into cells selectively block PKC translocation and function [186–188]. PKCα may be the most important PKC for mediating calcium induced differentiation. During the first 48 hr after the calcium switch in mouse keratinocytes, the translocation of PKCα from the cytosol to the membrane paralleled in time the induction of loricrin and profilaggrin better than did the changes in the other PKC isozymes [190]. Downregulation of PKCα by bryostatin-1 and 12-deoxyphorbol 13 phenylacetate (DPP) also correlated with the inhibition of calcium-induced loricrin and profilaggrin expression better than did the effects of these phorbol esters on the other isozymes [190,191]. More compelling is that when PKCα production is reduced by transfecting mouse keratinocytes with an antisense construct to the PKCα transcript, the ability of calcium to increase the expression of late differentiation markers is substantially reduced [192]. In contrast, calcium does not increase the level of these isozymes in SCC4 cells, consistent with the lack of calcium-induced differentiation in this cell line.

2. AP-1 Factors

Although a mechanism involving transcription factors in the fos and jun families acting on their AP-1 sites in the promoter regions of the genes involved with differentiation seems likely, the actual mechanism by which PKC induces differentiation is not clear [193–196]. PKC activation leads to a rapid increase in c-fos and c-jun [197–199] and increased binding to AP-1 sites as assessed by gel retardation studies [200]. A similar increase in c-fos was seen in SCCF12 following phorbol ester administration, but involucrin mRNA was not increased, unlike the increase seen in NHK [197]. However, c-fos and c-jun are not the only transcription factors capable of binding to AP-1 sites. Other members of the fos and jun families [fra-1, fra-2, jun B, jun D] have been found in keratinocytes [200] and are differentially distributed throughout the epidermis. Calcium increases the levels of fra-2, junB, and junD in the nucleus of mouse keratinocytes in a manner blocked by inhibitors of PKC [201]. The AP-1 site from the involucrin gene was found to bind fra-1, jun B, and jun D on gel retardation analysis [202]. In our own studies with a dominant negative mutant of c-jun [203], a mutant which blocks c-jun/fos regulated transcriptional activity in AP-1–regulated genes such as prolactin, we showed that cotransfection with this mutant markedly stimulated transcriptional activity of involucrin gene constructs. This surprising result suggests that c-jun plays an inhibitory rather than a stimulatory role in involucrin gene transcription. Regulation of the levels of these transcriptional factors is not the only means by which calcium and PKC can control their activity. C-jun, for example, is phosphorylated on five sites. The three sites near the DNA-binding region in the C-terminal region (thr239, ser243, ser249) when phosphorylated reduce DNA binding [204], whereas the two sites in the N-terminal domain (ser63, ser73) when phosphorylated increase the transactivation function of c-jun [205]. PKC activation results in a decrease in phosphorylation of the C-terminal region of c-jun, whereas jun N-terminal kinase (JNK) phosphorylates the N-terminal sites. In contrast, the C-terminal phosphorylation of fra-1 and fra-2 [206] increases their ability to bind to DNA. Furthermore, a number of proteins (e.g., jif-1, ref-1, ip-1) have been found in the nucleus and cytoplasm which can block or promote binding of members of the fos/jun family to AP-1 sites [207–209]. At least one of these inhibitory proteins (ip-1) works only in the dephosphorylated state, such that phosphorylation following PKC activation renders it inactive. Thus, calcium and PKC can exert control of differentiation by a number of mechanisms. As detailed below, $1,25(OH)_2D$ interacts with calcium and PKC in these actions.

E. $1,25(OH)_2D$ Regulated Differentiation

The observation that $1,25(OH)_2D$ induces keratinocyte differentiation was first made by Hosomi et al. [210] and provided a rationale for the previous and unexpected finding of $1,25(OH)_2D$ receptors in the skin. As discussed earlier, $1,25(OH)_2D$ is likely to be an autocrine or paracrine factor for epidermal differentiation, since it is produced by the keratinocyte. The receptors for and the production of $1,25(OH)_2D$ vary with differentiation [29,211,212] in a manner suggesting feedback regulation; both are reduced in the later stages of differentiation.

1,25(OH)$_2$D increases involucrin, transglutaminase activity, and cornified enve-lope formation at subnanomolar concentrations in preconfluent keratinocytes [40,133,210,213,214]. The rise in involucrin and transglutaminase following 1,25(OH)$_2$D administration is accompanied by a rise in their respective mRNAs and increased transcription of their genes [127]. At these concentrations, 1,25(OH)$_2$D has been found to promote proliferation in some studies [215–217], although the antiproliferative actions are most frequently observed, especially when concentrations above 10^{-9}M are employed. The mechanisms underlying the proproliferative actions are not known. The antiproliferative effects are likely due to a reduction in c-myc and stimulation of TGF-β, p21^{wafl} and p27^{kipl} [89,90].

The mechanisms by which 1,25(OH)$_2$D alters keratinocyte differentiation involve both genomic and nongenomic pathways. The 1,25(OH)$_2$D receptor (VDR) may be critical for some or all pathways. No studies have been reported using keratinocytes from patients or animals with defective or missing VDR, al-though alopecia is a feature of humans with inactivating VDR mutations [218] and the mouse knockout model of the VDR gene [219]. An acute increase in Cai as-sociated with an acute increase in phosphoinositide turnover (producing a rise in both IP$_3$ and DAG) has been observed in several studies [220–224]. Not all in-vestigators (including ourselves) have been able to reproduce these acute effects of 1,25(OH)$_2$D [161], although a gradual rise in Cai and cornified envelope for-mation is observed [133]. Furthermore, vitamin D metabolites that do not induce differentiation and bind poorly to the VDR [1αOHD and 24,25(OH)$_2$D] have been reported to increase both Cai and IP$_3$ acutely [220,223]. The rise in Cai, IP$_3$, and DAG is accompanied by translocation of PKC to the membrane [223,225]. Down-regulation of PKC and inhibition of its activity have been reported to block the ability of 1,25(OH)$_2$D to stimulate cornified envelope formation [223]. However, the role of PKC in mediating or interacting with 1,25(OH)$_2$D in its effects on ker-atinocyte differentiation remains virtually unexplored, even though PKC stimu-lated AP-1 factors are well known to modulate 1,25(OH)$_2$D regulated gene ex-pression and differentiation in other cells [226].

1,25(OH)$_2$D and calcium interact in their ability to inhibit proliferation and stimulate involucrin and transglutaminase gene expression [127]. The higher the Cao, the more sensitive is the keratinocyte to the antiproliferative effect of 1,25(OH)$_2$D (and vice versa) [214]. The interaction on gene expression is more complex. Both calcium (in the absence of 1,25(OH)$_2$D) and 1,25(OH)$_2$D (at 0.03 mM calcium) raise the mRNA levels for involucrin and transglutaminase in a dose-dependent fashion. The stimulation is synergistic at intermediate concentra-tions of calcium (0.1 mM) and 1,25(OH)$_2$D (10^{-10} M), but inhibition is observed in combination at higher concentrations. The synergism is more apparent at ear-lier times after the calcium switch (4 hr) than later (24–72 hr), when inhibition of gene expression by the higher combined concentrations of calcium and 1,25(OH)$_2$D becomes dominant. Reductions in K1/K10 keratins, involucrin, transglutaminase, and filaggrin were similarly observed in immunolocalization studies of keratinocytes grown at the air-liquid interface when treated with high concentrations of $1,25(OH)_2D$ ($10^{-6}M$) in the presence of calcium [227]. The molecular mechanisms underlying this complex dose- and time-dependent interaction between calcium and $1,25(OH)_2D$ on keratinocyte differentiation are being actively investigated, and may underlie some of the side effects when $1,25(OH)_2D$ analogs are used topically for the management of psoriasis.

F. Clinical Implications

These actions of $1,25(OH)_2D$ defined primarily at the level of tissue culture have physiological implications. Humans with mutations in their VDR often are completely bald. This phenotype has received little study and is not seen in vitamin D deficiency. On the other hand, rats maintained in the dark on a vitamin D–deficient diet that is otherwise normal demonstrate striking changes in gross appearance, including matted hair, patchy alopecia, scaling and erythema, and a variable but significant defect in the barrier to transcutaneous water loss [228]. These changes are not due to gross alterations in cutaneous sterologenesis [229] but suggest a more subtle abnormality in differentiation. Histologically, the skin from such rats is thinner, with fewer granular cell layers and increased nuclei in the basal cell layer [228]. Such changes are similar to the changes observed in psoriasis. In fact, the antiproliferative, prodifferentiating effects of $1,25(OH)_2D$ and its analogs have been put to clinical use in the management of psoriasis, as discussed more fully in the chapters in Part III.

Whether other dysplastic or malignant lesions can be successfully treated or prevented with $1,25(OH)_2D$ analogs remains for future investigation.

REFERENCES

1. Bikle DD, Nemanic MK, Whitney JO, Ellas PW. Neonatal human foreskin keratinocytes produce 1.25-dihydroxyvitamin D_3. Biochemistry 1986; 25:1545–1548.
2. Fu GK, Lin D, Zhang MYH, Bikle DD, Shackleton CHL, Miller WL, Portale AA. Cloning of the human 25-hydroxyvitamin D-1α-hydroxylase and mutations causing vitamin D-dependent rickets type 1. Mol Endocrinol 1997; 11:1961–1970.
3. Lehmann B, Pietzsch J, Kampf A, Wozel G, Meurer M. Human hacat keratinocytes metabolize 1 α-hydroxyvitamin D_3 and vitamin D_3 to 1 α,25-dihydroxyvitamin D_3. In: Norman AW, Bouillon R, Thomasset M, ed. Vitamin D Chemistry, Biology and Clinical Applications of the Steroid Hormone. Riverside, CA: University of California, 1997.
4. Rudolph T, Lehmann B, Pietzsch J, Kampf A, Wozel G, Meurer M. Normal human Keratinocytes in Organotypic Culture Metabolize Vitamin D_3 to 1 α,25-Dihydrox-

yvitamin D_3. In: Norman AW, Bouillon R, Thomasset M, ed. Vitamin D Chemistry, Biology and Clinical Applications of the Steroid Hormone Riverside, CA: University of California, 1997.

5. Ichikawa F, Sato K, Nanjo M, Nishii Y, Shinki T, Takahashi N, Suda T. Mouse primary osteoblasts express vitamin D_3 25-hydroxylase mRNA and convert 1 α-hydroxyvitamin D_3 into 1 α,25-dihydroxyvitamin D_3. Bone 1995; 16:129–135.

6. Guo YD, Strugnell S, Back DW, Jones G. Transfected human liver cytochrome P-450 hydroxylates vitamin D analogs at different side-chain positions. Proc Natl Acad Sci USA 1993; 90:8668–8672.

7. Bikle DD, Nemanic MK, Gee E, Elias P. 1,25-Dihydroxyvitamin D_3 production by human keratinocytes: Kinetics and regulation. J Clin Invest 1986; 78:557–566.

8. Matsumoto K, Azuma Y, Kiyoki M, Okumura H, Hashimoto K, Yoshikawa K. Involvement of endogenously produced 1,25-dihydroxyvitamin D-3 in the growth and differentiation of human keratinocytes. Biochim Biophys Acta 1991; 1092: 311–318.

9. Barbour GL, Coburn JW, Slatoposky E, Norman AW, Horst RL. Hypercalcemia in an anephric patient with sarcoidosis: evidence for extrarenal generation of 1,25-dihydroxyvitamin D_3. N Engl J Med 1981; 305:440–443.

10. Lambert PW, Stern PH, Avioli RC, Brackett NC, Turner RT, Green A, Fu I, Bell NH. Evidence for extrarenal production of 1α,25-dihydroxyvitamin D in man. J Clin Invest 1982; 69:722–725.

11. Littledike ET, Horst RL. Metabolism of vitamin D_3 in nephrectomized pigs given pharmacological amounts of vitamin D_3. Endocrinology 1982; 111:2008–2013.

12. Bikle DD, Halloran BP, Riviere JE. Production of 1,25 dihydroxyvitamin D_3 by perfused pig skin. J Invest Dermatol 1994; 102:796–798.

13. Usui E, Noshiro M, Okuda K. Molecular cloning of cDNA for vitamin D_3 25-hydroxylase from rat liver mitochondria. FEBS Lett 1990; 262:135–138.

14. Ohyama Y, Noshiro M, Okuda K. Cloning and expression of cDNA encoding 25-hydroxyvitamin D_3 24-hydroxylase. FEBS Lett 1991; 278:195–198.

15. Takeyama K, Kitanaka S, Sato T, Kobori M, Yanagisawa J, Kato S. 25-Hydroxyvitamin D_3 1 α-hydroxylase and vitamin D synthesis. Science 1997; 277:1827–1830.

16. St-Arnaud R, Messerlian S, Moir JM, Omdahl JL, Glorieux FH. The 25-hydroxyvitamin D 1 α-hydroxylase gene maps to the pseudovitamin D-deficiency rickets (PDDR) disease locus. J Bone Min Res 1997; 12:1552–1559.

17. Shinki T, Shimada H, Wakino S, Anazawa H, Hayashi M, Saruta T, DeLuca HF, Suda T. Cloning and expression of rat 25-hydroxyvitamin D_3-1 α-hydroxylase cDNA. Proc Natl Acad Sci USA 1997; 94:12920–12925.

18. Monkawa T, Yoshida T, Wakino S. Molecular cloning of cDNA and genomic DNA for human 25-hydroxyvitamin D_3 1 α-hydroxylase. Biochem Biophys Res Commun 1997; 239:527–533.

19. Rasmussen H, Wong M, Bikle DD, Goodman DB. Hormonal control of the renal conversion of 25-hydroxycholecalciferol to 1,25-dihydroxycholecalciferol. J Clin Invest 1972; 51:2502–2504.

20. Rost CR, Bikle DD, Kaplan RA. In vitro stimulation of 25-hydroxycholecalciferol 1 α-hydroxylation by parathyroid hormone in chick kidney evidence for a role for adenosine 3′,5′-monophosphate. Endocrinology 1981; 108:1002–1006.

21. Brenza HL, Kimmel-Jehan C, Jehan F, Shinki T, Wakino S, Anazawa H, Suda T, DeLuca HF. Parathyroid hormone activation of the 25-hydroxyvitamin D_3-1 α-hydroxylase gene promoter. Proc Natl Acad Sci USA 1998; 95:1387–1391.

22. Kerry DM, Dwivedi PP, Hahn CN, Morris HA, Omdahl JL, May BK. Transcriptional synergism between vitamin D-responsive elements in the rat 25-hydroxyvitamin D_3 24-hydroxylase (CYP24) promoter. J Biol Chem 1996; 271:29715–29721.

23. Henry HL. Response of chick kidney cell cultures to 1,25 dihydroxyvitamin D_3. In: Norman AW, Schaefer K, Herrath DV, eds. Vitamin D, Basic Research and Its Clinical Application. Berlin: de Gruyter, 1979:467–474.

24. Bikle DD, Gee E. Free, and not total, 1,25-dihydroxyvitamin D regulates 25-hydroxyvitamin D metabolism by keratinocytes. Endocrinology 1989; 124:649–654.

25. Spanos E, Barrett DD, Chong KT, MacIntyre I. Effect of oestrogen and 1,25-dihydroxycholecalciferol metabolism in primary chick kidney cell cultures. Biochem J 1978; 174:231–236.

26. Trechsel U, Bonjour J-P, Fleisch H. Regulation of the metabolism of 25-hydroxyvitamin D_3 in primary cultures of chick kidney cells. J Clin Invest 1979; 64:206–217.

27. Reeve L, Tanaka Y, DeLuca HF. Studies on the site of 1,25-dihydroxyvitamin D_3 synthesis in vivo. J Biol Chem 1983; 258:3615–3617.

28. Shultz TD, Fox J, Health III H, Kumar R. Do tissues other than the kidney produce 1,25-dihydroxyvitamin D_3 in vivo? A re-examination. Proc Natl Acad Sci USA 1983; 80:1746–1750.

29. Pillai S, Bikle DD, Elias PM. 1,25-Dihydroxyvitamin D production and receptor binding in human keratinocytes varies with differentiation. J Biol Chem 1988; 263:5390–5395.

30. Pillai S, Bikle DD, Hincenbergs M, Elias PM. Biochemical and morphological characterization of growth and differentiation of normal human neonatal keratinocytes in a serum-free medium. J Cell Physiol 1988; 134:229–239.

31. Bikle DD, Pillai S, Gee E, Hincenbergs M. Regulation of 1,25-dihydroxyvitamin D production in human keratinocytes by interferon-gamma. Endocrinology 1988; 124:655–660.

32. Van Ruissen F, Van de Kerkhof PC, Schalkwijk J. Signal transduction pathways in epidermal proliferation and cutaneous inflammation. Clin Dermatol 1995; 13: 161–190.

33. Chen TC, Persons K, Liu WW, Chen ML, Holick MF. The antiproliferative and differentiative activities of 1,25 dihydroxyvitamin D_3 are potentiated by epidermal growth factor and attenuated by insulin in cultured human keratinocytes. J Invest Dermatol 1995; 104:113–117.

34. Pillai S, Bikle DD, Eessalu TE, Aggarwal BB, Elias PM. Binding and biological effects of tumor necrosis factor alpha on cultured human neonatal foreskin keratinocytes. J Clin Invest 1989; 83:816–821.

35. Bikle DD, Pillai S, Gee EA, Hincenbergs M. Tumor necrosis factor-alpha regulation of 1,25-dihydroxyvitamin D production by human keratinocytes. Endocrinology 1991; 129:33–38.

36. Lehmann B. HaCaT cell line as a model system for vitamin D_3 metabolism in human skin. J Invest Dermatol 1997; 108:78–82.

37. Trefzer U, Brockhaus M, Lotscher H, Parlow F, Budnik A, Grewe M, Christoph H, Kapp A, Schoff E, Lug. The 55-KD tumor necrosis factor receptor is regulated by tumor necrosis factor-alpha and by ultraviolet B irradiation. J Clin Invest 1993; 92: 462–470.

38. Wood LC, Elias PM, Sequeira-Martin SM, Grunfeld C, Feingold KR. Occlusion lowers cytokine mRNA levels in essential fatty acid-deficient and normal mouse epidermis, but not after acute barrier disruption. J Invest Dermatol 1994; 103: 834–838.

39. Rheinwald JG, Beckett MA. Defective terminal differentiation in culture as a consistent and selectable character of malignant human keratinocytes. Cell 1980; 22:629–632.

40. Bikle DD, Pillai S, Gee E. Squamous carcinoma cell lines produce 1,25 dihydroxyvitamin D_3, but fail to respond to its prodifferentiating effect. J Invest Derm 1991; 97:435–441.

41. Ratnam AV, Bikle DD, Su M-J, Pillai S. Squamous carcinoma cell lines fail to respond to the prodifferentiation actions of 1,25-dihydroxyvitamin D despite normal levels of the vitamin D receptor. J Invest Dermatol 1996; 106:522–525.

42. Halloran BP, Schaefer P, Lifshcitz M, Levens M, Goldsmith RS. Plasma vitamin D metabolite concentration in chronic renal failure: Effect of oral administration of 25-hydroxyvitamin D_3. J Clin Endocrinol Metab 1984; 59:1063–1069.

43. Marchisio PC, Bondanza S, Cremona O, Cancedda R, DeLuca M. Polarized expression of integrin receptors ($\alpha_6\beta_4$, $\alpha_2\beta_1$, $\alpha_3\beta_1$, and $\alpha_v\beta_5$) and their relationship with the cytoskeleton and basement membrane matrix in cultured human keratinocytes. J Cell Biol 1991; 112:761–773.

44. Peltonen J, Larjava J, Jaakkola S. Localization of integrin receptors for fibronectin, collagen and laminin in human skin: Variable expression in basal and squamous cell carcinomas. J Clin Invest 1989; 84:1916–1923.

45. Guo M, Kim LT, Akiyama SK, Gralnick HR, Yamada KM, Grinnell F. Altered processing of integrin receptors during keratinocyte activation. Exp Cell Res 1991; 195: 315–322.

46. Moll R, Franke WW, Schiller DL, Geiger B, Krepler R. The catalog of human cytokeratins: Patterns of expression in normal epithelia, tumors and cultured cells. Cell 1982; 31:11–24.

47. Eichner R, Sun TT, Aebi U. The role of keratin subfamilies and keratin pairs in the formation of human epidermal intermediate filaments. J Cell Biol 1986; 102:1767–1777.

48. Warhol MJ, Roth J, Lucocq JM, Pinkus GS, Rice RH. Immuno-ultrastructural localization of involucrin in squamous epithelium and cultured keratinocytes. J Histochem Cytochem 1985; 33:141–149.

49. Thacher SM, Rice RH. Keratinocyte-specific transglutaminase of cultured human epidermal cells: relation to cross-linked envelope formation and terminal differentiation. Cell 1985; 40:685–695.

50. Steven AC, Bisher ME, Roop DR, Steinert PM. Biosynthetic pathways of filaggrin and loricrin—two major proteins expressed by terminally differentiated epidermal keratinocytes. J Struct Biol 1990; 104:150–162.

51. Dale BA, Resing KA, Lonsdale-Eccles JD. A keratin filament associated protein. Ann NY Acad Sci 1985; 455:330–342.
52. Mehrel T Hohl D, Rothnagel JA, Longley MA, Bundman D, Cheng C, Lichti U, Bisher ME, Steven AC, St. Identification of a major keratinocyte cell envelope protein, loricrin. Cell 1990; 61:1103–1112.
53. Elias PM, Menon GK, Grayson S, Brown BE. Membrane structural alterations in murine stratum corneum: Relationship to the localization of polar lipids and phospholipases. J Invest Dermatol 1988; 91:3–10.
54. Hohl D. Cornified cell envelope. Dermatologica 1990; 180:201–211.
55. Rheinwald JG, Green H. Serial cultivation of strains of human epidermal keratinocytes: The formation of keratinizing colonies from single cells. Cell 1975; 6:331–344.
56. Wolbach SB, Howe PR. Tissue changes following deprivation of fat-soluble A vitamin. J Exp Med 1925; 43:753–777.
57. Fell HB, Mellanby E. Metaplasia produced in cultures of chick ectoderm by high vitamin A. J Physiol 1953; 119:470–488.
58. Wolbach SB, Howe PR. Epithelial repair in recovery from vitamin A deficiency. J Exp Med 1933; 57:511–526.
59. Fuchs E, Green H. Regulation of terminal differentiation of cultured human keratinocytes by vitamin A. Cell 1981; 25:617–625.
60. Gilfix BM, Eckert RL. Coordinate control by vitamin A of keratin gene expression in human keratinocytes. J Biol Chem 1981; 260:14026–14029.
61. Choi Y, Fuchs E. TGF-β and retinoic acid: regulators of growth and modifiers of differentiation in human epidermal cells. Cell Reg 1990; 1:791–809.
62. Kline PR, Rice RH. Modulation of involucrin and envelope competence in human keratinocytes by hydrocortisone, retinyl acetate and growth arrest. Cancer Res 1983; 43:3203–3207.
63. Rubin AL, Parenteau NL, Rice RH. Coordination of keratinocyte programming in human SCC-13 carcinoma and normal epidermal cells. J Cell Physiol 1989; 138:208–214.
64. Hohl D, Lichti U, Breitkreutz D, Steinert PM, Roop DR. Transcription of the human loricrin gene in vitro is induced by calcium and cell density and suppressed by retinoic acid. J Invest Dermatol 1991; 96:414–418.
65. Fleckman P, Dale BA, Holbrook KA. Profilaggrin, a high molecular-weight precursor of filaggrin in human epidermis and cultured keratinocytes. J Invest Dermatol 1985; 85:507–512.
66. Segaert S, Garmyn M, Degreef H, Bouillon R. Retinoic acid modulates the anti-proliferative effect of 1,25-dihydroxyvitamin D_3 in cultured human epidermal keratinocytes. J Invest Dermatol 1997; 109:46–54.
67. Vollberg TM Sr, Nervi C, George MD, Fujimoto W, Krust A, Jetten AM. Retinoic acid receptors as regulators of human epidermal keratinocyte differentiation. Mol Endocrinol 1992; 6:667–676.
68. Kastner P, Krust A, Mendelsohn C, Garnier JM, Zelent A, Leroy P, Staub A, Chambon P. Murine isoforms of retinoic acid receptor gamma with specific patterns of expression. Proc Natl Acad Sci USA 1990; 87:2700–2704.

69. Elder JT, Astrom A, Pettersson U, Tavakkol A, Krust A, Kastner P, Chambon P, Voorheer JJ. Retinoic acid receptors and binding proteins in human skin. J Invest Dermatol 1992; 98:36S–41S.

70. Saitou M, Sugai S, Tanaka T, Shimouchi K, Fuchs E, Narumiya S, Kakizuka A. Inhibition of skin development by targeted expression of a dominant-negative retinoic acid receptor. Nature 1995; 374:159–162.

71. Hu L, Crowe DL, Rheinwald JG, Chambon P, Gudas LJ. Abnormal expression of retinoic acid receptors and keratin 19 by human oral and epidermal squamous cell carcinoma cell lines. Cancer Res 1991; 51:3972–3981.

72. Finzi E, Blake MJ, Celano P, Skouge J, Diwan R. Cellular localization of retinoic acid receptor-gamma expression in normal and neoplastic skin. Am J Pathol 1992; 140:1463–1471.

73. Torma H, Rollman O, Vahlquist A. Detection of mRNA transcripts for retinoic acid, vitamin D_3, and thyroid hormone (c-erb-A) nuclear receptors in human skin using reverse transcription and polymerase chain reaction. Acta Derm Venereol 1993; 73:102–107.

74. Schule R, Umesono K, Mangelsdorf DJ, Bolado J, Pike JW, Evans RM. Jun-Fos and receptors for vitamin A and D recognize a common response element in the human osteocalcin gene. Cell 1990; 61:497–504.

75. Xie Z, Bikle DD. Cloning of the human phospholipase Cγ1 promoter and identification of a DR-6 type vitamin D responsive element. J Biol Chem 1997; 272:6573–6577.

76. Li X-Y, Xiao J-H, Feng X, Qin L, Voorhees JJ. Retinoid X receptor-specific ligands synergistically upregulate 1,25-dihydroxyvitamin D_3-dependent transcription in epidermal keratinocytes in vitro and in vivo. J Invest Dermatol 1997; 108:506–512.

77. Kliewer SA, Umesono K, Mangelsdorf DJ, Evans RM. Retinoid X receptor interacts with nuclear receptors in retinoic acid, thyroid hormone and vitamin D_3 signalling. Nature 1992; 355:446–449.

78. Yu VC, Delsert C, Andersen B, Holloway JM, Devary OV, Naar AM, Kim SY, Boutin J-M, Glass CK, Ro. RXRβ: a coregulator that enhances binding of retinoic acid, thyroid hormone, and vitamin D receptors to their cognate response elements. Cell 1991; 67:1251–1266.

79. Forman BM, Casanova J, Raaka BM, Ghysdael J, Samuels HH. Half-site spacing and orientation determines whether thyroid hormone and retinoic acid receptors and related factors bind to DNA response elements as monomers, homodimers, or heterodimers. Mol Endocrinol 1992; 6:429–442.

80. Glass CK, Devary OV, Rosenfeld MG. Multiple cell type-specific proteins differentially regulate target sequence recognition by the α retinoic acid receptor. Cell 1990; 63:729–738.

81. Xie Z, Bikle DD. Differential regulation of vitamin D-responsive elements in normal and transformed keratinocytes. J Invest Dermatol 1998; 110:730–733.

82. Kang S, Li XY, Duell EA, Voorhees JJ. The retinoid X receptor agonist 9-cis-retinoic acid and the 24-hydroxylase inhibitor ketoconazole increase activity of 1,25-dihydroxyvitamin D_3 in human skin in vivo. J Invest Dermatol 1997; 108: 513–518.

83. McKay IA, Leigh IM. Epidermal cytokines and their roles in cutaneous wound healing. Br J Dermatol 1991; 124:513–518.

84. Ansel J, Perry P, Brown J. Cytokine modulation of keratinocyte cytokines. J Invest Dermatol 1990; 94:101S–107S.

85. Coffey Robert Jr, Derynck Rik, Wilcox Josiah N. Letters to Nature: Production and auto-induction of transforming growth factor-alpha in human keratinocytes. Nature 1987; 328:817–820.

86. Glick AB, Danielpour DD, Morgan D, Sporn MB, Yuspa SH. Induction and autocrine receptor binding of transforming growth factor-β2 during terminal differentiation of primary mouse keratinocytes. Mol Endocrinol 1990; 4:46–52.

87. Coffey RJ, Sipes NJ, Bascom CC, Graves-Deal R, Pennington CY, Weissman BE, Moses HL. Growth modulation of mouse keratinocytes by transforming growth factors. Cancer Res 1988; 48:1596–1602.

88. Shipley GD, Pittelkow MR, Willie JJ, Scott RE, Moses HL. Reversible inhibition of normal human prokeratinocyte proliferation by type-B transforming growth factor-growth inhibitor in serum free medium. Cancer Res 1986; 46:2068–2071.

89. Kim HJ, Abdelkader N, Katz M, McLane JA. 1,25-Dihydroxy-vitamin-D$_3$ enhances antiproliferative effect and transcription of TGF-β1 on human keratinocytes in culture. J Cell Physiol 1992; 151:579–587.

90. Koli K, Keski-Oja, J. Vitamin D$_3$ and calcipotriol enhance the secretion of transforming growth factor-β1 and -β2 in cultured murine keratinocytes. Growth Factors 1993; 8:153–163.

91. Vollberg TM, George MD, Jetten AM. Induction of extracellular matrix gene expression in normal human kerotinocytes by transforming growth factor B is altered by cellular differentiation. Exp Cell Res 1991; 193:93–100.

92. George MD, Vollberg TM, Floyd E, Stein JP, Jetten AM. Regulation of transglutaminase type II by transforming growth factor-β1 in normal and transformed human epidermal keratinocytes. J Biol Chem 1990; 265:11098–11104.

93. Pietenpol JA, Holt JT, Stein RW, Moses HL. Transforming growth factor β1 suppression of c-myc gene transcription: Role in inhibition of keratinocyte proliferation. Proc Natl Acad Sci USA 1990; 87:3758–3762.

94. Halaban R, Langdon R, Birchall N, Cuono C, Baird A, Scott G, Moellmann G, McGuire J. Basic fibroblast growth factor from human keratinocytes is a natural mitogen for melanocytes. J Cell Biol 1988; 107:1611–1619.

95. O'Keefe EJ, Chiu ML, Payne RE. Stimulation of growth of keratinocytes by bFGF. J Invest Dermatol 1988; 90:767–769.

96. Bottaro DP, Rubin JS, Ron D, Finch PW, Florio C, Aaronson SA. Characterization of the receptor for keratinocyte growth factor. J Biol Chem 1990; 265:12767–12770.

97. Rubin JS, Osada H, Finch PW, Taylor WG, Rudikoff S, Aaronson SA. Purification and characterization of a newly identified growth factor specific for epithelial cells. Proc Natl Acad Sci USA 1989; 86:802–806.

98. DeLapp NW, Dieckman BS. Effect of basic fibroblast growth factor (bFGF) and insulin-like growth factors type I (IGF-I) and type II (IGF-II) on adult human keratinocyte growth and fibronectin secretion. J Invest Dermatol 1990; 94:777–780.

99. Misra P, Nickoloff BJ, Morhenn VB, Hintz RL, Rosenfeld RG. Characterization of insulin-like growth factor-I/somatomedin-C receptors on human keratinocyte monolayers. J Invest Dermatol 1986; 87:264–267.

100. Nickoloff BJ. Binding of ^{125}I-gamma interferon to cultured human keratinocytes. J Invest Dermatol 1987; 89:132–135.

101. Morhenn VB, Wood GS. Gamma interferon-induced expression of class II major histocompatibility complex antigens by human keratinocytes: Effects of conditions of culture. In: Milstone LM, Edelson RL, eds. Endocrine, Metabolic and Immunologic Functions of Keratinocytes. Ann NY Acad Sci 1988:321–330.

102. Nickoloff BJ, Griffiths CEM, Barker JNWN. The role of adhesion molecule, chemotactic factors and cytokines in inflammatory and neoplastic skin disease—1990 update. J Invest Dermatol 1990; 94:151S–157S.

103. Merendino JJ Jr, Insogna KL, Milstone LM, Broadus AE, Stewart AF. Parathyroid hormone-like protein from cultured human keratinocytes. Science 1986; 231: 388–390.

104. Hanafin NM, Chen TC, Heinrich G, Segre GV, Holick MF. Cultured human fibroblasts and not cultured human keratinocytes express a PTH/PTHrP receptor mRNA. J Invest Dermatol 1995; 105:133–137.

105. Orloff JJ, Kats Y, Urena P, Schipani E, Vasavada RC, Philbrick WM, Behal A, Abou-Samra AB, Segre G. Further evidence for a novel receptor for amino-terminal parathyroid hormone-related protein on keratinocytes and squamous carcinoma cell lines. Endocrinology 1995; 136:3016–3023.

106. Holick MF, Ray S, Chen TC, Tian X, Persons KS. A parathyroid hormone antagonist stimulates epidermal proliferation and hair growth in mice. Proc Natl Acad Sci USA 1994; 91:8014–8016.

107. Whitfield JF, Isaacs RJ, Jouishomme H, MacLean S, Chakravarthy BR, Morley P, Barisoni D, Regalia E,A. C-terminal fragment of parathyroid hormone-related protein, PTHrP-(107–111), stimulates membrane-associated protein kinase C activity and modulates the proliferation of human and murine skin keratinocytes. J Cell Physiol 1996; 166:1–11.

108. Luger TA, Stadler BM, Luger BM, Sztein MB, Schmidt JA, Hawley-Nelson P, Grabner G, Oppenheim JJ. Characteristics of an epidermal cell thymocyte-activating factor (ETAF) produced by human epidermal cells and a human squamous cell carcinoma line. J Invest Dermatol 1983; 81:187–193.

109. Kupper TS, Ballard DW, Chau AO, McGuire JS, Flood PM, Horowitz MC, Langdon R, Lightfoot L, Gubler U. Human keratinocytes contain mRNA indistinguishable from monocyte interleukin 1α and B mRNA. J Exp Med 1986; 164:2095–2100.

110. Luger TA, Kock A, Kirnbauer R, Scharwarz T, Ansel JC. Keratinocyte-derived interleukin 3: Endocrine, metabolic, and immunologic functions of keratinocytes. Ann NY Acad Sci 1988:253–261.

111. Grossman RM, Krueger J, Yourish D, Granelli-Piperno A, Murphy DP, May LT, Kupper TS, Sehgal PB, Gottlieb AB. Interleukin 6 is expressed in high levels in psoriatic skin and stimulates proliferation of cultured human keratinocytes. Proc Natl Acad Sci USA 1989; 86:6367–6371.

112. Larsenk CG, Anderson AO, Oppenheim JJ, Matsushima K. Production of inter-leukin-8 by human dermal fibroblasts and keratinocytes in response to interleukin-1 or tumor necrosis factor. Immunology 1989; 68:31–36.

113. Kupper TS, Lee F, Coleman D, Chodakewitz J, Flood P, Horowitz M. Keratinocyte derived T-cell growth factor (KTGF) is identical to granulocyte macrophage colony stimulation factor (GM-CSF). J Invest Dermatol 1988; 91:185–188.

114. Chodakewitz JA, Lacy J, Edwards SE. Macrophage colony-stimulating factor production by murine and human keratinocytes. Immunology 1990; 144:2190–2196.

115. Kupper TS, Horowitz M, Birchall N, Mizutani H, Coleman D, McGuire J, Flood P, Dower S, Lee F. Hematopoietic, lymphopoietic, and proinflammatory cytokines produced by human and murine keratinocytes: Endocrine, metabolic and immunologic functions of keratinocytes. NY: Ann NY Acad Sci 1988:262–270.

116. Menon GK, Grayson S, Elias PM. Ionic calcium reservoirs in mammalian epidermis: Ultrastructural localization by ion-capture cytochemistry. J Invest Dermatol 1985; 84:508–512.

117. Mauro T, Rassner U, Bench G, Feingold KR, Elias PM, Cullander C. Acute barrier disruption causes quantitative changes in the calcium gradient. J Invest Dermatol 1996; 106:919.

118. Lee SH, Elias PM, Feingold KR, Mauro T. A role for ions in barrier recovery after acute perturbation. J Invest Dermatol 1994; 102:976–979.

119. Menon GK, Price LF, Bommannan B, Elias PM, Feingold KR. Selective obliteration of the epidermal calcium gradient leads to enhanced lamellar body secretion. J Invest Dermatol 1994; 102:789–795.

120. Lee SH, Elias PM, Proksch E, Menon GK, Mao-Luiang M, Feingold KR. Calcium and potassium are important regulators of barrier homeostasis in murine epidermis. J Clin Invest 1992; 89:530–538.

121. Menon GK, Elias PM, Lee SH, Feingold KR. Localization of calcium in murine epidemiology following disruption and repair of the permeability barrier. Cell Tiss Res 1992; 270:503–512.

122. Hennings H, Michael D, Cheng C, Steinert P, Holbrook K, Yuspa SH. Calcium regulation of growth and differentiation of mouse epidermal cells in culture. Cell 1980; 19:245–254.

123. Hennings H, Holbrook KA. Calcium regulation of cell-cell contact and differentiation of epidermal cells in culture: An ultrastructural study. Exp Cell Res 1983; 143:127–142.

124. Zamnsky GB, Nguyen U, Chou I-N. An immunofluorescence study of the calcium-induced coordinated reorganization of microfilaments and microtubules in cultured human epidermal keratinocytes. J Invest Dermatol 1991; 97:984–995.

125. Inohara S, Tatsumi Y, Cho H, Tanaka Y, Sagami S. Actin filament and desmosome formation in cultured human keratinocytes. Arch Dermatol Res 1990; 282:210–212.

126. Pillai S, Bikle DD, Mancianti ML, Cline P, Hincenbergs M. Calcium regulation of growth and differentiation of normal human keratinocytes: modulation of differentiation competence by growth and extracellular calcium. J Cell Physiol 1990; 143:294–302.

127. Su M-J, Bikle DD, Mancianti ML, Pillai S. 1,25-Dihydroxyvitamin D_3 potentiates the keratinocyte response to calcium. J Biol Chem 1994; 269:14723–14729.

128. Yuspa SH, Kilkenny AE, Steinert PM, Roop DR. Expression of murine epidermal differentiation markers is regulated by restricted extracellular calcium concentrations in vitro. J Cell Biol 1989; 109:1207–1217.

129. Ng DC, Su M-J, Kim R, Bikle DD. Regulation of involucrin gene expression by calcium in normal human keratinocytes. Front Biosci 1996; 1:16–24.

130. Huff CA, Yuspa SH, Rosenthal D. Identification of control elements 3' to the human keratin 1 gene that regulate cell type and differentiation-specific expression. J Biol Chem 1993; 268:377–384.

131. Ryynanen J, Jaakkola S, Engvall E, Peltonen J, Uitto J. Expression of B4 integrins in human skin: Comparison of epidermal distribution with β1-integrin epitopes, and modulation by calcium and vitamin D_3 in cultured keratinocytes. J Invest Dermatol 1991; 97:562–567.

132. Glick AB, Sporn MB, Yuspa SH. Altered regulation of TGF-β1 and TGF-α in primary keratinocytes and papillomas expressing v-Ha-ras. Mol Carcin 1991; 4:210–219.

133. Pillai S, Bikle DD. Role of intracellular free calcium in the cornified envelope formation of keratinocytes: Differences in the mode of action of extracellular calcium and 1,25-dihydroxyvitamin D. J Cell Physiol 1991; 146:94–100.

134. Hennings H, Kruszewski FH, Yuspa SH, Tucker RW. Intracellular calcium alterations in response to increased external calcium in normal and neoplastic keratinocytes. Carcinogenesis 1989; 10:777–780.

135. Sharpe GR, Gillespie JI, Greenwell JR. An increase in intracellular free calcium is an early event during differentiation of cultured human keratinocytes. FEBS Lett 1989; 254:25–28.

136. Bikle DD, Ratnam AV, Mauro T, Harris J, Pillai S. Changes in calcium responsiveness and handling during keratinocyte differentiation: Potential role of the calcium receptor. J Clin Invest 1996; 97:1085–1093.

137. Kruszewski FH, Hennings H, Yuspa SH, Tucker RW. Regulation of intracellular free calcium in normal murine keratinocytes. Am J Physiol 1991; 261:C767–C773.

138. Pillai S, Bikle DD, Mancianti M-L, Hincenbergs M. Uncoupling of the calcium-sensing mechanism and differentiation in squamous carcinoma cell lines. Exp Cell Res 1991; 192:576–573.

139. Kruszewski FH, Hennings H, Tucker RW, Yuspa SH. Differences in the regulation of intracellular calcium in normal and neoplastic keratinocytes are not caused by ras gene mutations. Cancer Res 1991; 51:4206–4212.

140. Jaken S, Yuspa SH. Early signs for keratinocyte differentiation: role of Ca^{2+}-mediated inositol lipid metabolism in normal and neoplastic epidermal cells. Carcinogenesis 1988; 9:1033–1038.

141. Reiss M, Lipsey L, Zhou Z-L. Extracellular calcium-dependent regulation of transmembrane calcium fluxes in murine keratinocytes. J Cell Physiol 1991; 147:281–291.

142. Oda Y, Tu C-L, Pillai S, Bikle DD. The calcium sensing receptor and its alternatively spliced form in keratinocyte differentiation. J Biol Chem 1998; 273:23344–23352 .

143. Clapham DE. Calcium signaling. Cell 1995; 80:259–268.

144. Punnonen K, Denning M, Lee E, Li L, Rhee SG, Yuspa SH. Keratinocyte differentiation is associated with changes in the expression and regulation of phospholipase C isoenzymes. J Invest Dermatol 1993; 101:719–726.

145. Pillai S, Bikle DD. ATP stimulates phosphoinositide metabolism, mobilizes intracellular calcium and inhibits terminal differentiation of human epidermal keratinocytes. J Clin Invest 1992; 90:42–51.

146. Jones KT, Sharpe GR. Thapsigargin raises intracellular free calcium levels in human keratinocytes and inhibits the coordinated expression of differentiation markers. Exp Cell Res 1994; 210:71–76.

147. Pillai S, Bikle DD. Lanthanum influx into cultured human keratinocytes: Effect on calcium flux and terminal differentiation. J Cell Physiol 1992; 151:623–629.

148. Li L, Tucker RW, Hennings H, Yuspa SH. Chelation of intracellular Ca^{2+} inhibits murine keratinocyte differentiation in vitro. J Cell Physiol 1995; 163:105–114.

149. Galietta LJV, Barone V, De Luca M, Romeo G. Characterization of chloride and cation channels in cultured human keratinocytes. Eur J Physiol 1991; 418:18–25.

150. Mauro TM, Pappone PA, Rivkah Isseroff R. Extracellular calcium affects the membrane currents of cultured human keratinocytes. J Cell Physiol 1990; 143:13–20.

151. Mauro TM, Rivkah Isseroff R, Lasarow R, Pappone PA. Ion channels are linked to differentiation in keratinocytes. J Membr Biol 1993; 132:201–209.

152. Grando SA, Horton RM, Mauro TM, Kist DA, Lee TX, Dahl MV. Activation of keratinocyte nicotinic cholinergic receptors stimulates calcium influx and enhances cell differentiation. J Invest Dermatol 1996; 107:412–418.

153. Liu M, Chen TY, Ahamed B, Li J, Yau KW. Calcium-calmodulin modulation of the olfactory cyclic nucleotide-gated cation channel [published erratum appears in Science 1994 Dec 23;266(5193):1933]. Science 1994; 266:1348–1354.

154. Hoth M, Penner R. Depletion of intracellular calcium stores activates a calcium current in mast cells. Nature 1992; 355:353–356.

155. Putney Jr JW. Capacitative calcium entry revisited. Cell Calc 1990; 11:611–624.

156. Oda Y, Timpe LC, McKenzie RC, Sauder DN, Largman C, Mauro T. Alternatively spliced forms of the cGMP-gated channel in human keratinocytes. FEBS Lett 1997; 414:140–145.

157. Nemeth EF, Scarpa A. Rapid mobilization of cellular calcium in bovine parathyroid cells evoked by extracellular divalent cations. J Biol Chem 1987; 262:5188–5196.

158. Brown EM, Gamba G, Riccardi D. Cloning and characterization of an extracellular Ca^{2+}-sensing receptor from bovine parathyroid. Nature 1993; 366:575–580.

159. Garrett JE, Capuano IV, Hammerland LG. Molecular cloning and functional expression of human parathyroid calcium receptor cDNAs. J Biol Chem 1995; 270:12919–12925.

160. Hebert SC, Brown EM. The extracellular calcium receptor. Curr Opin Cell Biol 1995; 7:484–492.

161. Pillai S, Bikle DD, Su M-J, Ratnam A, Abe J. 1,25 dihydroxyvitamin D upregulates the phosphatidyl inositol signalling pathway in human keratinocytes by increasing phospholipase C levels. J Clin Invest 1995; 96:602–609.

162. Hawley-Nelson P, Stanley JR, Schmidt J, Gullino M, Yuspa SH. The tumor promoter 12-O-tetradecanoylphorbol-13-acetate accelerates keratinocyte differentiation and stimulates growth of an unidentified cell type in cultured human epidermis. Exp Cell Res 1982; 137:155–167.

163. Yuspa SH, Ben T, Hennings H, Lichti U. Divergent responses in epidermal basal cells exposed to the promoter 12-O-tetradecanoylphorbol-13-acetate. Cancer Res 1982; 42:2344–2349.

164. Kitajima Y, Inoue S, Nagao S, Nagata K, Yaoita H, Nozawa Y. Biphasic effects of 12-O-tetradecanoylphorbol-13-acetate on the cell morphology of low calcium-grown human epidermal carcinoma cells: Involvement of translocation on down regulation of protein kinase C[1]. Cancer Res 1988; 48:964–970.

165. Rice RH, Rong XH, Chakravarty R. Suppression of keratinocyte differentiation in SSC-9 human carcinoma cells by benzo[a]pyrene, 12-O-tetradecanoylphorbol-13-acetate and hydroxyurea. Carcinogenesis 1988; 9:1885–1890.

166. Sheu H, Kitajima Y, Yaoita H. Involvement of protein kinase C in translocation of desmoplakins from cytosol to plasma membrane during desmosome formation in human squamous cell carcinoma cells grown in low to normal calcium concentration. Exp Cell Res 1989; 185:176–190.

167. Nagao S, Kitajima Y, Nagata K, Inoue S, Yaoita H, Nozawa Y. Correlation between cell-cell contact formation and activation of protein kinase C in a human squamous cell carcinoma cell line. J Invest Dermatol 1989; 92:175–178.

168. Yuspa SH, Ben T, Hennings H. The induction of epidermal transglutaminase and terminal differentiation by tumor promoters in cultured epidermal cells. Carcinogenesis 1983; 4:1413–1418.

169. Dlugosz AA, Yuspa SH. Protein kinase C regulates keratinocyte transglutaminase (TGK) gene expression in cultured primary mouse epidermal keratinocytes induced to terminally differentiate by calcium. J Invest Dermatol 1994; 102:409–414.

170. Matsui MS, Illarda I, Wang N, DeLeo VA. Protein kinase C agonist and antagonist effects in normal human epidermal keratinocytes. Exp Dermatol 1993; 2:247–256.

171. Dlugosz AA, Yuspa SH. Coordinate changes in gene expression which mark the spinous to granular cell transition in epidermis are regulated by protein kinase C. J Cell Biol 1993; 120:217–225.

172. Lu B, Rothnagel JA, Longley MA, Tsai SY, Roop DR. Differentiation-specific expression of human keratin 1 is mediated by a composite AP-1/steroid hormone element. J Biol Chem 1994; 269:7443–7449.

173. Disepio D, Jones A, Longley MA, Bundman D, Rothnagel JA, and Roop DA. The proximal promoter of the mouse loricrin gene contains a functional AP-1 element and directs keratinocyte specific but not differentiation specific expression. J Biol Chem 1995; 270:10792–10799.

174. Moscat J, Flemming TP, Molloy CJ, Lopez-Barahona M, Aaronson SA. The calcium signal for Balb 1 MK keratinocyte terminal differentiation induces sustained alterations in phosphoinositide metabolism without detectable protein kinase C activation. J Biol Chem 1989; 264:11228–11235.

175. Filvaroff E, Stern D, Dotto G. Tyrosine phosphorylation is an early an specific event involved in primary keratinocyte differentiation. Mol Cell Biol 1990; 10:1164–1173.

176. Chakravarthy BR, Isaacs RJ, Morley P, Durkin JP, Whitfield JF. Stimulation of protein kinase C during Ca(2+)-induced keratinocyte differentiation: Selective blockade of MARCKS phosphorylation by calmodulin. J Biol Chem 1995; 270:1362–1368.

177. Hepler JR, Earp HS, Harden TK. Long-term phorbol ester treatment down-regulates protein kinase C and sensitizes the phosphoinositide signaling pathway to hormone and growth factor stimulation: Evidence for a role of protein kinase C in agonist-induced desensitization. J Biol Chem 1988; 263:7610–7619.

178. Kojima I, Shibata H, Ogata E. Phorbol ester inhibits angiotensin-induced activation of phospholipase C in adrenal glomerulosa cells: Its implication in the sustained action of angiotensin. Biochem J 1986; 237:253–258.

179. Dlugosz AA, Mischak H, Mushinski JF, Yuspa SH. Transcripts encoding protein kinase C-alpha, -delta, -epsilon, -zeta, and -eta are expressed in basal and differentiating mouse keratinocytes in vitro and exhibit quantitative changes in neoplastic cells. Mol Carcinog 1992; 5:286–292.

180. Denning MF, Dlugosz AA, Howett MK, Yuspa SH. Expression of an oncogenic rasHa gene in murine keratinocytes induces tyrosine phosphorylation and reduced activity of protein kinase C delta. J Biol Chem 1993; 268:26079–26081.

181. Reynolds NJ, Baldassare JJ, Henderson PA. Translocation and downregulation of protein kinase C isoenzymes-alpha and -epsilon by phorbol ester and bryostatin-1 in human keratinocytes and fibroblasts. J Invest Dermatol 1994; 103:364–369.

182. Fisher GJ, Tavakkol A, Leach K. Differential expression of protein kinase C isoenzymes in normal and psoriatic adult human skin: reduced expression of protein kinase C-beta II in psoriasis. J Invest Dermatol 1993; 101:553–559.

183. Geiges D, Marks F, Gschwendt M. Loss of protein kinase C delta from human HaCaT keratinocytes upon ras transfection is mediated by TGF alpha. Exp Cell Res 1995; 219:299–303.

184. Denning MF, Kazanietz MG, Blumberg PM, Yuspa SH. Cholesterol sulfate activates multiple protein kinase C isoenzymes and induces granular cell differentiation in cultured murine keratinocytes. Cell Growth Differ 1995; 6:1619–1626.

185. Mochly-Rosen D. Localization of protein kinases by anchoring proteins: a theme in signal transduction. Science 1995; 268:247–251.

186. Ron D, Luo J, Mochly-Rosen D. C2 region-derived peptides inhibit translocation and function of beta protein kinase C in vivo. J Biol Chem 1995; 270: 24180–24187.

187. Johnson JA, Gray MO, Chen CH, Mochly-Rosen D. A protein kinase C translocation inhibitor as an isozyme-selective antagonist of cardiac function. J Biol Chem 1996; 271:24962–24966.

188. Hundle B, McMahon T, Dadgar J, Chen CH, Mochly-Rosen D, Messing RO. An inhibitory fragment derived from protein kinase C epsilon prevents enhancement of nerve growth factor responses by ethanol and phorbol esters. J Biol Chem 1997; 272:15028–15035.

189. Goodnight J, Mischak H, Mushinski JF. Selective involvement of protein kinase C isozymes in differentiation and neoplastic transformation. Adv Cancer Res 1994; 64:159–209.

190. Denning MF, Dlugosz AA, Williams EK, Szallasi Z, Blumberg PM, Yuspa SH. Specific protein kinase C isozymes mediate the induction of keratinocyte differentiation markers by calcium. Cell Growth Differ 1995; 6:149–157.

191. Szallasi Z, Kosa K, Smith CB, et al. Differential regulation by anti-tumor-promoting 12-deoxyphorbol-13-phenylacetate reveals distinct roles of the classical and novel protein kinase C isozymes in biological responses of primary mouse keratinocytes. Mol Pharmacol 1995; 47:258–265.

192. Lee YS, Dlugosz AA, McKay R, Dean NM, Yuspa SH. Definition by specific antisense oligonucleotides of a role for protein kinase C alpha in expression of differ-

entiation markers in normal and neoplastic mouse epidermal keratinocytes. Mol Carcinog 1997; 18:44–53.

193. Downward J, Waterfield MD, Parker PJ. Autophosphorylation and protein kinase C phosphorylation of the epidermal growth factor receptor. Effect on tyrosine kinase activity and ligand binding affinity. J Biol Chem 1985; 260: 14538–14546.

194. Goode N, Hughes K, Woodgett JR, Parker PJ. Differential regulation of glycogen synthase kinase-3 beta by protein kinase C isotypes. J Biol Chem 1992; 267: 16878–16882.

195. Schlessinger J. Allosteric regulation of the epidermal growth factor receptor kinase. J Cell Biol 1986; 103:2067–2072.

196. Kolch W, Heidecker G, Kochs G. Protein kinase C alpha activates RAF-1 by direct phosphorylation. Nature 1993; 364:249–252.

197. Yaar M, Gilani A, DiBenedetto PJ, Harkness DD, Gilchrest BA. Gene modulation accompanying differentiation of normal versus malignant keratinocytes. Exp Cell Res 1993; 206:235–243.

198. Holladay K, Fujiki H, Bowden GT. Okadaic acid induces the expression of both early and secondary response genes in mouse keratinocytes. Mol Carcinog 1992; 5:16–24.

199. Bollag WB, Xiong Y, Ducote J, Harmon CS. Regulation of fos-lacZ fusion gene expression in primary mouse epidermal keratinocytes isolated from transgenic mice. Biochem J 1994; 300:263–270.

200. Welter JF, Eckert RL. Differential expression of the fos and jun family members c-fos, fosB, Fra-1, Fra-2, c-jun, junB and junD during human epidermal keratinocyte differentiation. Oncogene 1995; 11:2681–2687.

201. Rutberg SE, Saez E, Glick A, Dlugosz AA, Spiegelman BM, Yuspa SH. Differentiation of mouse keratinocytes is accompanied by PKC-dependent changes in AP-1 proteins. Oncogene 1996; 13:167–176.

202. Welter JF, Crish JF, Agarwal C, Eckert RL. Fos-related antigen (Fra-1), junB, and junD activate human involucrin promoter transcription by binding to proximal and distal AP1 sites to mediate phorbol ester effects on promoter activity. J Biol Chem 1995; 270:12614–12622.

203. Bowden GT, Schneider B, Domann R, Kulesz-Martin M. Oncogene activation and tumor suppressor gene inactivation during multistage mouse skin carcinogenesis. Cancer Res 1994; 54:1882s–1885s.

204. Boyle WJ, Smeal T, Defize LHK. Activation of protein kinase C decreases phosphorylation of c-Jun at sites that negatively regulate its DNA-binding activity. Cell 1991; 64:573–584.

205. Smeal T, Binetruy B, Mercola D. Oncoprotein-mediated signalling cascade stimulates c-Jun activity by phosphorylation of serines 63 and 73. Mol Cell Biol 1992; 12:3507–3513.

206. Gruda MC, Kovary K, Metz R, Bravo R. Regulation of Fra-1 and Fra-2 phosphorylation differs during the cell cycle of fibroblasts and phosphorylation in vitro by MAP kinase affects DNA binding activity. Oncogene 1994; 9:2537–2547.

207. Xanthoudakis S, Curran T. Identification and characterization of Ref-1, a nuclear protein that facilitates AP-1 DNA-binding activity. EMBO J 1992; 11:653–665.

208. Monteclaro FS, Vogt PK. A Jun-binding protein related to a putative tumor suppressor. Proc Natl Acad Sci USA 1993; 90:6726–6730.

209. Auwerx J, Sassone-Corsi P. IP-1: A dominant inhibitor of Fos/Jun whose activity is modulated by phosphorylation. Cell 1991; 64:983–993.

210. Hosomi J, Hosoi J, Abe E, Suda T, Kuroki T. Regulation of terminal differentiation of cultured mouse epidermal cells by $1\alpha,25$-dihydroxyvitamin D_3. Endocrinology 1983; 113:1950–1957.

211. Merke J, Schwittay D, Furstenberger G, Gross M, Marks F, Ritz E. Demonstration and characterization of 1,25-dihydroxyvitamin D_3 receptors in basal cells of epidermis of neonatal and adult mice. Calcif Tissue Int 1985; 37:257–267.

212. Horiuchi N, Clemens TL, Schiller AL, Holick MF. Detection and developmental changes of the 1,25-(OH)2-D_3 concentration in mouse skin and intestine. J Invest Dermatol 1985; 84:461–464.

213. Smith EL, Walworth NC, Holick MF. Effect of $1\alpha,25$-dihydroxyvitamin D_3 on the morphologic and biochemical differentiation of cultured human epidermal keratinocytes grown in serum-free conditions. J Invest Dermatol 1986; 86:709–714.

214. McLane JA, Katz M, Abdelkader N. Effect of 1,25-dihydroxyvitamin D_3 on human keratinocytes grown under different culture conditions. In Vitro Cell Dev Biol 1990; 26:379–387.

215. Bollag WB, Ducote J, Harmon CS. Biphasic-Effect of 1,25-dihydroxyvitamin D_3 on primary mouse epidermal keratinocyte proliferation. J Cell Physiol 1995; 163:248–256.

216. Itin PH, Pittelkow MR, Kumar R. Effects of vitamin D metabolites on proliferation and differentiation of cultured human epidermal keratinocytes grown in serum-free or defined culture medium. Endocrinology 1994; 135:1793–1798.

217. Gniadecki R. Stimulation versus inhibition of keratinocyte growth by 1,25-dihydroxyvitamin D_3: Dependence on cell culture conditions. J Invest Dermatol 1996; 106:510–516.

218. Feldman D, Malloy PJ. Hereditary 1,25-dihydroxyvitamin D resistant rickets: Molecular basis and implications for the role of 1,25(OH) 2D_3 in normal physiology. Mol Cell Endocrinol 1990; 72:C57–C62.

219. Yoshizawa T, Handa Y, Uematsu Y, Takeda S, Sekine K, Yoshihara Y, Kawakami T, Arioka K, Sato H, Uchiy. Mice lacking the vitamin D receptor exhibit impaired bone formation, uterine hypoplasia and growth retardation after weaning. Nature Genet 1997; 16:391–396.

220. Bittiner B, Bleehen SS, MacNeil S. $1\alpha,25(OH)_2$ vitamin D_3 increased intracellular calcium in human keratinocytes. Br J Dermatol 1991; 124:230–235.

221. Tang W, Ziboh VA, Isseroff R. Novel regulatory action of 1,25-dihydroxyvitamin D on the metabolism of polyphosphoinositides in murine epidermal keratinocytes. J Cell Physiol 1987; 132:131–136.

222. McLaughlin JA, Cantley LC, Holick MF. $1,25(OH)_2D_3$ increased calcium and phosphatidylinositol metabolism in differentiating cultured human keratinocytes. J Nutr Biochem 1990; 1:81–87.

223. Yada Y, Ozeki T, Meguro S, Mori S, Nozawa Y. Signal transduction in the onset of terminal keratinocyte differentiation induced $1\alpha,25$-dihydroxyvitamin D_3: Role of

protein kinase C translocation. Biochem Biophys Res Commun 1989; 163: 1517–1522.

224. Tang W, Ziboh VA. Agonist/inositol trisphosphate-induced release of calcium from murine keratinocytes: A possible link with keratinocyted differentiation. J Invest Dermatol 1991; 96:134–138.

225. Hanafin NM, Persons KS, Holick MF. Increased PKC activity in cultured human keratinocytes and fibroblasts after treatment with 1 ∝,25-dihydroxyvitamin D_3. J Cell Biochem 1995; 57:362–370.

226. Lian JB, Stein GS, Bortell R, Owen TA. Phenotype suppression: A postulated molecular mechanism for mediating the relationship of proliferation and differentiation by Fos/Jun interactions at AP-1 sites in steroid responsive promoter elements of tissue-specific genes. J Cell Biochem 1991; 45:9–14.

227. Regnier M, Darmon M. 1,25-dihydroxyvitamin D_3 stimulates specifically the last steps of epidermal differentiation of cultured human keratinocytes. Differentiation 1991; 47:173–188.

228. Pavlovitch JH, Galoppin L, Rizk M, Didierjean L, Balsan S. Alterations in rat epidermis provoked by chronic vitamin D deficiency. Am J Physiol 1984; 247: E228–E233.

229. Feingold KR, Williams ML, Pillai S, Menon GK, Bikle DD, Elias PM. The effect of vitamin D status on cutaneous sterologenesis in and in vitro. Biochim Biophys Acta 1987; 930:193–200.

6

Vitamin D and the Hair Follicle

Jörg Reichrath
University of the Saarland, Homburg, Germany

I. INTRODUCTION

The hair follicle is a highly hormone-sensitive organ [1]. The regulatory mechanisms governing hair cycling, starting from a resting state (telogen) and progressing to a state of rapid growth (anagen), are still obscure [1,2]. Several clinical and laboratory observations suggest that 1,25-dihydroxyvitamin D_3 [1,25$(OH)_2D_3$, calcitriol], endogenously produced or therapeutically applied may be an interesting candidate as a hair growth–regulatory factor. First, patients with hereditary 1,25-dihydroxyvitamin D_3–resistant rickets type II (HVDRR [3]) and vitamin D receptor (VDR) knockout mice [4,5] exhibit a phenotype that includes alopecia totalis. Second, experimental chemotherapy–induced alopecia in neonatal rats can be prevented by topical 1,25-dihydroxyvitamin D_3 application [6]. Third, pigs suffering from acute to subacute vitamin D toxicosis were reported to develop a rough hair coat [7].

Vitamin D (calciferol) is a hormone that is involved in not only calcium homeostasis [8] but also in immune regulation, cell growth, and differentiation [9–11]. The biologically most active vitamin D metabolite, 1,25-dihydroxyvitamin D_3, is enzymatically synthesized in skin—e.g., by keratinocytes that were shown to possess 1α- and 25-hydroxylase activity [10,12,13] or by successive hydroxylation of vitamin D at the 1- and 25-positions in kidney and liver [11].

II. MODE OF ACTION OF VITAMIN-D ANALOGS

A. Genomic Effects

Like classical steroid hormones, 1,25-dihydroxyvitamin D_3 exerts its genomic effects by binding to an intranuclear receptor (VDR) belonging to the superfamily of *trans*-acting transcriptional factors, which includes the estrogen, progesterone, glucocorticoid, thyroxine, aldosterone, and retinoic acid receptors [14]. Like all classical steroid hormone receptors, VDR is essentially made up of two functional domains, a hormone-binding domain and a DNA-binding domain, which consists of two zinc fingers. The mechanism of vitamin D action involves binding of 1,25-dihydroxyvitamin D_3 to the hormone-binding domain of the VDR. The DNA-binding domain of the VDR, in turn, associates with specific DNA sequence elements located upstream of vitamin D–responsive gene promoters and modulates transcription of vitamin D–responsive target genes [14]. Recently, it has been shown that VDR requires auxiliary proteins for effective DNA binding to their responsive elements in target genes, thus regulating transcriptional activity [15]. These proteins were identified as the retinoid-X receptors (RXR-α,-β,-γ) forming heterodimeric complexes with VDR and the classical retinoic acid receptors (RAR-α,-β,-γ) [15,16]. It has been shown that there are at least two different classes of vitamin D–responsive elements that are activated either by the VDR alone or by heterodimers of VDR and RXR-α [17]. Thus, the RXR ligand and the nature of the responsive element determine whether VDR is regulated by RXR-α [17].

B. Nongenomic Effects

Nongenomic effects of 1,25-dihydroxyvitamin D_3 and analogs are related to effects on intracellular calcium [18]. In keratinocytes and other cell types, 1,25-dihydroxyvitamin D_3 elevates free cytosolic calcium levels [18,19], at least in part by increasing the activity of plasma membrane L-type Ca^{2+} channels and phospholipase C.

III. EXPRESSION OF VDR IN KEY STRUCTURES OF THE HAIR FOLLICLE

Numerous studies have analyzed expression of VDR in epidermis and hair follicle using hormone-binding studies or immunohistochemistry [20–25]. Applying ^3H-1,25(OH)$_2D_3$ and autoradiographic techniques, Stumpf et al. in 1979 showed, for the first time, the presence of VDR in cells of the hair bulb sheath [20]. In both adult and neonatal rat skin, the strongest labeling was observed in that study in cells of the outer root sheath. Near the hair bulb, the cells of the inner hair sheath and of the hair medulla of coarse hair were weakly and variably labeled, as were the cells of the hair bulb. Cells of the hair dermal papilla were generally unlabeled with ^3H-1,25(OH)$_2D_3$, although an occasionally weakly labeled cell was reported. Cells of the epithelial hair sheath of involuting catagen and telogen stages of the hair cycle showed variable nuclear labeling with ^3H-1,25(OH)$_2D_3$, similar to that of adjacent anagen hairs.

Detection of VDR in the hair follicle by immunohistochemical techniques [23–25] largely corresponds to results using ^{3}H-1,25(OH)$_2$D$_3$ and autoradiographic techniques [20–22]. Using mAb 9A7γ, VDR in the human hair follicle are most markedly detected in the nuclei of keratinocytes of the outer root sheath, while the labeling intensity of the cells of the inner root sheath is very heterogeneous, some nuclei staining strongly, others rather weakly [24] (Figure 6.1A, see color insert). Interestingly, expression of VDR has been demonstrated by immunohistochemistry in dermal papilla cells of human and murine hair follicles [24] (Figure 6.1B, see color insert), that had not been detected before by autoradiographic techniques.

The analysis of depilation-induced hair growth in the C57 BL-6 mouse is a particularly useful model for hair research and enables the study of hair cycle-dependent interactions between keratinocytes, fibroblasts, melanocytes, and skin immune cells. When the entire depilation-induced hair cycle was investigated immunohistochemically in C 57 BL-6 mice using mAb 9A7γ, hair cycle–associated changes in VDR expression became apparent [24,26]. It has been demonstrated that VDR immunoreactivity in keratinocytes and dermal papillary fibroblasts of telogen hair follicles is very weak. However, the nuclear immunoreactivity of these cell populations increases during early anagen and midanagen, reaching a maximum in mature anagen VI follicles [24,26]. With catagen development, follicular VDR immunoreactivity slightly decreases again, but remains distinctly above telogen levels [24,26]. This suggests that VDR expression may be differentially regulated during distinct hair cycle stages and that, correspondingly, the sensitivity of VDR-expressing follicular cell populations to stimulation with endogenous 1,25-dihydroxyvitamin D$_3$ changes with the hair cycle. Because keratinocytes and perifollicular macrophages are capable of synthesizing 1,25-dihydroxyvitamin D$_3$, the controlled local synthesis of 1,25-dihydroxyvitamin D$_3$ and the regulated expression of its corresponding receptor in key cell populations of the hair follicle may be integral components of the obscure mechanisms controlling hair cycling. The rather weak immunoreactivity in hair matrix keratinocytes of early anagen follicles which display the highest proliferative activity of epithelial follicular cells during the hair cycle [27] and the strong VDR expression of outer root sheath keratinocytes and dermal papillary fibroblasts during anagen, with their relatively low proliferative activity, are in agreement with the concept that VDR expression reflects cell proliferation and differentiation [28].

Using immunohistochemical techniques, it has been demonstrated that RXR-α and VDR are strongly expressed in key structures of human and murine hair follicles [24–26,29,30], including root sheath keratinocytes and cells of the dermal papillae. RXR-α immunoreactivity in these key structures of the hair follicle in C 57 BL-6 mice was shown during the depilation-induced hair cycle to be stronger in anagen IV–VI and catagen as compared with anagen I–III or telogen [26]. Hair cycle–dependent differences in the expression of RXR-α and VDR are obviously caused not only by the altered proliferative activity, for staining patterns of VDR and RXR-α are not concordant with the staining pattern of a mAb (clone PC10) directed against proliferating cell nuclear antigen (PCNA) [26]. Furthermore, these findings indicate that the expression of VDR and RXR-α is regulated similarly during the hair cycle, supporting the hypothesis that RXR-α is involved in hair growth via modulation of vitamin D signaling pathways. It deserves further systematic exploration whether the RXR-ligand 9-*cis* retinoic acid may modulate effects of 1,25-dihydroxyvitamin D_3 on hair growth. The sensitivity of RXR-α- and VDR-expressing follicular cell populations to stimulation with endogenous 1,25-dihydroxyvitamin D_3 or 9-*cis* retinoic acid may change with the hair cycle [26].

IV. THE HVDRR SYNDROME AND VDR KNOCKOUT MICE

VDR knockout mice [4,5] and patients with hereditary 1,25-dihydroxyvitamin D_3–resistant rickets type II (HVDRR) [3] exhibit, after weaning, a striking phenotype that includes alopecia totalis (Figure 6.2, see color insert). HVDRR is a human syndrome that arises as a result of heterogeneous molecular defects in the VDR and is characterized by elevated levels of 1,25-dihydroxyvitamin D_3, hypocalcemia, secondary hyperparathyroidism, early-onset rickets, and—in the most severe cases—alopecia [3]. Investigations using fibroblasts and/or lymphocytes derived from HVDRR individuals have revealed that these cells are biologically unresponsive to calcitriol treatment [3,31]. Defective VDR from patients with HVDRR have been classified into three groups: hormone-binding defects, DNA-binding defects, and nuclear-transfer or nuclear-localization defects [31]. Single unique point mutations have been identified—e.g., within the second or third exons that encode the DNA-binding domain of the VDR gene [3]. The majority of HVDRR children have sparse body hair, and some have total scalp and body alopecia. Patients with severe alopecia in most cases lack eyebrows and sometimes eyelashes. The onset of hair loss usually occurs during the first year of life, several month before biochemical and radiological manifestations of the disease are observed. An analysis of HVDRR patients has shown that there may be a correlation between the severity of rickets and the presence of alopecia. In addition, patients with alopecia generally have more severe resistance to 1,25-dihydroxyvitamin D_3 than those without alopecia. In families with a prior history of the disease, the onset of hair loss during the first year of life provides initial diagnostic evidence for HVDRR. If one member of a kindred develops alopecia, all affected members can be expected to do so as well [32]. Conflicting results obtained by the histological examination of hair follicles in HVDRR patients are reported in the literature. Hochberg et al. [33] stated that a scalp biopsy specimen of one affected child showed that the number and appearance of the hairs were normal as seen by light microscopic examination. However, absent or sparse hair follicles have also been reported in the scalp skin in two HVDRR patients from another study [34].

It has been shown that HVDRR patients have an absolute or partial resistance to the action of calcitriol analogs. However, even in patients who respond favorably to pharmacological doses of calcitriol, as proved by a return to calcium homeostasis and the healing of the bone disease, the alopecia does not improve [32]. It is known that children with vitamin D–deficiency rickets or vitamin D–dependent rickets type I, who have marked hypocalcemia and hypophosphatemia, usually have normal hair growth [32]. Therefore, it can be speculated that the absence of 1,25-dihydroxyvitamin D_3 per se does not appear to cause alopecia [32].

V. REGULATION OF HAIR GROWTH BY 1,25-DIHYDROXYVITAMIN D_3 IN VITRO

The effect of 1,25-dihydroxyvitamin D_3 on human hair follicle growth and hair fiber production has been investigated using a whole-organ culture system [35]. In that study, relatively low concentrations (1–10 nm) of 1,25-dihydroxyvitamin D_3 stimulated the cumulative growth of hair follicles and hair fibers by 52 and 36%, respectively [35]. The initial rates of follicle and fiber growth were increased, whereas the respective growth periods were unaffected. Higher concentrations of 1,25-dihydroxyvitamin D_3 inhibited dose-dependently both follicle and fiber growth (EC_{50} values of 100 nm), in part due to reduction of the growth periods. There was a marked delay between the onset of 1,25-dihydroxyvitamin D_3–induced hair follicle and hair fiber growth inhibition. Incubation of hair follicles with 100 nm 1,25-dihydroxyvitamin D_3 resulted in a rapid, transient inhibition of DNA synthesis (55% inhibition at 24 hr), followed by a gradual return to control levels at day 4. Prolonged (>5 hr) incubation in the presence of 100 nm of 1,25-dihydroxyvitamin D_3 was required for follicle growth to be manifest. Interestingly, Ro 31-7549, a selective inhibitor of protein kinase C, did not prevent 1,25-dihydroxyvitamin D_3–induced inhibition of hair follicle growth [35]. The authors concluded that 1,25-dihydroxyvitamin D_3 may play a physiological role in maintaining optimal hair follicle activity, and that elevation of 1,25-dihydroxyvitamin D_3 may inhibit hair growth in vivo. This biphasic effect of 1,25-dihydroxyvitamin D_3 reflects the situation in cultured epidermal keratinocytes, where it has been shown that, depending on the culture conditions (including concentration of calcium and epidermal growth factor), 1,25-dihydroxyvitamin D_3 at low doses stimulates and at higher doses inhibits the proliferation of keratinocytes [36,37].

Limat and coworkers have analyzed the effects of 1,25-dihydroxyvitamin D_3 and a vitamin D analog (calcipotriol) on cultured outer root sheath cells [38]. In organotypic outer root sheath cultures, incubation with 1,25-dihydroxyvitamin D_3 or calcipotriol resulted in a thinning of the living cell compartment concomitant with a thickening of the horny layer. They found reduced expression of differentiation markers—such as keratin 10, involucrin, and filaggrin—that paralleled the thinning of the malpighian rete. No alteration in the expression of the alpha 6 and beta 1 integrin chains was found. As determined by quantification of BrdU-positive cells, proliferation of outer root sheath cells was apparently not affected by 1,25-dihydroxyvitamin D_3 or calcipotriol. They concluded that vitamin D analogs may affect the growth of these cells mainly by accelerating the differentiation pathway within the suprabasal living cell compartment of the hair follicle.

VI. PROTECTION FROM CHEMOTHERAPY-INDUCED ALOPECIA BY 1,25-DIHYDROXYVITAMIN D_3

In 1992, Jimenez and Yunis [6] reported their findings that 1,25-dihydroxyvitamin D_3 protected neonatal rats from chemotherapy-induced alopecia (CIA). In three separate experiments, 0.2 μg of topical 1,25-dihydroxyvitamin D_3 protected rats from alopecia induced by etoposide, cytoxan, and a doxorubicin cytosan combination. In another experiment, 0.1 μg of topical 1,25-dihydroxyvitamin D_3 protected rats from etoposide-induced alopecia at the site of application. The authors concluded that 1,25-dihydroxyvitamin D_3 may offer a new and exciting approach to the prevention of CIA. However, one has to mention that the neonatal rat model they used does not mimic the situation in humans particularly well. Using a murine model that closely mimics CIA in humans, Paus et al. showed that calcitriol does not prevent CIA in adolescent mice but enhances the regrowth of normally pigmented hair shafts [39,40]. When—prior to injecting 1×120 mg/kg cyclophosphamide IP—0.2 μg calcitriol or vehicle alone was administered topically to the back skin of C 57/BL-6 mice with all hair follicles in anagen, no significant macroscopic differences in the onset and severity of CIA were seen [39,40]. However, hair shaft regrowth after CIA, which is often retarded and patchy, thus displaying severe and sometimes persistent pigmentation disorders, was significantly accelerated, enhanced, and qualitatively improved in test compared with control mice. Histomorphometric analysis suggests that this phenomenon is related to the fact that 1,25-dihydroxyvitamin D_3–pretreated follicles favor the "dystrophic catagen pathway" of response to chemical injury—i.e., a follicular repair strategy allowing for the unusually fast reconstruction of a new, undamaged anagen hair bulb [40]. Therefore, it cannot be expected that topical 1,25-dihydroxyvitamin D_3 or analogs can prevent human CIA, but topical calcitriols may well modulate and enhance the regrowth of normal hair coat. Recently, it was shown that calcitriol modulates cyclophosphamide-induced apoptosis in murine hair follicles in vivo [41]. This study provides evidence that vitamin D analogs—directly or indirectly—inhibit rather that induce the apoptosis of normal epithelial cells in vivo.

It remains to be analyzed whether the downregulation of cyclophosphamide-induced apoptosis parameters by topical calcitriols reflects direct interactions of vitamin D analogs with VDR of follicular keratinocytes or with those of other resident cell populations, which subsequently may modulate follicular apoptosis [41]. It is as yet unknown to what extend the hair follicle, which exhibits abundant vitamin D–receptors and expresses them in a hair cycle-dependent fashion, employs locally synthesized calcitriols to control its rate of keratinocyte apoptosis during physiological hair follicle regression. Additionally, it has to be examined whether topical calcitriols that suppress hair follicle apoptosis may be used therapeutically to protect growing hair follicles from chemotherapy-induced hair damage without inhibiting the efficacy of cytostatic drugs in the elimination of malignant cells, particularly of extrafollicular scalp skin metastases [41].

VII. SUMMARY AND CONCLUSIONS

Several clinical and laboratory observations convincingly show that endogenously produced or therapeutically applied 1,25-dihydroxyvitamin D_3 or analogs may be interesting candidates as regulatory factors of hair growth. Patients with hereditary 1,25-dihydroxyvitamin D_3–resistant rickets type II (HVDRR) [3] and vitamin D receptor (VDR) knockout mice [4,5] exhibit a phenotype that includes alopecia totalis. Additionally, experimental chemotherapy-induced alopecia (CIA) in neonatal rats can be prevented by topical 1,25-dihydroxyvitamin D_3 application [6], and pigs suffering from acute to subacute vitamin D toxicosis were reported to develop a rough hair coat [7].

Laboratory investigations have shown expression of VDR and its nuclear cofactor RXR-α in key structures of the hair follicle that is differentially regulated during distinct hair cycle stages [24,26]. These findings support the hypothesis that the hair follicle may be a sensitive target organ for endogenously produced or therapeutically applied 1,25-dihydroxyvitamin D_3 and suggest that the sensitivity of VDR-expressing follicular cell populations to stimulation with 1,25-dihydroxyvitamin D_3 changes with the hair cycle. Because keratinocytes and perifollicular macrophages are capable of synthesizing 1,25-dihydroxyvitamin D_3, the controlled local synthesis of 1,25-dihydroxyvitamin D_3 and the regulated expression of its corresponding receptor in key cell populations of the hair follicle may be integral components of the obscure mechanisms controlling hair cycling.

In conclusion, it can be postulated that 1,25-dihydroxyvitamin D_3 and its corresponding nuclear receptor (VDR) are of great importance for the physiology of hair follicles and that therapeutically applied 1,25-dihydroxyvitamin D_3 may modulate hair growth in vivo. However, one has to mention that patients treated topically with large doses of the 1,25-dihydroxyvitamin D_3 analog calcipotriol for the skin disease psoriasis do not show changes in hair growth. Additionally, it is known that children with vitamin D–deficiency rickets or vitamin D–dependent rickets type I, who lack 1,25-dihydroxyvitamin D_3, usually have normal hair growth. Therefore, it can be speculated that the absence of 1,25-dihydroxyvitamin D_3 per se does not appear to cause alopecia or to profoundly modulate hair growth.

Future studies will have to clarify the physiological function of vitamin D analogs as hair growth modulatory factors and their potential clinical applications. New strategies to evaluate the modulation of hair growth by vitamin D analogs will include in vivo studies with new vitamin D analogs that exert less systemic side effects as well as combination therapy of 1,25-dihydroxyvitamin D_3 with possibly synergistically acting agents such as 9-*cis* retinoic acid, the ligand of the retinoid-X receptor.

Furthermore, target genes of 1,25-dihydroxyvitamin D_3 that are involved in the regulation of hair growth still have to be identified. The regulatory mechanisms governing hair cycling, starting from a resting state (telogen) and progressing to a state of rapid growth (anagen), are still obscure. It will have to be examined whether genes that may be of high importance for the regulation of hair growth, such as the genes for TGF-β [42], patched [43], sonic hedgehog [44], or the hairless gene [45] are specifically regulated by 1,25-dihydroxyvitamin D_3. The molecular mechanisms that mediate the biological effects of vitamin D analog on hair growth still have to be identified and deserve systematic exploration. Additionally, it is not known whether vitamin D analog administered in hair follicle–targeting liposome preparations are therapeutically effective in the treatment of various hair diseases such as androgenetic alopecia or distinct variants of scarring alopecia, including lichen planopilaris, lupus erythematosus, or pseudopelade Brocq. However, it can be speculated that new vitamin D analog exerting less systemic side effects may represent promising new drugs for the modulation of hair growth and the treatment of various hair diseases.

REFERENCES

1. Ebling FG, Hale PA, Randall VA. Hormones and hair growth. In: Goldsmith LA, ed. Physiology, Biochemistry and Molecular Biology of the Skin, 2^d ed. Oxford, UK: Oxford University Press, 1991:660–696.
2. Paus R, Handjiski B, Czarnetzki BM, Eichmüller S. Biology of the hair follicle. Hautarzt 1994; 45:808–825.
3. Malloy PJ, Pike JW, Feldman D. Hereditary, 1,25-dihydroxyvitamin D_3 resistant rickets. In: Feldman D, Glorieux FH, Pike JW, eds. Vitamin D. San Diego, CA: Academic Press, 1997:765–787.
4. Li YC, Pirro AE, Amling M, Delling G, Baron R, Bronson R, Demay MB. Targeted ablation of the vitamin D receptor: An animal model of vitamin D–dependent rickets type II with alopecia. Proc Natl Acad Sci USA 1997; 94:9831–9835.
5. Yoshizawa T, Handa Y, Uematsu Y, Takeda S, Sekine K, Yoshihara Y, Kawakami

T, Arioka K, Sato H, Uchiyama Y, Masuchige S, Fukamizu A, Matsumoto T, Kato S. Mice lacking the vitamin D receptor exhibit impaired bone formation, uterine hypoplasia and growth retardation after weaning. Nature Genet 1997; 16:391–396.

6. Jimenez JJ, Yunis AA. Protection from chemotherapy-induced alopecia by 1,25-dihydroxyvitamin D_3. Cancer Res 1992; 52:5123–5125.

7. Hulsman HG, Stockhofe-Zurwieden N, Ganter M, Müller E. Clinical findings in vitamin D poisoning of swine. Tierärztl Prax 1991; 19:488–492.

8. DeLuca HF. The vitamin D system in the regulation of calcium and phosphorus metabolism. Nutr Rev 1979; 37:161–193.

9. Rigby WFC. The immunobiology of vitamin D. Immunol Today 1988; 9:54–58.

10. Bikle DD, Pillai S. Vitamin D, calcium, and epidermal differentiation. Endocrinol Rev 1993; 14:3–19.

11. Holick MF. Photobiology, physiology, and clinical applications for vitamin D. In: Goldsmith LA, ed. Physiology, Biochemistry and Molecular Biology of the Skin, 2^d ed. Vol 1. Oxford, UK: Oxford University Press, 1991:928–956.

12. Rudolph T, Lehmann B, Pietzsch J, Kämpf A, Wozel G, Meurer M. Normal human keratinocytes in organotypic culture metabolize vitamin D_3 to $1\alpha,25$-dihydroxyvitamin D_3. In: Norman AW, Bouillon R, Thomasset M, eds. Vitamin D: Chemistry, Biology and Clinical applications of the Steroid Hormone. Riverside, CA: University of California, 1994:581–582.

13. Lehmann B, Pietsch J, Kämpf A, Wozel G, Meurer M. Human HaCaT keratinocytes metabolize $1\alpha,25$-dihydroxyvitamin D_3. In: Norman AW, Bouillon R, Thomasset M, eds. Vitamin D: Chemistry, Biology and Clinical Applications of the Steroid Hormone. Riverside, CA: University of California, 1994:583–584.

14. Haussler MR. Vitamin D receptors: Nature and function. Annu Rev Nutr 1986; 6:527–562.

15. Yu VC, Delsert C, Andersen B, Holloway JM, Devary OV, Näär AM, Kim SY, Boutin JM, Glass CK, Rosenfeld MG. $RXR\beta$: A coregulator that enhances binding of retinoic acid, thyroid hormone and vitamin D receptors to their cognate response elements. Cell 1991; 67:1251–1266.

16. Leid M, Kastner P, Lyons R, Nakshatri H, Saunders M, Zacharewski T, Chen J, Staub A, Garnier J, Mader S, Chambon P. Purification, cloning and RXR identity of the HaLa cell factor with which RAR or TR heterodimerizes to bind target sequences efficiently. Cell 1992; 68:377–395.

17. Carlberg C, Bendik I, Wyss A, Meier E, Sturzenbecker LJ, Grippo LJ, Hunzicker W. Two nuclear signaling pathways for vitamin D. Nature 1993; 361:657–660.

18. Bouillon R, Okamura WH, Norman AW. Structure-function relationship in the vitamin D endocrine system. Endocrinol Rev 1995; 16:200–257.

19. Bittiner B, Bleehen SS, MacNeil S. 1α-25(OH)$_2$ Vitamin D_3 increases intracellular calcium in human keratinocytes. Br J Dermatol 1991; 124:230–235.

20. Stumpf WE, Sar M, Reid FA, Tanaka Y, DeLuca HF. Target cells for 1,25-dihydroxyvitamin D_3 in intestinal tract, stomach, kidney, skin, pituitary, and parathyroid. Science 1979; 206:1188–1190.

21. Stumpf WE, Clark SA, Sar M, DeLuca HF. Topographical and developmental studies on target sites of 1,25(OH)$_2$ vitamin D_3 in skin. Cell Tissue Res 1984; 238:489–496.

22. Stumpf WE, Koike N, Hayakawa N, Tokuda K, Nishimiya K, Hirate J, Okazaki A,

Kumaki K. Distribution of 1,25-dihydroxyvitamin D_3[22-oxa] in vivo receptor bindung in adult and developing skin. Arch Dermatol Res 1995; 287:294–303.

23. Milde P, Hauser U, Simon T, Mall G, Ernst V, Haussler MR, Frosch P, Rauterberg EW. Expression of 1,25-dihydroxyvitamin D_3 receptors in normal and psoriatic skin. J Invest Dermatol 1991; 97:230–239.

24. Reichrath J, Schilli M, Kerber A, Bahmer FA, Czarnetzki BM, Paus R. Hair follicle expression of 1,25-dihydroxyvitamin D_3 receptors during the murine hair cycle. Br J Dermatol 1994; 131:477–482.

25. Reichrath J, Collins ED, Epple S, Kerber A, Norman AW, Bahmer FA. Immunohistochemical detection of 1,25-dihydroxyvitamin D_3 receptors (VDR) in human skin: A comparison of five antibodies. Pathol Res Pract 1996; 192:281–289.

26. Paus R, Jung M, Schilli M, Kerber A, Egly C, Chambon P, Bahmer FA, Reichrath J. Hair follicle expression of 1,25-dihydroxyvitamin D_3 receptors (VDR) and retinoid-X receptor-α (RXR-α). In: Norman AW, Bouillon R, Thomasset M, eds. Vitamin D: A Pluripotent Steroid Hormone: Structural Studies, Molecular Endocrinology and Clinical Applications. Berlin & New York: de Gruyter, 1994:617–618.

27. Paus R. Hair growth inhibition by heparin in mice: a model system for studying the modulation of epithelial cell growth by glycosaminoglycans? Br J Dermatol 1991; 124:415–422.

28. Pillai S, Bikle DD, Elias PM. 1,25-Dihydroxyvitamin D_3 production and receptor binding in human keratinocytes varies with differentiation. J Biol Chem 1988; 263:5390–5395.

29. Reichrath J, Münßinger T, Kerber A, Rochette-Egly C, Chambon P, Bahmer FA, Baum HP. In situ detection of retinoid-X receptor expression in normal and psoriatic skin. Br J Dermatol 1995; 133:168–175.

30. Reichrath J, Mittmann M, Kamradt J, Müller SM. Expression of retinoid-X receptors (-α, -β, -γ) and retinoic acid receptors (-α, -β, -γ) in normal human skin: An immunohistological evaluation. Histochem J 1997; 29:127–133.

31. Liberman UA, Eil C, Marx SJ. Resistance to 1,25-dihydroxyvitamin D_3. J Clin Invest 1983; 71:192–200.

32. Holick MF. Vitamin D resistance and alopecia. Arch Dermatol 1985; 121:601–603.

33. Hochberg Z, Gilhar A, Haim S, Friedman-Birnbaum R, Levy J, Benderly A. Calcitriol-resistant rickets with alopecia. Arch Dermatol 1985; 121:646–647.

34. Rosen JF, Fleischman AR, Finberg L, Hamstra A, DeLuca HF. Rickets with alopecia: An inborn error of vitamin D metabolism. J Pediatr 1979; 94:729–735.

35. Harmon CS, Nevins TD. Biphasic effect of 1,25-dihydroxyvitamin D_3 on human hair follicle growth and hair fiber production in whole organ cultures. J Invest Dermatol 1994; 103:318–322.

36. Gniadecki R. Stimulation versus inhibition of keratinocyte growth by 1,25-dihydroxyvitamin D_3: Dependence on cell culture conditions. J Invest Dermatol 1996; 106:510–516.

37. Smith EL, Walworth NC, Holick MF. Effect of 1α,25-dihydroxyvitamin D_3 on the morphological and biochemical differentiation of cultured human epidermal keratinocytes grown in serum-free conditions. J Invest Dermatol 1986; 86:709–714.

38. Limat A, Hunziker T, Braathen LR. Effects of 1 alpha, 25-dihydroxyvitamin D_3 and

calcipotriol on organotypic cultures of outer root sheath cells: A potential model to evaluate antipsoriatic drugs. Arch Dermatol Res 1993; 285:402–409.

39. Paus R, Schilli MB, Plonka P, Menrad A, Reichrath J, Czarnetzki BM, Handjiski B. Topical calcitriol, calcipotriol and KH 1060 do not prevent chemotherapy-induced alopecia in mice, but accelerate hair re-growth and re-pigmentation. J Invest Dermatol 1995; 104:659a.

40. Paus R, Schilli MB, Handjiski B, Menrad A, Henz BM, Plonka P. Topical calcitriol enhances normal hair regrowth but does not prevent chemotherapy-induced alopecia in mice. Cancer Res 1996; 56:4438–4443.

41. Schilli MB, Paus R, Menrad A. Reduction of intrafollicular apoptosis in chemotherapy-induced alopecia by topical calcitriol-analogs. J Invest Dermatol 1998; 111:598–604.

42. Paus R, Foitzik K, Welker P, Bulfone-Paus S, Eichmüller S. Transforming growth factor-beta receptor type I and II expression during murine hair follicle development and cycling. J Invest Dermatol 1997; 109:518–526.

43. Dahmane N, Lee J, Robins P, Heller P, Ruiz i Altaba A. Activation of the transcription factor Gli1 and the Sonic hedgehog signalling pathway in skin tumours. Nature 1997; 389:876–881.

44. St-Jacques B, Dassule HR, Karavanova I, Botchkarev VA, Li J, Danielian PS, McMahon JA, Lewis PM, Paus R, McMahon AP. Sonic hedgehog signaling is essential for hair development. Curr Biol 1998; 24:1058–1068.

45. Ahmad W, Irvine AD, Lam H, Buckley C, Bingham EA, Panteleyev AA, Ahmad M, McGrath JA, Christiano AM. A missense mutation in the zinc-finger domain of the human hairless gene underlies congenital atrichia in a family of irish travellers. Am J Hum Genet 1998; 63:984–991.

7

Effect of Vitamin D on Melanocytes and Its Role in Melanogenesis

Rebecca S. Mason
University of Sydney, Sydney, New South Wales, Australia

I. MELANOCYTES AND MELANOGENESIS

Melanocytes are derived from the neural crest and migrate to the epidermis, where they are normally found in close proximity to the basement membrane, with their dendritic processes in contact with keratinocytes. This epidermal-melanin unit consists of keratinocytes and melanocytes in a ratio of approximately 36:1 [1]. It is clear that there is considerable interdependence between the two cell types [2,3] and between melanocytes and the underlying dermal fibroblasts [4]. Melanocytes tend to be mainly quiescent in skin but may proliferate or become functionally active and may increase pigment synthesis and transfer to keratinocytes under a variety of conditions, including ultraviolet (UV) exposure [1].

Pigment synthesis, which occurs in melanosomes, is controlled by the rate-limiting enzyme tyrosinase, which catalyses at least two steps: the conversion of tyrosine to dihydroxyphenylalanine (dopa) and of dopa to dopa-quinone [1,3]. The remaining steps in melanin synthesis may occur spontaneously, but in the melanosome they are regulated and involve auxiliary enzymes such as dopachrome tautomerase and peroxidase. Tyrosinase interacts with at least two related proteins—tyrosinase-related proteins 1 and 2 (TRP-1 and TRP-2), whose functions are not entirely clear, though TRP-2 may function as a dopachrome tautomerase. Together, however, they seem to form a complex with tyrosinase, which modulates tyrosinase activity [5]. Melanosomes are transported to melanocyte dendrites and transferred to keratinocytes. As the keratinocytes migrate upward in the epidermis, the melanin contained in them provides protection from further UV damage, often forming a protective cap above the nucleus [3].

II. VITAMIN D FORMATION AND SKIN PIGMENTATION

Since increased skin pigmentation has long been known to reduce UV penetration and to reduce the production of vitamin D in skin, it has been proposed by Loomis [6] and others that the distribution of skin pigmentation according to latitude resulted, at least in part, from evolutionary pressures related to vitamin D formation. It was hypothesised that dark skin color near the equator would reduce the risk of vitamin D intoxication due to excess sun exposure, while light pigmentation would allow vitamin D synthesis at high latitudes despite limited availability of UV radiation. As discussed in Chapter 3, it is now accepted that the prevention of vitamin D intoxication due to continued UV exposure seems to occur mainly as a result of conversion of previtamin D_3 to the relatively inactive "overirradiation products" [7] rather than to reduced penetration of UV in pigmented skin. There does seem to be some support, however, for the proposal that light skin color may facilitate sufficient vitamin D synthesis at high latitudes to prevent the bone-deforming aspects of rickets [8].

At a more immediate level, although vitamin D compounds are mainly involved in bone and mineral metabolism, reports of the widespread distribution of vitamin D receptors in many cell types in skin raised the possibility that these compounds might have a range of actions in skin [9]. The similarity of action spectra for UV-induced production of previtamin D_3 from 7-dehydrocholesterol and UV-induced tanning has contributed to speculation that 7-dehydrocholesterol might be one of the chromophores involved in UV-associated pigmentation [3,10]. Despite these tantalizing suggestions, whether the actions of vitamin D compounds in skin include a role in modulating melanogenesis is as yet unclear.

III. VITAMIN D RECEPTORS IN PIGMENT CELLS

There is good evidence that the classic intracellular vitamin D receptor is present in many melanoma cell lines and in melanocytes. There have been several reports of the presence of vitamin D receptors, with classical binding affinities and sucrose density gradient sedimentation characteristics, in a majority of rodent and human melanoma cell lines [11–14]. In at least one case, where binding of the active hormone 1,25 dihydroxyvitamin D_3 [$1,25(OH)_2D_3$] was not able to be demonstrated in Cloudman S91 cells [15], the presence of a smaller than normal, presumably mutated receptor was demonstrated in studies using a vitamin D receptor antibody [16]. Although one group could detect no specific binding of $1,25(OH)_2D_3$ to cultured human melanocytes [15], data consistent with the presence of a classical vitamin D receptor in human melanocytes has been presented by Abdel-Malek et al. [16] on the basis of immunohistochemistry and gel electrophoresis, showing the expected protein size, and by Ranson et al. [17], who demonstrated appropriate binding affinity and analog specificity.

IV. WHOLE ANIMAL STUDIES

Because of evidence of interactions between keratinocytes, fibroblasts and melanocytes, experiments in living animals may have theoretical advantages over some cell culture models at least. There have been two significant in vivo studies published, both in rodents. In 1982, Pavlovitch and colleagues [18] reported that when rats were maintained on a vitamin D-deficient diet, their skin tyrosinase response to UV irradiation measured 20 hr after UV exposure was impaired compared with that of rats of normal vitamin D status (Table 1). Rats whose blood calcium concentrations were maintained in the normal range despite vitamin D deficiency, by supplementation with calcium and lactose, still showed an impaired tyrosinase response after UV exposure. Basal levels of skin tyrosinase were unaffected by vitamin D status. Skin cyclic AMP (cAMP) concentrations (in picomoles per milligram of wet weight) were significantly higher in vitamin D sufficient rats under basal conditions and rose to a greater extent after UV exposure compared with D-deficient animals, whether or not the D-deficient animals were supplemented with calcium and lactose. The significance of the cAMP results is uncertain, in view of evidence that cAMP is not a major mediator of UV-induced pigmentation [19]. The implication of the study is that very low vitamin D levels prior to exposure may compromise the ability of skin to pigment in a normal way after UV.

The second study was reported some years later by the Nordlund group [16]. Their mice, which were apparently of normal vitamin D status, were treated topi-

Table 1 The Effect of Vitamin D Status and Different Dietary Level of Calcium on Change in Rat Skin Tyrosinase Activity in Response to UV Exposure[a]

	Skin tyrosinase activity (counts per minute/mg of soluble proteins)		
	Before UV exposure	After UV exposure	
Diet		3 hr	20 hr
0.4% calcium	1980 ± 200	2070 ± 258	5500 ± 320[b]
30 IU of vitamin D/day	(13)	(13)	(13)
0.4% calcium,	1900 ± 200	2120 ± 230	3800 ± 400
no vitamin D	(14)	(14)	(14)
2% calcium, 20% lactose,	2327 ± 213	2500 ± 320	3572 ± 139
no vitamin D	(8)	(8)	(8)

[a] Values are means ± SEM. Number of animals in parentheses.
[b] $p < 0.001$ for the difference in skin tyrosinase activity before and 20 hr after UV exposure of vitamin D–fed and vitamin D–deficient rats.
Source: From Ref. 18.

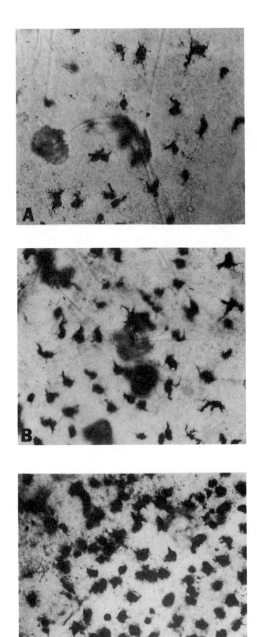

cally on each ear with vitamin D_3 (cholecalciferol) up to 100 μg/day or with 1 μg/day 1,25(OH)$_2$D$_3$. Some mice were also exposed to daily UV irradiation prior to vitamin D treatment. After 10 days, in the mice treated with 100 μg vitamin D_3 but not with UV, dopa-positive cells (a marker of melanocytes) were increased by 50% above vehicle control. In sets of mice that received UV irradiation, dopa-positive cells in animals receiving vitamin D_3 were twofold higher than in vehicle-treated controls (Figure 1). No significant effects were noted with smaller doses of vitamin D_3. There was a small increase in dopa-positive cells in mouse ears exposed to 1,25(OH)$_2$D$_3$ at one time point (10 days), but there were no results reported of mice exposed to 1,25(OH)$_2$D$_3$ and UV. The two studies, though limited and not directly comparable, are important, because, as indicated below, melanocytes are difficult to examine in an isolated environment. The papers provide evidence that, at least in rodents, vitamin D deficiency or supplementation may affect parameters relating to pigmentation in skin, especially after UV exposure.

V. CELL CULTURE MODELS

The first evidence that vitamin D compounds might modulate melanogenesis emerged from studies in mouse melanoma cells in 1974. Oikawa and Nakayasu [20] reported that both vitamin D_3 (cholecalciferol) and vitamin D_2 (ergocalciferol) but not their precursors enhanced tyrosinase activity in a subline of mouse B16 melanoma cells and speculated that vitamin D might be involved in the tanning signal mechanism. This remained an isolated observation for some years. Most of the early studies in melanoma cells were concerned with the newly discovered anti-proliferative, prodifferentiating effects of 1,25(OH)$_2$D$_3$ in a variety of cell lines. The anti-proliferative effects of the vitamin D compound were demonstrated in several melanoma cell lines [11,13,14]. Growth suppression of solid tumor xenografts of vitamin D receptor positive melanoma cells, but not of a receptor-negative melanoma line was also reported [21]. More recently, analogs of 1,25(OH)$_2$D$_3$ with reduced calcemic activity have also been shown to inhibit the proliferation of the mouse melanoma B16 cell line [22].

In melanoma cells, an antiproliferative, prodifferentiation effect implies a possible stimulation of pigmentary activity. Dose-dependent stimulation of tyrosinase activity and melanin synthesis in B16 melanoma cells by 1,25(OH)$_2$D$_3$

Figure 1 Photographic representation of the effects of topical application of 100 μg cholecalciferol, with or without prior UVB irradiation, on the murine pinnal epidermal melanocytes after 10 days of treatment. A. Ethanol control. B. Pinnal epidermis treated with 100 μg cholecalciferol/ear. C. The effect of concomitant treatment with 10 mJ/cm^2 UVB and 100 μg cholecalciferol/ear. (From Ref. 16.)

was reported by Hosoi et al. [13] and in two human melanoma cell lines by Mason et al. [14]. Whether this represents merely a push in the direction of differentiated function or a true regulation of pigmentary activity cannot easily be determined.

Considerably less clear is whether vitamin D compounds alter melanogenesis in cultured melanocytes. Tomita and co-workers [10] reported increased immunoreactive tyrosinase activity and increased cell area in cultured human melanocytes derived from suction blisters in the presence of micromolar concentrations of vitamin D_3, similar to those used by Oikawa and Nakayasu [20], but no effect of 7-dehydrocholesterol, vitamin D_2 or 10 nmol/L $1,25(OH)_2D_3$. Abdel-Malek and colleagues [16], who had noted an increase in dopa-positive cells in the ears of mice treated with vitamin D_3, reported inhibition rather than stimulation of tyrosinase activity in human foreskin melanocytes cultured in the presence of 10 nmol/L $1,25(OH)_2D_3$ with less effect of $25(OH)D_3$ and little effect of vitamin D_3. No effect of small concentrations (1μmol/L) of vitamin D_3 was seen in melanocytes in organ culture by Iwata et al. [23], though other metabolites were not tested. Treatment of human melanocytes with a variety of D metabolites including $25(OH)D$ and $1,25(OH)_2D_3$ by Mansur et al. [15] also did not apparently alter melanin content of neonatal melanocytes or alter the increase in melanin content noted after seven daily irradiations. Ranson et al. [17] reported dose-dependent but modest stimulation (1.4 to 1.6-fold) of tyrosinase activity in human foreskin melanocytes after 48 hr of treatment with $1,25(OH)_2D_3$. In these experiments, treatment with $1,25(OH)_2D_3$ also reduced melanocyte numbers in culture. As with many other agents, there was some variability in response from donor to donor [23–25]. More recently, hybrid analogs of $1,25(OH)_2D_3$, which are less calcemic but show greater bioactivity than $1,25(OH)_2D_3$ in epidermal cell models, were also shown to be more effective in stimulating human melanocyte tyrosinase activity than $1,25(OH)_2D_3$, though even these compounds caused only modest increases in tyrosinase activity [26].

The data are inconsistent, but the nature of the culture system needs to be considered in order to interpret the results. Melanocytes are notoriously difficult to grow in sufficient numbers for experiments. In general, most melanocyte culture systems require the presence of phorbol 12-myristate-13-acetate, cholera toxin, bovine pituitary extract or basic fibroblast growth factor to stimulate melanocyte proliferation [27]. If these agents remain during experiments, however, the melanocytes are hardly in an unstimulated, quiescent state. Agents that increase intracellular cyclic AMP, such as cholera toxin, stimulate tyrosinase message and/or activity in melanoma cells [28,29] and in some melanocyte cultures [23,30]. Under some circumstances, phorbol ester has also been shown to increase melanocyte tyrosinase activity [25,31,32]. In the culture systems described by Tomita et al. [10], Ranson et al. [17] and Holliday et al. [26], all of which showed stimulation of tyrosinase by vitamin D compounds, media containing melanocyte mitogens was used to stimulate melanocyte proliferation but these agents were removed for 3 days prior to experiments. This may allow time for any chronic upregulation of cAMP-dependent pathways or chronic downregulation of the protein kinase C pathways to recover [25,30,32]. None of these agents were used in the organ cultures of Iwata et al. [23], but the authors did not examine $1,25(OH)_2D_3$ or high doses of vitamin D_3 in their model.

The melanocytes used by Abdel-Malek et al. [16] were maintained for experiments in the presence of phorbol ester, isobutylmethylxanthine, and cholera toxin. The latter agents both increase intracellular cAMP. In the studies of Mansur et al. [15], the melanocytes were cultured in the presence of cholera toxin and bovine hypothalamic extract, which appears to contain a range of melanocyte mitogens [27].

If there is any involvement of vitamin D compounds in pigmentation in vivo, the studies provide little information on the effective vitamin D metabolite(s). Vitamin D itself has little bioactivity in most systems, though this is by no means certain in skin. In some reports [10,16,33], vitamin D_3 has been shown to be more biologically active than the active hormone, $1,25(OH)_2D_3$. The signal pathway may not involve the classical vitamin D receptor which has little affinity for vitamin D itself. In the whole animal studies, any vitamin D provided may have been converted systematically to $1,25(OH)_2D_3$ or other metabolites, though the production of $1,25(OH)_2D_3$ is tightly regulated. It is also possible that vitamin D_3 is converted to other metabolites by epidermal cells. Evidence for 1-hydroxylase activity [conversion of $25(OH)D$ to $1,25(OH)_2D$] in skin cells is well established [34,35] and has been recently confirmed by data showing expression of the 1 alpha-hydroxylase gene in keratinocytes [36]. The skin 1-hydroxylase is also tightly regulated and is greatly product inhibited [35]. Evidence for an earlier metabolic step, conversion of vitamin D to $25(OH)D$ by skin cells has been elusive. Part of the difficulty relates to the poor water solubility of the substrate, vitamin D. In a recent report, Rudolph et al. [37] provided data apparently demonstrating 25-hydroxylase activity in keratinocytes using a system with large concentrations of bovine serum albumin to improve substrate solubility. It is conceivable that any vitamin D provided to skin cells may be gradually converted to $1,25(OH)_2D_3$, providing a constant source of this biologically active compound, which is the natural ligand for the vitamin D receptor. The possibility that other biologically relevant metabolic pathways exist in skin cannot be excluded [38].

VI. CONCLUSIONS

The question of whether vitamin D compounds can be shown to influence melanogenesis or melanocyte numbers thus rests on very limited and conflicting reports. No two experimental systems have been comparable. On balance, it could be argued that there is evidence that vitamin D receptors are present in pigment cells, along with most other nucleated cells, and that vitamin D compounds may modulate melanogenesis under some conditions. On the other hand, reduced pigmentation and/or impaired pigmentary response to UV irradiation are not recognized features of either vitamin D deficiency or vitamin D resistance due to receptor mutations in humans [39]. It could be argued, however, that many cell types and systems which are targets of accepted nonclassical actions of vitamin D compounds are not generally noted to be abnormal in vitamin D deficiency or resistance.

Experience with the use of $1,25(OH)_2D_3$ and analogs of this compound as topical agents for the treatment of psoriasis has now extended over several years [40]. Increased pigmentation with this treatment, with or without UV exposure, has not apparently been reported. Recently, topical treatment with $1,25(OH)_2D_3$ was shown to enhance regrowth of normally pigmented hair in mice after chemotherapy-induced alopecia [41]. The authors concluded that this response was more likely due to an effect of $1,25(OH)_2D_3$ on fast reconstruction of undamaged anagen hair follicle bulbs than to a direct effect on hair pigmentation.

From a teleological viewpoint, it is tempting to speculate that vitamin D compounds have intrinsic functions in skin. From the evidence to date, it is not clear that melanogenesis is a major target.

REFERENCES

1. Quevedo WC Jr, Fitzpatrick TB, Pathak MA, Jimbow K. Role of light in human skin colour variation. Am J Phys Anthropol 1975; 43:393–408.
2. Halaban R, Langdon R, Birchall N, Cuono C, Baird A, Scott G, Moellman G, McGuire J. Basic fibroblast growth factor from human keratinocytes is a natural mitogen for melanocytes. J Cell Biol 1988; 107:1611–1619.
3. Gilchrest BA, Park H-Y, Eller MS, Yaar M. Mechanisms of ultraviolet light–induced pigmentation. Photochem Photobiol 1996; 63:1–10.
4. Archambault M, Yaar M, Gilchrest BA. Keratinocytes and fibroblasts in a human skin equivalent model enhance melanocyte survival and melanin synthesis after ultraviolet irradiation. J Invest Dermatol 1995; 104:859–867.
5. Orlow SJ, Zhou B-K, Chakraborty AK, Drucker M, Pifko-Hirst, Pawelek JM. High-molecular-weight forms of tyrosinase and the tyrosinase-related proteins: Evidence for a melanogenic complex. J Invest Dermatol 1994; 103:196–201.
6. Loomis WF. Skin-pigment regulation of vitamin-D biosynthesis in man. Science 1967; 157:501–506.
7. Holick MF, MacLaughlin JA, Doppelt SH. Regulation of cutaneous previtamin D_3 photosynthesis in man: Skin pigment is not an essential regulator. Science 1981; 211:590–593.
8. Neer RM. The evolutionary significance of vitamin D, skin pigment, and ultraviolet light. Am J Phys Anthropol 1975; 43:409–416.

9. Kragballe K. The future of vitamin D in dermatology. J Am Acad Dermatol 1997; 37:S72–S76.

10. Tomita Y, Torinuki W, Tagami H. Stimulation of human melanocytes by vitamin D$_3$ possibly mediates skin pigmentation after sun exposure. J Invest Dermatol 1988; 90:882–884.

11. Colston K, Colston MJ, Feldman D. 1,25-dihydroxyvitamin D$_3$ and malignant melanoma: the presence of receptors and inhibition of cell growth in culture. Endocrinology 1981; 108:1083–1086.

12. Frampton RJ, Suva LJ, Eisman JA, Findlay DM, Moore GE, Moseley JM, Martin TJ. Presence of 1,25-dihydroxyvitamin D$_3$ receptors in established human cancer cell lines in culture. Cancer Res 1982; 42:1116–1119.

13. Hosoi J, Abe E, Suda T, Kuroki T. Regulation of melanin synthesis of B16 melanoma cells by 1α,25-dihydroxyvitamin D$_3$ and retinoic acid. Cancer Res 1985; 45:1474–1478.

14. Mason RS, Pryke AM, Ranson M, Thomas HB, Posen S. Human melanoma cells: functional modulation by calciotropic hormones. J Invest Dermatol 1988; 90: 834–840.

15. Mansur CP, Gordon PR, Ray S, Holick MF, Gilchrest BA. Vitamin D, its precursors, and metabolites do not affect melanization of cultured human melanocytes. J Invest Dermatol 1988; 91:16–21.

16. Abdel-Malek ZA, Ross R, Trinkle L, Swope V, Pike JW, Nordlund JJ. Hormonal effects of vitamin D$_3$ on epidermal melanocytes. J Cell Physiol 1988; 136:273–280.

17. Ranson M, Posen S, Mason RS. Human melanocytes as a target tissue for hormones: In vitro studies with 1α,25-dihydroxyvitamin D$_3$, α-melanocyte stimulating hormone and beta-estradiol. J Invest Dermatol 1988; 91:593–598.

18. Pavlovitch JH. Rizk M. Balsan S. Vitamin D nutrition increases skin tyrosinase response to exposure to ultraviolet radiation. Mol Cell Endocrinol 1982; 25:295–302.

19. Friedmann PS, Gilchrest BA. Ultraviolet radiation directly induces pigment production by cultured human melanocytes. J Cell Physiol 1987; 133:88–94.

20. Oikawa A, Nakayasu M. Stimulation of melanogenesis in cultured melanoma cells by calciferols. FEBS Lett 1974; 42:32–35.

21. Eisman JA, Barkla DH, Tutton PJM. Suppression of in vivo growth of human cancer solid tumor xenografts by 1,25-dihydroxyvitamin D$_3$. Cancer Res 1987; 47:21–25.

22. Burke MD, White MC, Watts MC, Lee JK, Tyler BM, Posner GH, Brem H. Hybrid analogs of 1,25-dihydroxyvitamin D$_3$ having potent antiproliferative effects against murine tumor cell lines metastatic to the brain. In: Norman AW, Bouillon R, Thomasset M, eds. Vitamin D Chemistry, Biology and Clinical Applications of the Steroid Hormone. Riverside, CA: University of California, 1997:487–488.

23. Iwata M, Iwata S, Everett MA, Fuller BB. Hormonal stimulation of tyrosinase activity in human foreskin organ cultures. In Vitro Cell Dev Biol 1990; 26:554–560.

24. Friedmann PS, Wren FE, Matthews JNS. Ultraviolet stimulated melanogenesis by human melanocytes is augmented by di-acyl glycerol but not TPA. J Cell Physiol 1990; 142:334–341.

25. McLeod SD, Smith C, Mason RS. Stimulation of tyrosinase in human melanocytes by pro-opiomelanocortin-derived peptides. J Endocrinol 1995; 146:439–447.

26. Holliday C, Lee JK, Posner GH, Mason RS. Bioactivity of hybrid analogs of 1,25-di-hydroxyvitamin D_3 in skin cells. In: Norman AW, Bouillon R, Thomasset M, eds. Vitamin D Chemistry, Biology and Clinical Applications of the Steroid Hormone. Riverside, CA: University of California, 1997:95–96.

27. Yaar M, Gilchrest BA. Human melanocyte growth and differentiation: A decade of new data. J Invest Dermatol 1991; 97:611–617.

28. Abdel-Malek Z, Swope VB, Pallas J, Krug K, Nordlund JJ. Mitogenic, melanogenic, and cAMP responses of cultured neonatal human melanocytes to commonly used mitogens. J Cell Physiol 1992; 150:416–425.

29. Korner A, Pawelek J. Activation of melanoma tyrosinase by a cyclic AMP-dependent protein kinase in a cell-free system. Nature 1977; 267:444–447.

30. Hoganson GE, Ledwitz-Rigby F, Davidson RL, Fuller BB. Regulation of tyrosinase mRNA levels in mouse melanoma cell clones by melanocyte-stimulating hormone and cyclic AMP. Somatic Cell Mol Genet 1989; 15:255–263.

31. Maeda K, Tomita Y, Fukuda M, Tagami H. Effects of staurosporine, PMA and A23187 on human melanocyte cultures with dibutyryl cyclic AMP. Br J Dermatol 1992; 126:118–124.

32. Park H-Y, Russakovsky V, Ohno S, Gilchrest BA. The β isoform of protein kinase C stimulates human melanogenesis by activating tyrosinase in pigment cells. J Biol Chem 1993; 268:11742–11749.

33. Kanekura T, Laulederkind SJF, Kirtikara K, Goorha S, Ballou LR. Cholecalciferol induces prostaglandin E2 biosynthesis and transglutaminase activity in human keratinocytes. J Invest Dermatol 1998; 111:634–639.

34. Frankel TL, Mason RS, Hersey P, Murray E, Posen S. The synthesis of vitamin D metabolites by human melanoma cells. J Clin Endocrinol Metab 1983; 57:627–631.

35. Pillai S, Bikle DD, Elias PM. 1,25-Dihydroxyvitamin D production and receptor binding in human keratinocytes varies with differentiation. J Biol Chem 1988; 263:5390–5395.

36. Fu GK, Lin D, Zhang MY, Bikle DD, Shackelton CH, Miller WL, Portale AA. Cloning of the human 25-hydroxyvitamin D-1 alpha-hydroxylase and mutations causing vitamin D-dependent rickets type 1. Mol Endocrinol 1997; 11:1961–1970.

37. Rudolph T, Lehmann B, Pietzsch J, Kampf A, Wozel G, Meurer M. Normal human keratinocytes in organotypic culture metabolize vitamin D_3 to $1\alpha,25$-dihydroxyvitamin D_3. In: Norman AW, Bouillon R, Thomasset M, eds. Vitamin D Chemistry, Biology and Clinical Applications of the Steroid Hormone. Riverside, CA: University of California, 1997:581–582.

38. Norman AW, Bouillon R, Farach-Carson MC, Bishop JE, Zhou LX, Nemere I, Zhao J, Muralidharan KR, Okamura WH. Demonstration that 1 beta,25-dihydroxyvitamin D_3 is an antagonist of the nongenomic but not genomic biological responses and biological profile of the three A-ring diastereomers of 1 alpha,25-dihydroxyvitamin D_3. J Biol Chem 1993; 268:20022–20030.

39. Hochberg Z, Weisman Y. Calcitriol-resistant rickets due to vitamin D receptor defects. Trends Endocrinol Metab 1995; 6:216–219.

40. Kragballe K. Vitamin D_3 analogues. Dermatol Clin 1995; 13:835–839.

41. Paus R, Schilli MB, Handjiski B, Menrad A, Henz BM, Plonka P. Topical calcitriol enhances normal hair regrowth but does not prevent chemotherapy-induced alopecia in mice. Cancer Res 1996; 56:4438–4443.

8

Modulation of Immunocytes by Vitamin D

Lone Skov and Ole Baadsgaard
Gentofte Hospital, University of Copenhagen,
Hellerup, Denmark

Erik R. Hansen
Marselisborg Hospital, University of Aarhus, Aarhus, Denmark

I. INTRODUCTION

The immune system plays a critical role in the pathogenesis of psoriasis. Both antigen-presenting cells and T cells are found in the lesions and are involved in the development of the psoriatic skin lesion. Vitamin D_3 analogs demonstrate effect in the treatment of psoriasis. Vitamin D_3 has a strong immunomodulatory effect in vitro and inhibits autoimmune diseases in animal models in vivo. Immunocytes—including monocytes, Langerhans cells, and activated T cells—express the vitamin D_3 receptor. However, it is still unclear whether vitamin D_3 achieves its effect in psoriasis via a direct effect on the keratinocytes, immunocytes, or both (Figure 1). In the following we will discuss the effects of vitamin D_3 and the analogs as modulators of antigen-presenting cells and lymphocyte functions in vitro and in vivo.

II. IN VITRO EFFECTS OF VITAMIN D

A. Vitamin D and Monocyte Function

Monocytes continuously express vitamin D_3 receptors and have 1α-hydroxylase activity, which makes them able to convert the inactive form of vitamin D_3 [25-$(OH)D_3$] to the biologically active metabolite $1,25\text{-}(OH)_2D_3$ [1,2]. The hormone promotes the differentiation of human mononuclear cells in the direction of monocytes-macrophages [3,4]. $1,25\text{-}(OH)_2D_3$ treatment of freshly isolated mononu-

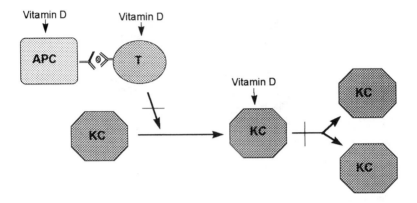

Figure 1 Possible mechanisms of action of vitamin D in psoriasis. Psoriasis is a hyper-proliferative disease characterized by increased keratinocyte proliferation and infiltration of leukocytes. Activated T cells are believed to initiate the psoriatic lesions. It is not known how the T cells achieve their activated state, but it may be through contact between the T-cell receptor and the MHC class II molecule on the antigen-presenting cell. Activated T cells then release factors that have been shown to stimulate keratinocyte hyperprolifera-tion. Vitamin D_3 analogs are effective in the treatment of psoriasis, but the mechanisms are not elucidated. Because of the in vitro effects of vitamin D_3 and analogs, one may specu-late whether the hormone acts directly on keratinocytes (KC), antigen-presenting cells (APC), T cells (T), or a combination. However, in vivo studies indicate that the effect of vitamin D in psoriasis is primarily due to an effect on keratinocyte proliferation.

clear cells and purified monocytes results in a decreased production of interleukin-1α (IL-1α), tumor necrosis factor-α (TNF-α), and IL-6 after stimulation [5–8]. This decrease in cytokine production was shown to be due to a decrease in the sta-bility of specific mRNA [7]. In contrast, when monocyte lines and long-term cul-tured monocytes were stimulated in the presence of vitamin D_3, increased pro-duction of IL-1 was the result [9]. Therefore the degree of differentiation of the monocytes may be critical for the effect of vitamin D_3. This correlates with the ef-fect of vitamin D_3 on differentiated and undifferentiated keratinocytes [10]. Re-cently, vitamin D_3 has been reported to inhibit IL-12 production by activated macrophages and blood dendritic cells cultured from mononuclear cells with the use of IL-4 and granulocyte-macrophage colony stimulating factor (GM-CSF) [11]. This is highly relevant, since IL-12 plays a pivotal role in the development of Th1 cells, and these cells may be involved in the pathogenesis of autoimmune disorders such as psoriasis. The vitamin D_3–induced decrease in monocyte/ macrophage IL-12 production seems to be due to a decrease in the mRNA tran-scription of both the IL-12 p35 and p40 subunits [11].

Only a few studies have looked at the effect of vitamin D_3 on monocyte ac-cessory cell function. These studies demonstrate that preincubation with 1,25-

$(OH)_2D_3$ decreased the monocyte accessory cell function, but it is not clear whether the decrease in the function was due to a direct effect on the monocytes or an indirect effect on the T cells because of carryover of vitamin D_3 [12]. Furthermore, vitamin D_3 treatment of monocytes led to a decreased HLA-DR expression on the monocytes, but this decrease did not correlate with the decreased accessory cell function [13].

B. Vitamin D and Lymphocyte Function

Activated T cells express vitamin D receptors while resting T cells do not. 1,25-D_3 inhibits proliferation of activated T cells in vitro by blocking the transition from the early to the late G_1 phase of the cell cycle [14]. Several groups have found that vitamin D_3 treatment of mononuclear cells, purified T cells, and T-cell clones reduced T-cell cytokines, including IL-2, interferon-γ (IFN-γ), and GM-CSF [9,15–17]; one group also found a reduction in lymphotoxin [18]. The transcription of the IL-2 and IFN-γ gene was unaffected by vitamin D_3 treatment, but the level of the mRNA was reduced, probably because of the decreased half life of mRNA [17,19]. The findings that vitamin D_3 is a potent inhibitor of the production of the Th1 cytokine IFN-γ and IL-2 and that it inhibits macrophage secretion of IL-12, a cytokine that stimulates activation and differentiation of Th1, lead to the hypothesis that vitamin D_3 preferentially inhibits Th1 functions. This is of potential interest, since psoriasis is considered to be mainly a Th1-type skin disease. To study the effect on psoriatic T cells, Barna et al. prepared T cell clones from psoriatic skin. They confirmed the in vitro inhibitory effect of vitamin D_3 on T-cell proliferation. However, in this system, the authors demonstrated that both Th1 (IFN-γ and IL-2) and Th2 (IL-4 and IL-5) cytokines were inhibited by vitamin D_3 analogs [20]. Furthermore, these authors were not able to reproduce the inhibitory effect of vitamin D_3 on GM-CSF values.

B-cell immunoglobulin production (IgG and IgM) in lectin-stimulated mononuclear cells was reduced by vitamin D [21]. In contrast, vitamin D_3 had no effect on the immunoglobulin production of B cells stimulated by Epstein-Barr virus, which is independent of T-cell participation or of highly purified B cells [22]. The decreased immunoglobulin production may therefore be indirectly mediated by an effect of vitamin D_3 on the monocytes and T cells.

III. IN VIVO EFFECTS OF VITAMIN D

A. Vitamin D and the Immunocytes

Treatment with $1,25(OH)_2D_3$ has demonstrated a beneficial effect in animal models of autoimmunity, such as experimental autoimmune encephalomyelitis and murine lupus, and in transplantation studies [23–25]. Hypercalcaemia caused by the hormone may confound the effect of vitamin D and limit the therapeutic application. Recently, new synthetic vitamin D_3 analogs with less pronounced hypercalcaemic effects in vivo have demonstrated efficiency in the prevention of autoimmune diseases and graft rejection, especially in combination with cyclosporin A [25–28]. In contrast to the animal studies, one short human study including 24 healthy volunteers treated with calcitriol tablets (2 μg/day), or placebo, for one week did not demonstrate any change in IL-1α and TNF-α concentration in supernatants or cell lysates from isolated mononuclear cells [29].

B. Vitamin D and the Number of Immunocytes in the Skin

Several immunohistochemical studies have looked at the effect of treatment with vitamin D_3 and the analogs (calcitriol, calcipotriol, and tacalcitol) on immunocytes in psoriatic skin. Skin biopsies have been taken after 1–12 weeks of treatment, and overall they demonstrate a marked reduction in the number of polymorphonuclear leukocytes. The effect starts as soon as after 1 week of treatment; a slight reduction in the number of T cells is first seen after 4 weeks of treatment; but there is no effect on the number of Langerhans cells [30–33]. The most pronounced effect on the immunocytes was after treatment with tacalcitol, which also reduces the number of monocytes in the skin [32]. Using flow cytometric quantification, we did not find any decrease in the number of CD45+ leukocytes in single cell suspensions obtained from psoriatic skin treated with calcipotriol for 7 days compared with vehicle-treated skin [34]. These results are in accordance with the immunohistochemical studies but in contrast to the strong antiproliferative effect of vitamin D_3 on T cells found in vitro.

Few studies have investigated the effect of vitamin D_3 and analogs on immunocytes in the skin of normal volunteers. Dam et al., using confocal laser scanning microscopy of epidermal suction blister roof, reported that calcipotriol treatment under occlusion for 4 days resulted in a decrease in the number of CD1a+ Langerhans cells [35]. In contrast, using flow cytometric quantification, we did not find any change in the number of CD1a+ Langerhans cells in epidermal cells either from normal skin or from psoriatic skin treated with calcipotriol, uncovered, twice daily for 7 days [34]. The difference between the results may be due to the sensitivity of detection of the CD1a+ Langerhans cells and the different vitamin D treatment protocols. In particular, treatment with calcipotriol under occlusion may lead to a toxic effect on the Langerhans cells.

In agreement with the decreased production of IL-6 in vitro by stimulated mononuclear cells and monocytes incubated with vitamin D_3, treatment of psoriatic plaque with calcipotriol led to a decline in the staining intensity of IL-6 but not of TNF-α [36]. However, the effect in vivo is probably due to an effect on the keratinocytes and not on the immunocytes. A recent study has demonstrated increased IL-10 protein concentration in biopsies from psoriatic skin treated with calcipotriol for few days [33]. The cells responsible for the increased IL-10 concentration have not been identified, but several cell types in the skin are capable of producing IL-10, including keratinocytes, Langerhans cells, and macrophages. IL-10 is a Th2 cytokine known to inhibits Th1 cytokines. Since psoriasis is a disease dominated by Th1 cells, increased IL-10 concentration in the lesions may have a beneficial effect in the treatment; however, further studies are needed. Furthermore the authors demonstrated a decreased concentration of IL-8 in psoriatic skin biopsies from lesions treated with calcipotriol for 7 days [33]. In agreement with these data $1,25$-$(OH)_2D_3$ has been shown to inhibited the IL-8 production from keratinocytes, fibroblasts, and peripheral blood monocytes in vitro [37]. IL-8 is chemotactic for both polymorphonuclear cells and T cells. However, if the decrease in the IL-8 concentration is one of the primarily mechanisms of action of vitamin D in psoriasis, one would expect that treatment would lead to a decrease not only in the number of polymorphonuclear cells but also in the number of T cells in the psoriatic lesions.

C. Vitamin D and the Antigen-Presenting Cell Function of Immunocytes from the Skin

Whether open application of vitamin D_3 and analogs on the skin has any immunosuppressive effect on the antigen-presenting capacity of epidermal cells is doubtful. Bagot et al. demonstrated that preincubation of epidermal cells with calcipotriol or $1,25(OH)_2D_3$ led to a pronounced inhibition of the human allogenic mixed epidermal cell-lymphocyte reaction [38]. After separating Langerhans cells and keratinocytes, preincubation of Langerhans cells with calcipotriol or $1,25(OH)_2D_3$ led to only a slight reduction in the mixed epidermal-lymphocyte reaction as compared with vehicle-treated Langerhans cells. As expected, Langerhans cell–depleted keratinocytes did not stimulate allogenic lymphocytes; but when added to untreated autologous epidermal cells, calcitriol-treated keratinocytes led to a marked inhibition of the mixed epidermal-lymphocyte reaction. This may be due to a direct effect of vitamin D_3 on keratinocytes, since the inhibitory effect of calcitriol was partly reversed by the addition of transforming growth factor-β (anti-TGF-β) neutralizing antibodies. However, the inhibition may also be due to an effect on the T cells of a simple carryover of vitamin D_3 and release of vitamin D_3 to the supernatant, since the authors in this study preincubated 25 times as many keratinocytes as Langerhans cells with vitamin D (10^5 keratinocytes compared with only 4×10^3 Langerhans cells) [38]. Using epidermal cells enriched with Langerhans cells, Dam et al. reported that calcipotriol and calcitriol induced a pronounced suppression of antigen-dependent T-cell proliferation [35]. The hormone was added directly to the cultures and the suppression was most likely due to a direct effect of the hormone on T cell proliferation, since T cells are very sensitive to vitamin D_3 in vitro.

We studied the effect of calcipotriol on the antigen-presenting capacity in the skin after in vivo treatment with calcipotriol. We treated normal volunteers and patients with psoriasis with calcipotriol and vehicle, and thereafter we isolated epidermal cells from the treated area. We found that calcipotriol had no effect on the ability of epidermal cells to effect the proliferation of autologous T cells either in the absence or in the presence of antigen [34]. This was found for both psoriatic and normal skin. A possible bias in this study is the risk of washing out calcipotriol from the epidermal cell during the isolation. However, treatment with a potent corticosteroid was included as a positive control and, as expected, this could abrogate the epidermal antigen-presenting capacity in this system.

IV. CONCLUSION AND FUTURE PROSPECTS

Vitamin D_3 and the synthetic vitamin D_3 analogs have been shown to be effective in the management of plaque psoriasis. The findings that psoriasis is a disease where the immune system plays an important role, that treatment with vitamin D_3 in animals with autoimmune disorders has demonstrated a beneficial effect, and that in vitro studies have demonstrated strong immunomodulatory properties of vitamin D_3, led us and others to speculate on whether one of the mechanisms of action of vitamin D_3 in psoriasis is due to an effect on immunocytes in the skin. The studies are still few and further studies are needed, but until now almost none of the studies support the hypothesis that the primary mechanism of action of the presently available vitamin D_3 analogs in vivo is on the immunocytes in the skin. In agreement with this finding, the vitamin D_3 analog calcipotriol has not demonstrated any effect in the treatment of other skin diseases where the immune system is known to play an important role, including atopic dermatitis and allergic contact dermatitis. Instead, the primary mechanism of action in psoriasis seems to be due to a direct effect on the hyperproliferative keratinocytes. However, new vitamin D_3 analogs may demonstrate more pronounced immunosuppressive properties and thereby extend the indications for use in the future.

REFERENCES

1. Provvedini DM, Tsoukas CD, Deftos LJ, Manolagas SC. 1,25-dihydroxyvitamin D_3 receptors in human leukocytes. Science 1983; 221:1181–1183.
2. Reichel H, Koeffler HP, Bishop JE, Norman AW. 25-Hydroxyvitamin D_3 metabolism by lipopolysaccharide-stimulated normal human macrophages. J Clin Endocrinol Metab 1987; 64:1–9.
3. Bar-Shavit Z, Teitelbaum SL, Reitsma P, Hall A, Pegg LE, Trial J, Kahn AJ. Induction of monocytic differentiation and bone resorption by 1,25-dihydroxyvitamin D_3. Proc Natl Acad Sci USA 1983; 80:5907–5911.

4. Kreutz M, Andreesen R, Krause SW, Szabo A, Ritz E, Reichel H. 1,25-dihydroxyvitamin D_3 production and vitamin D_3 receptor expression are developmentally regulated during differentiation of human monocytes into macrophages. Blood 1993; 82:1300–1307.

5. Muller K, Svenson M, Bendtzen K. 1 alpha,25-Dihydroxyvitamin D_3 and a novel vitamin D analogue MC 903 are potent inhibitors of human interleukin 1 in vitro. Immunol Lett 1988; 17:361–365.

6. Muller K, Diamant M, Bendtzen K. Inhibition of production and function of interleukin-6 by 1,25-dihydroxyvitamin D_3. Immunol Lett 1991; 28:115–120.

7. Muller K, Haahr PM, Diamant M, Rieneck K, Kharazmi A, Bendtzen K. 1,25-Dihydroxyvitamin D_3 inhibits cytokine production by human blood monocytes at the post-transcriptional level. Cytokine 1992; 4:506–512.

8. Tsoukas CD, Watry D, Escobar SS, Provvedini DM, Dinarello CA, Hustmyer FG, Manolagas SC. Inhibition of interleukin-1 production by 1,25-dihydroxyvitamin D_3. J Clin Endocrinol Metab 1989; 69:127–133.

9. Bhalla AK, Amento EP, Krane SM. Differential effects of 1,25-dihydroxyvitamin D_3 on human lymphocytes and monocyte/macrophages: Inhibition of interleukin-2 and augmentation of interleukin-1 production. Cell Immunol 1986; 98:311–322.

10. Gniadecki R. Stimulation versus inhibition of keratinocyte growth by 1,25-dihydroxyvitamin D_3: Dependence on cell culture conditions. J Invest Dermatol 1996; 106:510–516.

11. D'Ambrosio D, Cippitelli M, Cocciolo MG, Mazzeo D, Di Lucia P, Lang R, Sinigaglia F, Panina-Bordignon P. Inhibition of IL-12 production by 1,25-dihydroxyvitamin D_3: Involvement of NF-kappaB downregulation in transcriptional repression of the p40 gene. J Clin Invest 1998; 101:252–262.

12. Rigby WF, Waugh M, Graziano RF. Regulation of human monocyte HLA-DR and CD4 antigen expression, and antigen presentation by 1,25-dihydroxyvitamin D_3. Blood 1990; 76:189–197.

13. Rigby WF, Waugh MG. Decreased accessory cell function and costimulatory activity by 1,25-dihydroxyvitamin D_3-treated monocytes. Arthritis Rheum 1992; 35:110–119.

14. Rigby WF, Noelle RJ, Krause K, Fanger MW. The effects of 1,25-dihydroxyvitamin D_3 on human T lymphocyte activation and proliferation: A cell cycle analysis. J Immunol 1985; 135:2279–2286.

15. Tsoukas CD, Provvedini DM, Manolagas SC. 1,25-dihydroxyvitamin D_3: A novel immunoregulatory hormone. Science 1984; 224:1438–1440.

16. Lemire JM, Adams JS, Kermani-Arab V, Bakke AC, Sakai R, Jordan SC. 1,25-dihydroxyvitamin D_3 suppresses human T helper/inducer lymphocyte activity in vitro. J Immunol 1985; 134:3032–3035.

17. Tobler A, Gasson J, Reichel H, Norman AW, Koeffler HP. Granulocyte-macrophage colony-stimulating factor: Sensitive and receptor-mediated regulation by 1,25-dihydroxyvitamin D_3 in normal human peripheral blood lymphocytes. J Clin Invest 1987; 79:1700–1705.

18. Muller K, Rieneck K, Hansen MB, Bendtzen K. 1,25-Dihydroxyvitamin D_3–mediated suppression of T lymphocyte functions and failure of T cell-activating cytokines to restore proliferation. Immunol Lett 1992; 34:37–44.

19. Rigby WF, Denome S, Fanger MW. Regulation of lymphokine production and human T lymphocyte activation by 1,25-dihydroxyvitamin D_3: Specific inhibition at the level of messenger RNA. J Clin Invest 1987; 79:1659–1664.

20. Barna M, Bos JD, Kapsenberg ML, Snijdewint FG. Effect of calcitriol on the production of T-cell-derived cytokines in psoriasis. Br J Dermatol 1997; 136:536–541.

21. Lemire JM, Adams JS, Sakai R, Jordan SC. 1 alpha,25-dihydroxyvitamin D_3 suppresses proliferation and immunoglobulin production by normal human peripheral blood mononuclear cells. J Clin Invest 1984; 74:657–661.

22. Muller K, Heilmann C, Poulsen LK, Barington T, Bendtzen K. The role of monocytes and T cells in 1,25-dihydroxyvitamin D_3 mediated inhibition of B cell function in vitro. Immunopharmacology 1991; 21:121–128.

23. Lemire JM, Ince A, Takashima M. 1,25-Dihydroxyvitamin D_3 attenuates the expression of experimental murine lupus of MRL/l mice. Autoimmunity 1992; 12:143–148.

24. Lemire JM, Archer DC. 1,25-dihydroxyvitamin D_3 prevents the in vivo induction of murine experimental autoimmune encephalomyelitis. J Clin Invest 1991; 87:1103–1107.

25. Cantorna MT, Hayes CE, DeLuca HF. 1,25-Dihydroxyvitamin D_3 reversibly blocks the progression of relapsing encephalomyelitis, a model of multiple sclerosis. Proc Natl Acad Sci USA 1996; 93:7861–7864.

26. Casteels KM, Mathieu C, Waer M, Valckx D, Overbergh L, Laureys JM, Bouillon R. Prevention of type I diabetes in nonobese diabetic mice by late intervention with non-hypercalcemic analogs of 1,25-dihydroxyvitamin D_3 in combination with a short induction course of cyclosporin A. Endocrinology 1998; 139:95–102.

27. Veyron P, Pamphile R, Binderup L, Touraine JL. Two novel vitamin D analogues, KH 1060 and CB 966, prolong skin allograft survival in mice. Transpl Immunol 1993; 1:72–76.

28. Johnsson C, Binderup L, Tufveson G. The effects of combined treatment with the novel vitamin D analogue MC 1288 and cyclosporine A on cardiac allograft survival. Transpl Immunol 1995; 3:245–250.

29. Müller K. Immunoregulatory aspects of Vitamin D_3. Ph.D. disseration, University of Copenhagen, Copenhagen, Denmark, 1993.

30. de Jong EM, van de Kerkhof PC. Simultaneous assessment of inflammation and epidermal proliferation in psoriatic plaques during long-term treatment with the vitamin D_3 analogue MC903: Modulations and interrelations. Br J Dermatol 1991; 124:221–229.

31. Gerritsen MJ, Rulo HF, Van Vlijmen-Willems I, Van Erp PE, van de Kerkhof PC. Topical treatment of psoriatic plaques with 1,25-dihydroxyvitamin D_3: A cell biological study. Br J Dermatol 1993; 128:666–673.

32. Gerritsen MJ, Boezeman JB, van Vlijmen-Willems IM, van de Kerkhof PC. The effect of tacalcitol (1,24($OH)_2D_3$) on cutaneous inflammation, epidermal proliferation and keratinization in psoriasis: A placebo- controlled, double-blind study. Br J Dermatol 1994; 131:57–63.

33. Kang S, Yi S, Griffiths CE, Fancher L, Hamilton TA, Choi JH. Calcipotriene-induced improvement in psoriasis is associated with reduced interleukin-8 and increased interleukin-10 levels within lesions. Br J Dermatol 1998; 138:77–83.

34. Jensen AM, Børresen Lladó M, Skov L, Hansen ER, Larsen JK, Baadsgaard O. Calcipotriol inhibits the proliferation of hyperproliferative CD29+ keratinocytes in psoriatic epidermis in the absence of an effect on the function and number of antigen presenting cells. Br J Dermatol 1998; 139:984–991.

35. Dam TN, Møller B, Hindkjær J, Kragballe K. The vitamin D_3 analog calcipotriol suppresses the number and antigen-presenting function of Langerhans cells in normal skin. J Invest Dermatol 1996; S1:72–77.

36. Oxholm A, Oxholm P, Staberg B, Bendtzen K. Expression of interleukin-6-like molecules and tumour necrosis factor after topical treatment of psoriasis with a new vitamin D analogue (MC 903). Acta Derm Venereol 1989; 69:385–390.

37. Larsen CG, Kristensen M, Paludan K, Deleuran B, Thomsen MK, Zachariae C, Kragballe K, Matsushima K, Thestrup-Pedersen K. $1,25(OH)_2$-D_3 is a potent regulator of interleukin-1 induced interleukin-8 expression and production. Biochem Biophys Res Commun 1991; 176:1020–1026.

38. Bagot M, Charue D, Lescs MC, Pamphile RP, Revuz J. Immunosuppressive effects of 1,25-dihydroxyvitamin D_3 and its analogue calcipotriol on epidermal cells. Br J Dermatol 1994; 130:424–431.

9
Effect of Vitamin D on Langerhans Cells

Tomas Norman Dam
Marselisborg Hospital, University of Aarhus, Aarhus, Denmark

I. INTRODUCTION

A. History of Langerhans Cells

Epidermal Langerhans cells (LC) were discovered in 1868, when Paul Langerhans used a Cohnheim gold chloride staining method to demonstrate nerve fiber endings in the skin [1]. Based on the morphological information that could be obtained from the nonspecific stains available at that time, different theories about the function of LC emerged. Although investigators in the last century had already interpreted LC as leukocytes [2], it was not until the late 1960s that the discovery of Birbeck granules present in histiocytic cells of histiocytosis X lesions led to considerations about LC as a mesenchymal cell [3,4]. The idea of the epidermis as a purely ectodermal tissue needed revision, and strong evidence finally led to the conclusion that the epidermis constitutes an organ derived from ectodermal keratinocytes, neuroectodermal melanocytes, and mesenchymal LC [4]. Although LC were observed to be engaged in pinocytosis and phagocytosis in vivo, it was difficult to accept LC as antigen-presenting cells, because the in vivo phagocytic activity of keratinocytes was known to be higher than that of LC [5]. Techniques for enrichment of LC in epidermal cell suspensions and a large number of monoclonal antibodies became available during the 1970s, and studies of cell surface receptors on immune cells were applied to studies of the skin; this resulted in theories that LC were part of the immune system [6–8]. These theories received additional support because Silberberg et al. had previously discovered that lymphocytes were often seen in apposition to LC during challenge reactions in sensitized individuals; this phenomenon was not observed in irritant dermatitis [9,10]. Immunophenotyping and functional in vitro studies of LC demonstrated that LC express Fc and C3 receptors and class II major histocompatibility complex (MHC class II) on their surface [7–8]. When exposed to antigens, they undergo phenotypic and morphological changes and migrate to the regional lymph nodes, where antigens are presented along with MHC-class II determinants to resting T cells [11,12]. Streilein proposed the term *SALT* (skin-associated lymphoid tissues) to describe the scenario of potent antigen-presenting cells (APC), distinctive populations of T lymphocytes that preferentially infiltrate the epidermis, keratinocytes producing immunomodulatory cytokines, and draining peripheral lymph nodes [13]. Taken together, evidence from several studies suggested that LC can function as potent antigen-presenting cells in the generation of protective effector T-cell responses. LC play a critical role in the afferent limb of the skin immune system by acting as APC for a variety of antigens directly taken up by the LC or indirectly functioning as APC for haptens derived from keratinocytes and melanocytes [14].

B. Ontogeny and Tissue Distribution

As first described by Paul Langerhans, LC in the adult human are regularly spaced, suprabasally located dendritic cells within the epidermis [1]. The CD1a molecule selectively identifies LC, constituting 2–4% of the epidermal cells [15,16]. Resident human epidermal LC strongly express CD1a antigens, whereas CD1c antigens are expressed differently in epidermal LC and dermal dendritic cells (DDC) [17–19]. There has been much speculation about the function of the CD1 glycoproteins, which, like MHC class I molecules, are associated with the 12-kDa β2-microglobulin. The function of these molecules has been characterized in more detail only very recently [20–22]. Apparently the CD1 family comprises a third lineage of antigen-presenting molecules that presents a novel class of foreign and self antigens to MHC-unrestricted T cells. In immunohistochemical studies of human embryos, the expression of CD1a antigen on common leukocyte antigen-bearing (CD45$^+$) LC coincides with the initiation of bone marrow function at 11–12 weeks, and it has been concluded that LC migrate from the bone marrow into human embryonic skin during the first trimester [23]. Several studies have shown that LC originate from a mobile pool of precursor cells [24–27]. Furthermore, it has been found that epidermal LC are not only derived from but also continually repopulated by circulating precursor cells originating in the bone marrow [28–29]. The question whether dendritic cells originate from a separate lineage or belong to the monocyte macrophage family is still unresolved [30]. Despite the fact that a discrete dendritic cell colony–forming unit evidently exists in the bone marrow [31], evidence favors a basic myeloid differentiation program leading from early progenitors via blood monocytes to an early indeterminate type that can develop further into either a dendritic cell or a macrophage. It is possible that CD1c-positive dermal dendritic cells are LC precursors that increase CD1a and decrease CD1c expression upon taking up residence within the epidermis

[31a]. In addition, evidence of a monocytic origin emerged when it was shown that CD1a$^+$ cells could be generated from peripheral blood monocytes in vitro [32,33].

An average adult has a total of 2×10^9 LC, with some regional variation in the number of LC per unit area of skin, the range being 460–1000/mm^2 of body surface, with no difference in observed numbers between men and women [34,35]. There is considerable intersubject variation in the number of LC at a given site [36]. Therefore, the best control for investigation of changes in LC numbers is a subject's own adjacent skin [37]. Finally, insight into LC kinetics has been derived from studies in which a number of other physical or chemical treatments have been applied to the skin. Studies in rodents and humans [36] have shown that topical corticosteroids cause a dose-related, reversible decrease in costimulatory functions [38] and LC surface markers, including membrane ATPase and receptors for Fc-IgG (FcRII) and C3 [39].

C. Modulation of Immunocytes by Vitamin D

Local activation of T lymphocytes appears to play an important role in psoriasis and autoimmune skin diseases. Antigen-specific cutaneous immune responses require ligation of the T cell–receptor complex, with antigenic peptides bound to the MHC class II molecule and co-stimulatory signals provided by antigen-presenting cells (APC). The vitamin D receptor is expressed constitutively by many cells, including monocytes, LC, keratinocytes, and activated but not resting T lymphocytes [40–42]. Calcitriol [1,25(OH)$_2$D$_3$], the 1α-hydroxylated and biologically active metabolite of vitamin D$_3$, has been shown to inhibit activated CD45R0$^+$ T cells in vitro by blocking the transition from the early G1 phase to the late G1 phase of the cell cycle [43]. In addition, monocytes/macrophages have INF-γ inducible 1α-hydroxylase activity that makes them able to convert the inactive form of vitamin D$_3$ [25-(OH)$_2$D$_3$] to the active 1,25(OH)$_2$D$_3$ metabolite [44]. The stability of specific mRNA in freshly isolated activated human blood monocytes is reduced by 1,25(OH)$_2$D$_3$ [45], thereby reducing their ability to produce IL-1α, IL-6, and TNF-α [45–47]. Furthermore it has been demonstrated that the ability of monocytes to induce antigen-dependent T-cell proliferation is significantly reduced by 1,25(OH)$_2$-D$_3$ pretreatment for 24 hr [48,49]. Because the addition of IL-1, IL-6, or indomethacin does not restore antigen-dependent T-cell proliferation, these data suggest that 1,25(OH)$_2$D$_3$ treatment specifically modulates human monocytes phenotype and function, decreasing HLA-DR antigen expression and antigen presentation [50,51].

Surprisingly little is known about the secretory capacity of LC because it is virtually impossible to isolate pure LC from epidermal cell suspensions. Recently techniques for the generation of dendritic cells from CD34$^+$ progenitor cells have become available, and semiquantitative reverse-transcriptase polymerase chain reaction (PCR) analysis of dendritic cells generated in vitro has revealed distinct differences between the messenger RNAs displayed by CD1a- and CD14-derived dendritic cells [52]. $1,25(OH)_2D_3$ has been reported to decrease the mRNA transcription of both the IL-12 p35 and the (allergen) inducible p40 subunit production by activated macrophages and blood derived dendritic cells [53]. This finding might be particularly important, because IL-12 plays a key role in determining the development of Th1 cells that may be involved in the pathogenesis of psoriasis and autoimmune disorder. Although these findings clearly indicate that IL-12 is regulated by $1,25(OH)_2D_3$ in vitro, it is not yet clear if IL-12 secretion by epidermal keratinocytes [54] and LC is modulated by $1,25(OH)_2D_3$ in vivo.

II. EFFECTS OF VITAMIN D ON LANGERHANS CELLS IN NORMAL HUMAN SKIN

A. In Vivo Effects

There are only few studies of the effect of vitamin D in normal human skin. We have investigated the effect of the synthetic vitamin D_3 analog calcipotriol. In a dose-ranging study, calcipotriol cream was applied under occlusion using Finn chambers, then suction blisters were obtained from the treated areas and prepared for confocal laser scanning microscopy. The application of calcipotriol cream to normal human skin for 4 days resulted in a dose-dependent decrease in the number of $CD1a^+$ cells with a dendritic morphology and in the number of dendrites per cell. The change in the number of dendrites was detectable at lower calcipotriol concentrations than the decrease in the number of LC (Figure 9.1, see color insert). In a second study, without occlusion, calcipotriol at doses used clinically (50 $\mu g/g$) was compared with corticosteroid. It was found that the decrease in the number of LC induced by calcipotriol ointment 50 $\mu g/g$ was more pronounced than that induced by the potent topical corticosteroid mometasone furoate and that the combination of calcipotriol ointment and mometasone furoate did not further decrease the number of LC [41]. Furthermore, immunohistochemical staining of vertical cryosections from biopsies obtained after calcipotriol treatment of normal human skin for 4 days confirmed previous findings of decreased numbers of $CD1a^+/HLA-DR^+$ epidermal LC. Concomitantly, there was an increase in $CD1c^+$ cells arranged in clusters in the reticular dermis [55].

This latter finding suggests that complex phenomena are behind the observed net effect; it could be due to LC precursors migrating into the dermis or activated LC leaving the epidermis and changing their surface expression in the dermal microenvironment. These findings are in accordance with a study in mice showing that topically applied $1,25(OH)_2D_3$ decreases the number of LC during the first 3 days of the experiment. However, on day 5, the number of LC had completely normalized [56]. Migration of LC observed after broad-band ultraviolet B

(270–350 nm) is regulated by the synthesis of TNF-α in the epidermis [57], and it has been shown that local injection of TNF-α in mice induces LC migration [58,59]. Taken together with the inhibition of monocyte TNF-α production by 1,25(OH)$_2$D$_3$ [45], it is possible that calcipotriol might modify epidermal LC migration by changing epidermal concentrations of TNF-α. We believe that a migration of LC from epidermis into the dermis may be a likely explanation for the observed net reduction in LC by D$_3$ vitamins.

B. In Vitro Effects

The isolation of LC from the epidermis requires difficult and tedious procedures that yield only limited numbers of cells of varying purity [60]. Generation of large numbers of dendritic cells from circulating monocytes or CD34$^+$ progenitors has become an attractive alternative to the study of epidermal LC in vitro; they share many characteristics with cultured epidermal LC, including their ability to prime naive T cells [61,62]. However, freshly isolated human LC have unique functional properties and show varying phenotypic states within the epidermis [63,64]. Therefore, in vitro studies of freshly isolated LC may be particularly relevant to demonstrating LC-specific modulation and function in the human skin.

We have studied the effect of 1,25(OH)$_2$D$_3$ and calcipotriol on LC antigen presentation of purified protein derivative of tuberculin to primed autologous T lymphocytes. These experiments clearly indicated that addition of 1,25(OH)$_2$D$_3$ or calcipotriol to LC significantly decreased T-cell proliferation. Furthermore, this effect was not dependent on the purity of LC suspensions (60–97%), thus arguing against the hypothesis that the observed effect was mediated through lymphokines secreted by contaminating keratinocytes (3–40%). However, these results did not rule out the possibility that the observed effect was due to a direct effect on activated T cells [41]. To exclude this possibility, we pulsed LC with 1,25(OH)$_2$D$_3$ (10^{-8} M) for 1–48 hr prior to culture with T cells. It was found that more than 24 hr of LC preincubation was necessary to suppress antigen-presenting function of LC (Figure 2).

Other investigators have studied the effects of calcipotriol or 1,25(OH)$_2$D$_3$ in the allogenic human mixed epidermal cell lymphocyte reaction (allogenic MECLR) [65]. Addition of 1,25(OH)$_2$D$_3$ at the initiation of cultures was crucial for inducing a significant inhibition of proliferation. After separating LC and keratinocytes, preincubation of LC with calcipotriol or 1,25(OH)$_2$D$_3$ resulted in a 30% reduction in the allogenic MECLR compared with vehicle-treated LC. As expected, LC-depleted keratinocytes did not stimulate allogenic lymphocytes, but it was found that the addition of autologous keratinocytes pulsed with calcitriol for as little as 2 hr to untreated epidermal cells resulted in a marked inhibition of the MECLR. However, several other studies have indicated that it is necessary to pulse antigen-presenting cells for 24 hr (one study indicated 6 hr) to efficiently

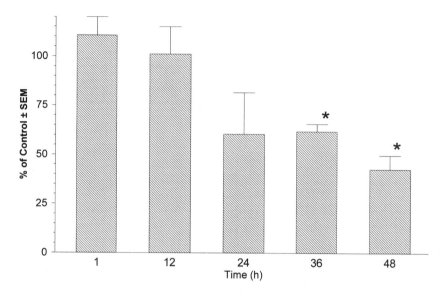

Figure 2 Time course of stimulatory capacity of LC and its inhibition by 1,25(OH)$_2$D$_3$. LC were purified from epidermal cell suspensions and cultured for 0, 1, 12, 36, and 48 hr with 1,25(OH)$_2$D$_3$ (10^{-7} M). After preincubation, LC were washed three times and then added to T cells and PPD 25 μg/mL for 72 hr. [3H]TdR was added during the final 16 hr and incorporation was determined by liquid scintillation. Statistical differences were calculated using Student's t-test and $p < 0.05$ was considered significant (*$p < 0.05$ versus control). Data are mean ± SEM.

reduce antigen presentation and accessory function [48–50]. Moreover, 1,25(OH)$_2$D$_3$ was used in concentrations at least 100-fold higher than required for inhibiting immunocytes. It is, therefore, likely that the effect of 1,25(OH)$_2$D$_3$ observed in this study is due to a rapid increase of intracellular free calcium in keratinocytes [66] or occurs through modulation of keratinocyte-secreted cytokines.

Another piece of information concerning the immunomodulatory effects of vitamin D$_3$ on LC has been derived from studies of the modulation of MHC class II expression by LC and monocytes. Immunohistochemistry and flow-cytometric analysis has revealed that HLA-DR but not the MHC class I expression is regulated by 1,25(OH)$_2$D$_3$ and calcipotriol in monocytes. In contrast, investigators unequivocally report unchanged expression of MHC class II products on LC [41,65]. The explanation for these findings is unknown; it may be that vitamin D cannot overcome the intrinsic ability of LC to quickly increase levels of class I and II MHC products almost fivefold during the first 12–18 hr after removal from the epidermal microenvironment [67].

III. LANGERHANS CELLS AS POSSIBLE TARGETS DURING VITAMIN D TREATMENT OF PSORIASIS VULGARIS

There is evidence indicating that the behavior of LC is changed in a number of skin diseases [68]. In analyzing a possible role of LC in the pathogenesis of various diseases, one has to take into account the delicate role these cells play in initiating and perpetuating a specific immunological response originating in the epidermis and possibly targeting the skin. Contact dermatitis, graft-versus-host disease, and rejection of skin allografts are examples in which LC exert their physiological role in the context of an intact immunosurveillance, leading to pathological conditions of the skin. However, most of the knowledge about LC in pathological processes rest on in vivo morphological or phenotypical observations or from in vitro studies. In considering the characteristic pathological changes of the epidermis in psoriasis, including a profoundly changed cytokine network [69], it appears that qualitative and/or quantitative changes of LC observed in developing and pharmacologically treated psoriatic lesions could be secondary to other (pathogenetic) mechanisms.

One series of experiments revealed that topical application of calcipotriol to psoriatic plaques resulted in normalization of the distribution of LC, associated with an increase in $CD1a^+$ epidermal LC [70,71], while others have found unchanged numbers of LC after treatment with tacalcitol [72]. Moreover, results exist regarding changes in the number and morphology of LC in developing psoriatic lesions [73,74]. However, these studies were performed using different methods for the enumeration of LC, and this may at least in part explain their discrepancy [75]. Infiltration of leukocytes, hyperproliferation, and parakeratosis are some pathological hallmarks of psoriasis (Figure 3, left). The primary events leading to T-cell activation and development of a psoriatic plaque are not known, but cross-linking of the T-cell receptor and MHC class II molecules on antigen-presenting cells by streptococcus- or staphylococcus-derived superantigens (SA) may result in activation of T cells (Th) secreting INF-γ but not IL-4 (Th1 cells). INF-γ can induce MHC class II expression in keratinocytes (KC), and contacts between trafficking T cells (Th) and LC could lead to further activation and transition from symptomless to lesional psoriatic skin. $1,25(OH)_2D_3$ and analogs are known to reduce the proliferation and enhance the differentiation of keratinocytes, to inhibit the proliferation of activated T cells and their production of IL-2 and INF-γ, and to reduce accessory cell function and production of IL-1α, IL-6, and TNF-α in freshly isolated activated human blood monocytes. Recently $1,25(OH)_2D_3$ has been reported to inhibit IL-12 production by activated macrophages. Therefore, it is tempting to speculate that vitamin D analogs might improve psoriasis by direct inhibition of LC antigen-presenting capacity and by skewing the lymphokine response toward a Th2 profile, probably by inhibiting IL-12 secretion by LC.

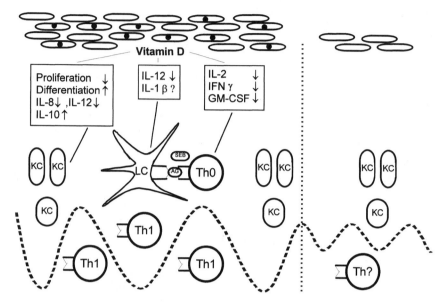

Figure 3 Graphic representation of possible actions of vitamin D in psoriasis. Infiltration of leukocytes, hyperproliferation, parakeratosis, and elongated rete ridges are some pathological hallmarks of psoriasis (left); reduced leukocytic infiltration and hyperproliferation after vitamin D treatment (right); bold stipulated line represents the basement membrane; superantigens (SA); antigens (AG); Langerhans cell (LC); T cells (Th0, Th1); keratinocytes (KC). Increased/decreased production ($\uparrow/\downarrow$). Costimulatory signals have been omitted for simplicity. IL, interleukin; KC, keratinocytes; LC, Langerhans cells; MECLR, mixed epidermal cell lymphocyte reaction; MHC, major histocompatibility complex; SA, superantigens.

Indirect evidence of the role of LC during calcipotriol-induced improvement in psoriasis has emerged from a study showing that improvement is associated with reduced IL-8 and increased IL-10 levels within treated lesions [76]. IL-10 pretreatment of LC has been demonstrated to inhibit the antigen-specific T-cell proliferation in Th1 clones but to have no effect on responses in Th2 clones [77]. Thus, it may well be that $1,25(OH)_2D_3$ can modulate LC antigen-presenting functions indirectly through IL-10 produced by activated keratinocytes [78]. The relative importance of LC, keratinocytes, and lymphocytes during vitamin D treatment of psoriasis has yet to be determined and could also depend on the route of administration and the specific characteristics of the vitamin D analog. In conclusion, a large body of evidence indicates that LC participate in the immunologic responses of psoriasis, but only a few studies suggests a primary pathogenic role of LC in this disease [79–82].

IV. CONCLUSION AND FUTURE PROSPECTS

Calcipotriol at doses used clinically changes the morphology of LC and suppresses the number of LC as well as their ability to stimulate T-cell proliferation in normal human skin. Together with the constitutive expression of the VDR by LC, these results indicate that human LC are direct targets of $1,25(OH)_2D_3$. There is some evidence to suggest that LC may be involved directly or indirectly in the pathogenesis of psoriasis. Within normal human skin, LC are antigen-presenting cells that acquire accessory cell function upon "activation." In the psoriatic epidermis however, the cytokine microinvironment is changed, leading to increased expression of costimulatory molecules on LC. As a result, LC within the psoriatic epidermis are able to present costimulatory signals together with yet unknown antigens precipitating psoriasis and resulting in the activation of cell-mediated immune mechanisms. The suppression of LC by vitamin D_3, together with the change in secretion of proinflammatory cytokines by epidermal cells and lymphocytes, may serve to inhibit the immunological component of psoriasis. These properties of $1,25(OH)_2D_3$ and analogs may be utilized for the pharmacological manipulation of the immune response in the skin. Studies of the relative importance of LC, keratinocytes, and lymphocytes during vitamin D treatment of skin diseases are, however, warranted.

REFERENCES

1. Langerhans P. Über die Nerven der menchlichen Haut. Virchows Arch A Pathol Anat Histopathol 1868; 44:325.
2. Herxheimer K. Über Pemphigus vegetans nebst Bemerkungen über die Natur der Langerhansschen Zellen. Arch Derm Syph (Berlin) 1896; 36:140.
3. Breathnach AS. The cell of Langerhans. Int Rev Cytol 1965; 18:1.
4. Wolff K. The Langerhans cell. In: Karger S, ed. Current Problems in Dermatology. Basel: Mali JWH, 1972.
5. Wolff K, Höningsmann H. Permeability of the epidermis and phagocytic activity of keratinocytes. Ultrastr Res 1971; 36:176.
6. Rowden G, Lewis MG, Sullivan AK. Ia antigen expression on human epidermal Langerhans cells. Nature 1977; 268:247.
7. Stingl G, Wolff-Schreiner EC, Pichler WJ, Gschnait F, Knapp W, Wolff K. Epidermal Langerhans cells bear Fc and C3 receptors. Nature 1977; 268:245–246.
8. Klareskog L, Tjernlund U, Forsum U, Peterson PA. Epidermal Langerhans cells express Ia antigens. Nature 1977; 268:248–250.
9. Silberberg I, Baer RL, Rosenthal SA. The role of Langerhans cells in contact allergy: I. An ultrastructural study in actively induced contact dermatitis in guinea pigs. Acta Derm Venereol 1974; 54:321–331.
10. Silberberg I. Apposition of mononuclear cells to langerhans cells in contact allergic reactions: An ultrastructural study. Acta Derm Venereol 1973; 53:1–12.

11. Poulter LW, Seymour GJ, Duke O, Janossy G, Panayi G. Immunohistological analysis of delayed-type hypersensitivity in man. Cell Immunol 1982; 74:358–369.
12. Scheynius A, Fischer T, Forsum U, Klareskog L. Phenotypic characterization in situ of inflammatory cells in allergic and irritant contact dermatitis in man. Clin Exp Immunol 1984; 55:81–90.
13. Streilein JW. Skin-associated lymphoid tissues (SALT): origins and functions. J Invest Dermatol 1983; 80(suppl):12s–16s.
14. Steiner G, Wolff K, Pehamberger H, Stingl G. Epidermal cells as accessory cells in the generation of allo-reactive and hapten-specific cytotoxic T lymphocyte (CTL) responses. J Immunol 1985; 134:736–741.
15. Fithian E, Kung P, Goldstein G, Rubenfeld M, Fenoglio C, Edelson R. Reactivity of Langerhans cells with hybridoma antibody. Proc Natl Acad Sci USA 1981; 78:2541–2544.
16. Murphy GF, Bhan AK, Sato S, Harrist TJ, Mihm MC Jr. Characterization of Langerhans cells by the use of monoclonal antibodies. Lab Invest 1981; 45:465–468.
17. Meunier L, Gonzalez Ramos A, Cooper KD. Heterogeneous populations of class II MHC$^+$ cells in human dermal cell suspensions: Identification of a small subset responsible for potent dermal antigen-presenting cell activity with features analogous to Langerhans cells. J Immunol 1993; 151:4067–4080.
18. Furue M, Nindl M, Kawabe K, Nakamura K, Ishibashi Y, Sagawa K. Epitopes for CD1a, CD1b, and CD1c antigens are differentially mapped on Langerhans cells, dermal dendritic cells, keratinocytes, and basement membrane zone in human skin. J Am Acad Dermatol 1992; 27:419–426.
19. Elder JT, Reynolds NJ, Cooper KD, Griffiths CE, Hardas BD, Bleicher PA. CD1 gene expression in human skin. J Dermatol Sci 1993; 6:206–213.
20. Beckman EM, Melian A, Behar SM, Sieling PA, Chatterjee D, Furlong ST, Matsumoto R, Rosat JP, Modlin RL, Porcelli SA. CD1c restricts responses of mycobacteria-specific T cells: Evidence for antigen presentation by a second member of the human CD1 family. J Immunol 1996; 157:2795–2803.
21. Bauer A, Huttinger R, Staffler G, Hansmann C, Schmidt W, Majdic O, Knapp W, Stockinger H. Analysis of the requirement for beta 2-microglobulin for expression and formation of human CD1 antigens. Eur J Immunol 1997; 27:1366–1373.
22. Zeng Z, Castano AR, Segelke BW, Stura EA, Peterson PA, Wilson IA. Crystal structure of mouse CD1: An MHC-like fold with a large hydrophobic binding groove (see comments). Science 1997; 277:339–345.
23. Miller I. Ontogenesis of immunity of the human fetus. In: The Immunity of the Human Fetus and Newborn Infant. The Hague/Boston/London: M Nijhoff, 1983.
24. Dam TN, Kang S, Nickoloff BJ, Voorhees JJ, Kragballe K. The induction and treatment of psoriasis in human skin grafts transplanted onto SCID mice is modified by 1,25-dihydroxyvitamin D$_3$. International Investigative Dermatology, Cologne, May 7–10, 1998.
25. Stingl G, Tamaki K, Katz SI. Origin and function of epidermal Langerhans cells. Immunol Rev 1980; 53:149–174.
26. Tamaki K, Katz SI. Ontogeny of Langerhans cells. J Invest Dermatol 1980; 75:12–13.
27. Tamaki K, Stingl G, Katz SI. The origin of Langerhans cells. J Invest Dermatol 1980; 74:309–311.

28. Katz SI, Tamaki K, Sachs DH. Epidermal Langerhans cells are derived from cells originating in bone marrow. Nature 1979; 282:324–326.
29. Volc-Platzer B, Stingl G, Wolff K, Hinterberg W, Schnedl W. Cytogenetic identification of allogeneic epidermal Langerhans cells in a bone-marrow-graft recipient. N Engl J Med 1984; 310:1123–1124.
30. Peters JH, Gieseler R, Thiele B, Steinbach F. Dendritic cells: From ontogenetic orphans to myelomonocytic descendants. Immunol Today 1996; 17:273–278.
31. Young JW, Szabolcs P, Moore MA. Identification of dendritic cell colony-forming units among normal human CD34$^+$ bone marrow progenitors that are expanded by c-kit-ligand and yield pure dendritic cell colonies in the presence of granulocyte/macrophage colony-stimulating factor and tumor necrosis factor alpha. J Exp Med 1995; 182:1111–1119.
31a. Murphy GF, Bhan AK, Harrist TJ, Mihm MC Jr. In situ identification of T6-positive cells in normal human dermis by immunoelectron microscopy. Br J Dermatol 1983; 108:423–431.
32. Rossi G, Heveker N, Thiele B, Gelderblom H, Steinbach F. Development of a Langerhans cell phenotype from peripheral blood monocytes. Immunol Lett 1992; 31:189–197.
33. Athanasas-Platsis S, Savage NW, Winning TA, Walsh LJ. Induction of the CD1a Langerhans cell marker on human monocytes. Arch Oral Biol 1995; 40:157–160.
34. Rowden G. The Langerhans cell. Crit Rev Immunol 1981; 3:95–180.
35. Berman B, Chen VL, France DS, Dotz WI, Petroni G. Anatomical mapping of epidermal Langerhans cell densities in adults. Br J Dermatol 1983; 109:553–558.
36. Ashworth J, Booker J, Breathnach SM. Effects of topical corticosteroid therapy on Langerhans cell antigen presenting function in human skin. Br J Dermatol 1988; 118:457–469.
37. Ashworth J, Turbitt ML, Mackie RM. The distribution and quantification of the Langerhans cell in normal human epidermis. Clin Exp Dermatol 1986; 11:153–158.
38. Aberer W, Stingl L, Pogantsch S, Stingl G. Effect of glucocorticosteroids on epidermal cell-induced immune responses. J Immunol 1984; 133:792–797.
39. Berman B, France DS, Martinelli GP, Hass A. Modulation of expression of epidermal Langerhans cell properties following in situ exposure to glucocorticosteroids. J Invest Dermatol 1983; 80:168–171.
40. Haussler MR, Norman AW. Chromosomal receptor for a vitamin D metabolite. Proc Natl Acad Sci USA 1969; 62:155–162.
41. Dam TN, Møller B, Hindkjær J, Kragballe K. The vitamin D$_3$ analog calcipotriol suppresses the number and antigen-presenting function of Langerhans cells in normal human skin. J Invest Dermatol 1996; 1:S72–S76.
42. Provvedini DM, Tsoukas CD, Deftos LJ, Manolagas SC. 1,25-dihydroxyvitamin D$_3$ receptors in human leukocytes. Science 1983; 221:1181–1183.
43. Rigby WF, Noelle RJ, Krause K, Fanger MW. The effects of 1,25-dihydroxyvitamin D$_3$ on human T lymphocyte activation and proliferation: A cell cycle analysis. J Immunol 1985; 135:2279–2286.
44. Koeffler HP, Reichel H, Bishop JE, Norman AW. Gamma-interferon stimulates production of 1,25-dihydroxyvitamin D$_3$ by normal human macrophages. Biochem Biophys Res Commun 1985; 127:596–603.

45. Muller K, Haahr PM, Diamant M, Rieneck K, Kharazmi A, Bendtzen K. 1,25-Dihydroxyvitamin D_3 inhibits cytokine production by human blood monocytes at the post-transcriptional level. Cytokine 1992; 4:506–512.

46. Muller K, Svenson M, Bendtzen K. 1 alpha,25-Dihydroxyvitamin D_3 and a novel vitamin D analogue MC 903 are potent inhibitors of human interleukin 1 in vitro. Immunol Lett 1988; 17:361–365.

47. Muller K, Diamant M, Bendtzen K. Inhibition of production and function of interleukin-6 by 1,25-dihydroxyvitamin D_3. Immunol Lett 1991; 28:115–120.

48. Tsoukas CD, Watry D, Escobar SS, Provvedini DM, Dinarello CA, Hustmyer FG, Manolagas SC. Inhibition of interleukin-1 production by 1,25-dihydroxyvitamin D_3. J Clin Endocrinol Metab 1989; 69:127–133.

49. Haq AU. 1,25-Dihydroxyvitamin D_3 (calcitriol) suppresses concanavalin A-stimulated human T cell proliferation through monocytes. Clin Immunol Immunopathol 1989; 50:364–373.

50. Rigby WF, Waugh M, Graziano RF. Regulation of human monocyte HLA-DR and CD4 antigen expression, and antigen presentation by 1,25-dihydroxyvitamin D_3. Blood 1990; 76:189–197.

51. Tokuda N, Mizuki N, Kasahara M, Levy RB. 1,25-Dihydroxyvitamin D_3 down-regulation of HLA-DR on human peripheral blood monocytes. Immunology 1992; 75:349–354.

52. de Saint-Vis B, Fugier-Vivier I, Massacrier C, Gaillard C, Vanbervliet B, Ait-Yahia S, Banchereau J, Liu YJ, Lebecque S, Caux C. The cytokine profile expressed by human dendritic cells is dependent on cell subtype and mode of activation. J Immunol 1998; 160:1666–1676.

53. D'Ambrosio D, Cippitelli M, Cocciolo MG, Mazzeo D, Di Lucia P, Lang R, Sinigaglia F, Panina-Bordignon P. Inhibition of IL-12 production by 1,25-dihydroxyvitamin D_3: Involvement of NF-kappaB downregulation in transcriptional repression of the p40 gene. J Clin Invest 1998; 101:252–262.

54. Muller G, Saloga J, Germann T, Bellinghausen I, Mohamadzadeh M, Knop J, Enk AH. Identification and induction of human keratinocyte-derived IL-12. J Clin Invest 1994; 94:1799–1805.

55. Dam TN, Møller B, Kragballe K. The morphology and activity of dermal dendritic cells in normal human skin is modified by the vitamin D_3 analogue calcipotriol. The European Society of Dermatological Research, 25 Annual meeting, Vienna, 23–26 September 1995.

56. Guo Z, Okamoto H, Imamura S. The effect of 1,25$(OH)_2$-vitamin D_3 on Langerhans cells and contact hypersensitivity in mice. Arch Dermatol Res 1992; 284:368–370.

57. Moodycliffe AM, Kimber I, Norval M. Role of tumour necrosis factor-alpha in ultraviolet B light-induced dendritic cell migration and suppression of contact hypersensitivity. Immunology 1994; 81:79–84.

58. Cumberbatch M, Kimber I. Dermal tumour necrosis factor-alpha induces dendritic cell migration to draining lymph nodes, and possibly provides one stimulus for Langerhans' cell migration. Immunology 1992; 75:257–263.

59. Kimber I, Cumberbatch M. Stimulation of Langerhans cell migration by tumor necrosis factor alpha (TNF-alpha). J Invest Dermatol 1992; 99:48S–50S.

60. Schmitt DA, Hanau D, Cazenave JP. Isolation of epidermal Langerhans cells. J Immunogenet 1989; 16:157–168.

61. Strunk D, Rappersberger K, Egger C, Strobl H, Kromer E, Elbe A, Maurer D, Stingl G. Generation of human dendritic cells/Langerhans cells from circulating CD34$^+$ hematopoietic progenitor cells. Blood 1996; 87:1292–1302.

62. Caux C, Massacrier C, Dezutter-Dambuyant C, Vanbervliet B, Jacquet C, Schmitt D, Banchereau J. Human dendritic Langerhans cells generated in vitro from CD34$^+$ progenitors can prime naive CD4$^+$ T cells and process soluble antigen. J Immunol 1995; 155:5427–5435.

63. Shibaki A, Meunier L, Ra C, Shimada S, Ohkawara A, Cooper KD. Differential responsiveness of Langerhans cell subsets of varying phenotypic states in normal human epidermis. J Invest Dermatol 1995; 104:42–46.

64. Inaba K, Schuler G, Witmer MD, Valinksy J, Atassi B, Steinman RM. Immunologic properties of purified epidermal Langerhans cells. Distinct requirements for stimulation of unprimed and sensitized T lymphocytes. J Exp Med 1986; 164:605–613.

65. Bagot M, Charue D, Lescs MC, Pamphile RP, Revuz J. Immunosuppressive effects of 1,25-dihydroxyvitamin D$_3$ and its analogue calcipotriol on epidermal cells. Br J Dermatol 1994; 130:424–431.

66. Bittiner B, Bleehen SS, MacNeil S. 1 alpha,25(OH)$_2$ vitamin D$_3$ increases intracellular calcium in human keratinocytes. Br J Dermatol 1991; 124:230–235.

67. Witmer-Pack MD, Valinsky J, Olivier W, Steinman RM. Quantitation of surface antigens on cultured murine epidermal Langerhans cells: rapid and selective increase in the level of surface MHC products (published erratum appears in J Invest Dermatol 1988; 91:286). J Invest Dermatol 1988; 90:387–394.

68. Wollenberg A, Wen S, Bieber T. Langerhans cell phenotyping: a new tool for differential diagnosis of inflammatory skin diseases (letter). Lancet 1995; 346:1626–1627.

69. Uyemura K, Yamamura M, Fivenson DF, Modlin RL, Nickoloff BJ. The cytokine network in lesional and lesion-free psoriatic skin is characterized by a T-helper type 1 cell-mediated response. J Invest Dermatol 1993; 101:701–705.

70. Mozzanica N, Cattaneo A, Schmitt E, Diotti R, Finzi AF. Topical calcipotriol for psoriasis-an immunohistologic study. Acta Derm Venereol Suppl (Stockh) 1994; 186:171–172.

71. de Jong EM, van de Kerkhof PC. Simultaneous assessment of inflammation and epidermal proliferation in psoriatic plaques during long-term treatment with the vitamin D$_3$ analogue MC903: Modulations and interrelations (see comments). Br J Dermatol 1991; 124:221–229.

72. Gerritsen MJ, Boezeman JB, van Vlijmen Willems IM, van de Kerkhof PC. The effect of tacalcitol (1,24(OH)$_2$D$_3$) on cutaneous inflammation, epidermal proliferation and keratinization in psoriasis: A placebo-controlled, double-blind study. Br J Dermatol 1994; 131:57–63.

73. Bieber T, Braun-Falco O. Distribution of CD1a-positive cells in psoriatic skin during the evolution of the lesions. Acta Derm Venereol 1989; 69:175–178.

74. Ashworth J, Mackie RM. A quantitative analysis of the Langerhans cell in chronic plaque psoriasis. Clin Exp Dermatol 1986; 11:594–599.

75. Bieber T, Ring J, Braun-Falco O. Comparison of different methods for enumeration of Langerhans cells in vertical cryosections of human skin. Br J Dermatol 1988; 118:385–392.

76. Kang S, Yi S, Griffiths CE, Fancher L, Hamilton TA, Choi JH. Calcipotriene-induced improvement in psoriasis is associated with reduced interleukin-8 and increased interleukin-10 levels within lesions. Br J Dermatol 1998; 138:77–83.

77. Enk AH, Angeloni VL, Udey MC, Katz SI. Inhibition of Langerhans cell antigen-presenting function by IL-10: A role for IL-10 in induction of tolerance. J Immunol 1993; 151:2390–2398.

78. Enk AH, Katz SI. Identification and induction of keratinocyte-derived IL-10. J Immunol 1992; 149:92–95.

79. Demidem A, Taylor JR, Grammer SF, Streilein JW. T-lymphocyte-activating properties of epidermal antigen-presenting cells from normal and psoriatic skin: Evidence that psoriatic epidermal antigen-presenting cells resemble cultured normal Langerhans cells. J Invest Dermatol 1991; 97:454–460.

80. Mier PD, Gommans JM, Roelfzema H. On the aetiology of psoriasis. Br J Dermatol 1980; 103:457–460.

81. Oxholm A, Oxholm P, Staberg B. Reduced density of T6-positive epidermal Langerhans' cells in uninvolved skin of patients with psoriasis. Acta Derm Venereol 1987; 67:8–11.

82. Barker JN. The immunopathology of psoriasis. Baillières Clin Rheumatol 1994; 8:429–438.

10
Interaction of Vitamin D and Retinoids

Sewon Kang
University of Michigan Medical Center, Ann Arbor, Michigan

I. INTRODUCTION

Like vitamin D, vitamin A and related molecules comprise an important group of therapeutic agents collectively referred to as retinoids. In terms of scope and history, retinoids have had greater impact in dermatology than vitamin D and its analogs, sometimes called deltanoids. Vitamins A and D, with distinct biological functions, are independently essential molecules of life. Our understanding of how retinoids and deltanoids mediate their respective cellular/biological effects was greatly enhanced by the discovery of their intranuclear receptors. Indeed, it was through the molecular study of structure and function of retinoid receptors and vitamin D receptors (VDRs) that the possibility of interaction between retinoids and deltanoids was revealed. This chapter highlights key observations germane to skin pharmacology that have advanced our understanding in this area.

II. RETINOIC ACID RECEPTORS IN HUMAN SKIN

In order to discuss the interaction of vitamin D and retinoids, an understanding of their receptors is necessary. For VDRs, Chapter 2 provides a thorough discussion. Here, a brief review of retinoic acid receptors (RARs) is presented.

Like VDRs, RARs belong to the steroid hormone receptor superfamily of ligand-activated transcription factors. First identified in 1987, three isoforms of RARs (α, β, and γ) have been characterized [1–3]. Retinoid X receptors (RXRs) represent another class of retinoid receptors for which there are also three isoforms (α, β, and γ) [3,4]. All-*trans* retinoic acid (*t*-RA) and its stereoisomer 9-*cis* retinoic acid (9-*c* RA) bind to RARs with similar high affinity [5]. The off rates for *t*-RA binding to RAR-α, RAR-β, and RAR-γ are similar [6]. However, for 9-*c* RA, the off rates differ in that they are fastest with RAR-γ and slowest with RAR-β. Because of this difference, in the presence of mixtures of *t*-RA and 9-*c* RA, RARs tend to prefer *t*-RA. This is especially the case for RAR-γ. To RXRs, *t*-RA does not bind, only 9-*c* RA does [7,8].

The relative expression of RARs and RXRs has been carefully examined in human skin. At the gene transcript level, RAR-α, RAR-γ, RXR-α, and RXR-β are readily detected in human epidermis [9]. Transcripts for the other isoforms (RAR-β and RXR-γ) are either very low or undetectable. This pattern is similarly observed in cultured human keratinocytes and fibroblasts [10]. Quantitation of the retinoid receptors at the protein level has been achieved utilizing keratome biopsy specimens from normal volunteers. The skin tissue obtained through this technique contains mostly epidermis with a small amount of papillary dermis. Analysis of the nuclear extract by ligand binding and immunological assays estimates the total RARs and RXRs per cell to be on average 1800 and 9400, respectively [5]. Of the RARs, RAR-γ is the predominant type, making up roughly 90%. The remaining 10% is RAR-α and no RAR-β is detectable. Compared to RARs, the fivefold more abundant RXRs are mostly of α subtype (90%), with the β subtype making up 10% [5]. These relative amounts of receptor proteins parallel the relative expression of the mRNAs.

A. Relevant Receptor Combination for Retinoid Response in Human Skin

As ligand-dependent transcription factors, members of the nuclear hormone receptor superfamily share other common features. First, they work as paired functional units (dimers). When the dimer is made up of two identical receptors, it is called a homodimer; whereas if it consists of two different receptors, it is called a heterodimer. Second, in the presence of the ligand, the receptor dimer binds to specific sequences of DNA in the enhancer region of gene promoter called the response element and regulates the transcription of the hormone-responsive genes. The response elements for retinoic acid (RAREs) consist of hexameric direct repeats (consensus sequence of -AGGTCA-) spaced by either two-(DR-2) or five-(DR-5) nucleotide base-pair spacing; for retinoid X response element (RXRE), the direct repeats are spaced by one nucleotide (DR-1). RARs and RXRs in nuclear extract isolated from normal human epidermis and cultured keratinocytes bind exclusively as heterodimers to RAREs (DR-2 and DR-5) and to RXRE (DR-1) [5,11,12]. No homodimers of either RARs or RXRs are detected in the gel shift studies. The RAR-RXR heterodimer binding to DNA is not dependent upon the presence of either *t*-RA or 9-*c* RA. However, to transactivate the RARE-containing responsive genes, RARE-bound RAR-RXR heterodimers require ligands.

Studies conducted in keratinocytes transfected with CAT reporter genes regulated by RAREs (DR-2 or DR-5) or RXRE (DR-1) have revealed ligand requirements for the reporter responsiveness. The RARE (DR-2 or DR-5) reporters are activated by t-RA, 9-c RA (by isomerization to t-RA), and the RAR-specific ligand CD367. They are not induced by RXR-specific SR-11237. The heterodimer requires the presence of RAR ligand only; the presence of RXR ligand does not confer additional transactivation. Transcription of RXRE (DR-1) reporter in keratinocytes, however, is not activated by any of the retinoids (even the RXR-specific SR-11237) unless RXRs are over-expressed. Only under such nonphysiological condition, normally absent RXR homodimer formation is promoted, which can respond to RXR ligands. In normal epidermal keratinocytes, however, RXRE is not activated by RXR ligand due to the lack of RXR homodimers and competitive formation of RAR/RXR heterodimers. Therefore, at their physiological levels in human skin epidermis, RARs and RXRs bind to RAREs as heterodimers and transactivate these elements in the presence of RAR ligands.

III. VITAMIN D SIGNALING IN HUMAN SKIN

Until the discovery that $1,25(OH)_2D_3$ was more than just a renal hormone involved in biological processes other than calcium homeostasis, the skin was simply viewed as the site of initiation of vitamin D biosynthesis under the influence of ultraviolet radiation. It is now well established that VDR is expressed and functionally active in human skin, making this a target tissue of vitamin D action. As was done for retinoid receptors, the specifics of VDR (the level of expression, identity of dimerizing receptor, and ligand responsiveness) in human skin have been examined. This is absolutely necessary for our understanding of vitamin D effects on human skin in vivo, because conflicting observations from different cell lines and in vitro conditions have indicated the tissue/cell-specific regulation of VDR signaling. For example, although VDREs identified in positively controlled genes such as human and rat osteocalcin [13–15], mouse osteopontin [16] and 24-hydroxylase [17,18] consist of hexanucleotide direct repeats with a spacer of three nucleotides (DR-3), VDR binding to the DR-5 type of VDRE as homodimers has been reported under extraordinarily high concentration of the receptors [19]. In transformed cell lines where VDR and RXR are both overexpressed, DR-3-containing reporter genes were synergistically activated by 9-c RA and $1,25(OH)_2D_3$ [20]. In contrast, in COS-7 and CV1 cells, $1,25(OH)_2D_3$ alone induced strong transactivation of VDRE (DR-3) by the heterodimers, and the addition of 9-c RA exerted an inhibitory effect on the $1,25(OH)_2D_3$-induced transactivation [21].

In human skin, the average number of VDRs per epidermal cell determined through ligand-binding assay is 220 [22]. This is far less than the retinoid receptors (RAR $\simeq$ 1800 and RXR $\simeq$ 9400) determined through the identical method

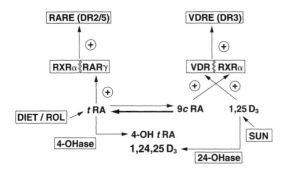

Figure 1   Metabolism and molecular action of retinoids and vitamin D. (From Ref. 37.)

[5]. When nuclear extract from normal human epidermis is mixed with a radiola-beled VDRE (DR-3) consensus sequence, the identity of the receptors that bound to the probe, identified through gel-shift assay, was VDR-RXR heterodimer with no VDR-VDR homodimer [23]. Therefore, similar to retinoid signaling, the vitamin D signaling in human skin occurs through VDR/RXR heterodimers. It is this dimerization of VDR with that of a retinoid receptor (RXR) for the functionality of VDR that provided the scientific rationale to consider a retinoid influence on the vitamin D signaling (Figure 1). The abundance of the RXRs (9400 per cell) in comparison to RARs (1800 per cell) or VDR (220 per cell) is consistent with their function as the key heterodimeric partners not only in the retinoid and vitamin D signaling but also in other hormone signaling (i.e., thyroid hormone, peroxisome proliferator–activated receptor).

IV. 24-HYDROXYLASE GENE AS THE MOLECULAR MARKER TO STUDY VITAMIN D SIGNALING IN HUMAN SKIN IN VIVO

Having established physical convergence of endogenous VDR and RXR from human skin on natural VDRE (DR-3), it was necessary to determine the responsiveness of the heterodimer to the respective ligands. For this purpose, one needs as a molecular tool, a gene whose expression in the tissue is tightly regulated and responsive to $1,25(OH)_2D_3$. Such is the 24-hydroxylase (OHase) gene, which contains VDRE of DR-3 type [24,25]. It is a cytochrome P-450 enzyme involved in the metabolism of vitamin D. It uses $25(OH)D_3$ and $1,25(OH)_2D_3$ as substrates to form $24,25(OH)_2D_3$ and $1,24,25(OH)_3D_3$, respectively. In human skin in vivo, topical applications of increasing concentration of $1,25(OH)_2D_3$ raise the mRNA

levels of 24-OHase [26]. This is accompanied by an increase in the level of enzyme activity. Application of 9-*c* RA alone to human skin has no effect on the 24-
OHase mRNA levels. However, coadministration of 9-*c* RA, with $1,25(OH)_2D_3$
synergistically enhances the mRNA expression of the gene [26] (Figure 2).

When *t*-RA is applied to human skin in vivo, small but significant amount
of 9-*c* RA, enough to activate retinoid receptors, is found in the viable epidermis
[27]. Therefore, similar to the situation where 9-*c* RA is applied with
$1,25(OH)_2D_3$, synergistic response of the 24-OHase gene transcript is expected,
and indeed observed, when *t*-RA (which can isomerize to 9-*c* RA) is coadminis-
tered with $1,25(OH)_2D_3$ [26]. Although receptor selectivity is an important feature
of both natural and synthetic retinoids that influences the efficiency/potency of inducing the desired retinoid effect, in clinical practice, the selectivity may not be as
relevant. For example, when individual human retinoid receptors are transfected
into CV-1 cells together with a chloramphenicol acetyltransferase (CAT) reporter
gene containing a RARE, concentrations required to obtain half-maximum induction (ED_{50}) of CAT activity are in the nanomolar range for *t*-RA and 13-*c* RA
[28,29]. Levels of *t*-RA in 0.1% *t*-RA–treated human skin in the viable layer are
significantly greater (micromolar range) than the ED_{50} values determined for all

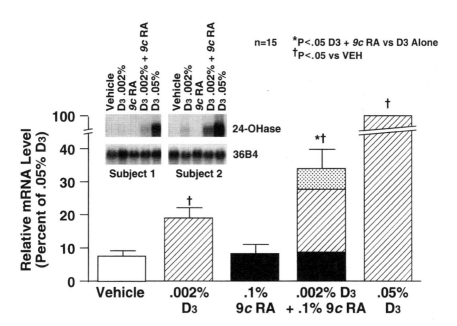

Figure 2 9-*c* RA and $1,25(OH)_2D_3$ synergistically increase 24-OHase gene expression
in human skin in vivo. Data represent mean ± SEM. Inset: Northern blot from two representative subjects. (From Ref. 26.)

three isoforms of RARs and for RXR-α [29]. Therefore, there are sufficient amounts of t-RA in treated skin to activate gene transcription over both RARs and RXR-α. Similarly, synthetic retinoids with a relative receptor selectivity, when used in a clinical setting, may penetrate into skin in such an amount as to act as panagonists for retinoid receptors.

Since 9-c RA is a panagonist for RXR and RAR and it can convert to t-RA, RXR-selective activation cannot be guaranteed with 9-c RA use. SR-11237 is a synthetic retinoid that activates RXRs but not RARs. Because adequate toxicity data to assure safe use in humans is lacking, SR-11237 could not be applied to normal research volunteers. However, in mouse skin, this synthetic RXR-specific retinoid synergizes with $1,25(OH)_2D_3$ to activate the transcription of 24-OHase gene [23]. Clearly, allosteric changes caused by VDR ligand in VDRE-bound VDR-RXR do not block access of ligands to RXR. In addition to RXR ligand binding, the presence of a transactivation function 2 (AF-2) domain of RXR is necessary to mediate maximal vitamin D signaling. A mutant RXR lacking the AF-2 domain inhibited endogenous VDR/RXR activity over DR-3 VDRE and, furthermore, showed reduced capacity to transactivate the enhancer element in response to $1,25(OH)_2D_3$ and SR-11237 [23]. Like 9-c RA on human skin, SR-11237 application alone to mouse skin is ineffective in inducing 24-OHase mRNA.

Since 9-c RA can also activate RARs, VDR/RAR heterodimer might be responsible in part for its synergism with $1,25(OH)_2D_3$ in inducing 24-OHase mRNA. This possibility was excluded by the use of CD-367, a RAR selective synthetic retinoid, on mouse skin. Unlike SR-11237, CD-367 when applied to mouse skin in combination with $1,25(OH)_2D_3$ demonstrated no synergistic increase in the 24-OHase mRNA.

In human skin, both vitamin D and retinoid signaling occur through respective hormone nuclear receptors heterodimerizing with RXR. However, they differ in terms of their responsiveness to RXR ligand. Whereas, for retinoids, only the ligand for RAR is sufficient to fully activate RAR-RXR heterodimer complex, for vitamin D the presence of RXR ligand can confer additional transactivation over what VDR ligand alone can induce. Therefore, RXR retinoids can positively influence vitamin D signaling in human skin.

A. Enhancing the Interaction of Retinoid and Vitamin D

Similar to the way in which $1,25(OH)_2D_3$ is metabolized to its inactive form by the 24-OHase, t-RA is inactivated by 4-OHase to 4-OH t-RA. This cytochrome P-450 enzyme is also inducible by t-RA in human skin [29]. Certain azols such as ketoconazole and liarozole possess inhibitory activity against the 4-OHase. Effective inhibition of the 4-OHase by either azoles can raise the endogenous levels of t-RA, thereby acting as retinoid-mimetic agents. Indeed, applying this pharmacological principle, both liarozole and ketoconazole have been used as monotherapy to successfully treat certain dermatological conditions that are retinoid-responsive (i.e., psoriasis, ichthyosis) [30–32]. Similarly, such azoles could be used in combination with low doses of *t*-RA to enhance the retinoid activity. A well-established retinoid bioassay in human skin in vivo is a 4 day patch test [33]. Continuous occlusive treatment of pharmacologically active doses of *t*-RA (e.g., 0.025–0.1%) to human buttock skin for 4 days consistently induces an erythema response clinically, epidermal hyperplasia and spongiosis histologically, and induction of 4-OHase activity biochemically [34–36]. In this bioassay, both 0.001% *t*-RA and 3% liarozole treatments alone do not cause clinical erythema or histological thickening of the epidermis [36]. The 4-OHase activity levels are slightly induced by each as compared with vehicle treatment. However, when liarozole and the low-dose *t*-RA are applied together, synergistic responses in both the clinical (erythema intensity) and histological (epidermal hyperplasia) parameters of the magnitude observed with 25× the dose of *t*-RA (0.025%) are seen (Figure 3) [36]. The induction in 4-OHase activity is similarly synergistic. Since topical application of *t*-RA together with 1,25(OH)$_2$D$_3$ can enhance the vitamin D activity in human skin, inhibiting the *t*-RA inactivating 4-OHase with an appropriate azole, either alone or in combination with low doses of the retinoid, is likely to have a similarly effect.

Following topical application of 9-*c* RA to human skin, *t*-RA makes up more than one-third of retinoic acid isomers extractable from the epidermis [27].

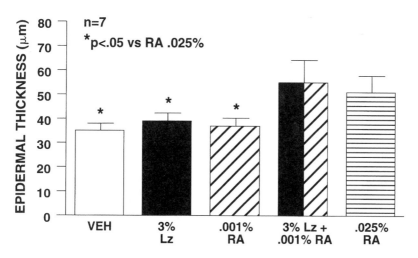

Figure 3 4-OHase inhibitor liarozole (Lz) induces epidermal hyperplasia response of human skin to low-dose *t*-RA in a 4-day patch test. Data represent mean ± SEM. (From Ref. 36.)

In addition, 9-*c* RA treatment induces only *t*-RA 4-OHase, which is unable to use 9-*c* RA as substrate for the hydroxylation reaction. The isomerization of 9-*c* RA to *t*-RA in the skin would explain the observed induction of the *t*-RA 4-OHase. The inability of 9-*c* RA to induce a hydroxylase activity in skin that would result in its inactivation suggests that there may not be a direct means of controlling 9-*c* RA levels after topical application. Rather, by first isomerizing to *t*-RA, which can then be inactivated by the *t*-RA 4-OHase or possibly by glucuronidation, 9-*c* RA is removed from skin. Therefore, azoles that inhibit *t*-RA 4-OHase used in combination with low doses of 9-*c* RA and $1,25(OH)_2D_3$ are likely to contribute positively in enhancing the vitamin D signaling in human skin. As for synthetic retinoids, unless they are inactivated by the 4-OHase, which for most is highly unlikely, the pharmacological principle with azoles described above would not be applicable.

V. IMPLICATIONS IN CLINICAL DERMATOLOGY

Although therapeutic benefits of vitamin D and its analog have been established in several dermatological conditions, one constant concern regarding the safety of their use is hypercalcemia and its sequelae. One obvious way to reduce the possibility of this side effect is to decrease the amount (i.e., concentration) of drug applied to the skin. Although this approach may improve the safety profile, such a method would suffer from reduced clinical efficacy or loss of it. Therefore, along with the dose reduction, a method to enhance the bioactivity of deltanoids must be introduced. The ability of RXR ligand to significantly enhance vitamin D signaling in human skin in vivo provides strong support for a combination treatment of RXR agonist and deltanoid as a pharmacological strategy to meet this objective. This type of enhancement in clinically relevant situations, however, still needs to be investigated.

REFERENCES

1. Petkovich M, Brand NJ, Krust A, Chambon P. A human retinoic acid receptor which belongs to the family of nuclear receptors. Nature 1987; 330:444–450.
2. Giguére V, Ong ES, Segui P, Evans RM. Identification of a receptor for the morphogen retinoic acid. Nature 1987; 330:624–629.
3. Mangelsdorf DJ, Thummel C, Beato M, Herrlich P, Schutz G, Umesono K, Blumberg B, Kastner P, Mark M, Chambon P, Evans RM. The nuclear receptor superfamily: The second decade. Cell 1995; 83:835–840.
4. Mangelsdorf DJ, Ong ES, Dyck JA, Evans RM. Nuclear receptor that identifies a novel retinoic acid-responsive pathway. Nature 1990; 345:224–229.

5. Fisher GJ, Talwar HS, Xiao JH, Datta SC, Reddy AP, Gaub MP, Rochette-Egly C, Chambon P, Voorhees JJ. Immunological identification and functional quantitation of retinoic acid and retinoid X receptor protein in human skin. J Biol Chem 1994; 269:20629–20635.

6. Allenby G, Bocquel MT, Saunder M, Kazmer S, Speck J, Rosenberger M, Lovey A, Kastner P, Grippo JF, Chambon P, Levin AA. Retinoic acid receptors and retinoid X receptors: Interaction with endogenous retinoic acids. Proc Natl Acad Sci USA 1993; 90:30–34.

7. Levin AA, Sturzenbecker LJ, Kazmer S, Bosakowski T, Huselton C, Allenby G, Speck J, Kratzeisen C, Rosenberger M, Lovey A, Grippo JF. 9-cis-retinoic acid steroisomer binds and activates the nuclear receptor RXRα. Nature 1992; 355:359–361.

8. Heyman RA, Mangelsdorf DJ, Dyck JA, Stein RB, Eichele G, Evans RM, Thaller C. 9-cis-retinoic acid is a high-affinity ligand for the retinoid X receptor. Cell 1992; 68:397–406.

9. Elder JT, Astrom A, Pettersson U, Tavakkol A, Griffiths CE, Krust A, Kaster P, Chambon P, Voorhees JJ. Differential regulation of retinoic acid receptors and binding proteins in human skin. J Invest Dermatol 1992; 98:673–679.

10. Elder JT, Fisher GJ, Zhang QY, Eisen D, Krust A, Kastner P, Chambon P, Voorhees JJ. Retinoic acid receptor gene expression in human skin. J Invest Dermatol 1991; 96:425–433.

11. Xiao JH, Durand B, Chambon P, Voorhees JJ. Endogeneous retinoic acid receptor–retinoid X receptor heterodimers are the major functional forms regulating retinoid-responsive elements in adult human keratinocytes. J Biol Chem 1995; 270:3001–3011.

12. Fisher GJ, Reddy AP, Datta SC, Kang S, Yi JY, Chambon P, Voorhees JJ. All-trans retinoic acid induces cellular retinol-binding protein in vivo. J Invest Dermatol 1995; 105:80–86.

13. Ozono K, Liao J, Kerner SA, Scott RA, Pike JW. The vitamin D–responsive element in the human osteocalcin gene: Association with a nuclear proto-oncogene enhancer. J Biol Chem 1990; 265:21881–21888.

14. Terpening CM, Haussler CA, Jurutka PW, Galligan MA, Komm BS, Haussler MR. The vitamin D–responsive element in the rat bone Gla protein gene is an imperfect direct repeat that cooperates with other cis-elements in 1,25-dihydroxyvitamin D$_3$–mediated transcriptional activation. Mol Endocrinol 1991; 5:373–385.

15. MacDonald PN, Haussler CA, Terpening CM, Galligan MA, Reeder MC, Whitfield GK, Haussler MR. Baculovirus-mediated expression of the human vitamin D receptor: Functional characterization, vitamin D response element interactions, and evidence for a receptor auxiliary factor. J Biol Chem 1991; 266:18808–18813.

16. Noda M, Vogel RL, Craig AM, Prahl J, DeLuca HF, Denhardt DT. Identification of a DNA sequence responsible for binding of the 1,25-dihydroxyvitamin D$_3$ receptor and 1,25-dihydroxyvitamin D$_3$ enhancement of mouse secreted phosphoprotein 1 (SPP-1 or osteopontin) gene expression. Proc Natl Acad Sci USA 1990; 87:9995–9999.

17. Zierold C, Darwish HM, DeLuca HF. Identification of a vitamin D-response element in the rat calcidiol (25-hydroxyvitamin D$_3$) 24-hydroxylase gene. Proc Natl Acad Sci USA 1994; 91:900–902.

18. Hahn CN, Kerry DM, Omdahl JL, May BK. Identification of a vitamin D responsive element in the promoter of the rat cytochrome P450(24) gene. Nucleic Acids Res 1994; 22:2410–2416.

19. Freedman LP, Arce V, Fernandez RP. DNA sequences that act as high affinity targets for the vitamin D_3 receptor in the absence of the retinoid X receptor. Mol Endocrinol 1994; 8:265–273.

20. Carlberg C, Bendik I, Wyss A, Meier E, Sturzenbecker LJ, Grippo JF, Hunziker W. Two nuclear signaling pathways for vitamin D. Nature 1993; 361:657–660.

21. MacDonald PN, Dowd DR, Nakajima S, Galligan MA, Reeder MC, Haussler CA, Ozato K, Haussler MR. Retinoid X receptors stimulate and 9-cis retinoic acid inhibits 1,25-dihydroxyvitamin D_3-activated expression of the rat osteocalcin gene. Mol Cell Biol 1993; 13:5907–5917.

22. Li XY, Boudjelal M, Xiao JH, Peng JH, Asuru A, Kang S, Fisher GJ, Voorhees JJ. 1,25-dihydroxyvitamin D_3 increases nuclear vitamin D receptors by blocking ubiquitin/proteasome-mediated degradation in human skin. Mol Endocrin (in press).

23. Li XY, Xiao JH, Feng X, Qin L, Voorhees JJ. Retinoid X receptor-specific ligands synergistically upregulate 1,25-dihydroxyvitamin D_3–dependent transcription in epidermal keratinocytes in vitro and in vivo. J Invest Dermatol 1997; 108:506–512.

24. Ohyama Y, Ozono K, Uchida M, Shinki T, Kato S, Suda Y, Yamamoto O, Noshiro M, Kato Y. Identification of a vitamin responsive element in the 5′-flanking region of the rat 25-hydroxyvitamin D_3 24-hydroxylase gene. J Biol Chem 1994; 269:10545–10550.

25. Zierold C, Darwish HM, DeLuca HF. Two vitamin D responsive elements function in the rat 1,25-dihydroxyvitamin D 24-hydroxylase promoter. J Biol Chem 1995; 270:1675–1678.

26. Kang S, Li XY, Duell EA, Voorhees JJ. The retinoid X receptor agonist 9-cis-retinoic acid and the 24-hydroxylase inhibitor ketoconazole increase activity of 1,25-dihydroxyvitamin D_3 in human skin in vivo. J Invest Dermatol 1997; 108:513–518.

27. Duell EA, Kang S, Voorhees JJ. Retinoic acid isomers applied to human skin in vivo each induce a 4-hydroxylase that inactivates only trans retinoic acid. J Invest Dermatol 1996; 106:316–320.

28. Astrom A, Pettersson U, Krust A, Chambon P, Voorhees JJ. Retinoic acid and synthetic analogs differentially activate retinoic acid receptor dependent transcription. Biochem Biophys Res Commun 1990; 173:339–345.

29. Duell EA, Åström A, Griffiths CEM, Chambon P, Voorhees JJ. Human skin levels of retinoic acid and cytochrome P-450-derived 4-hydroxyretinoic acid after topical application of retinoic acid in vivo compared to concentrations required to stimulate retinoic acid receptor-mediated transcription in vitro. J Clin Invest 1992; 90:1269–1274.

30. Dockx P, Decree J, Degreef H. Inhibition of the metabolism of endogenous retinoic acid as treatment for severe psoriasis: An open study with oral liarozole. Br J Dermatol 1995; 133:426–432.

31. Farr PM, Krause LB, Marks JM, Shuster S. Response of scalp psoriasis to oral ketoconazole. Lancet 1985; 2:921–922.

32. Lucker GP, Heremans AM, Boegheim PJ, van de Kerkhof PC, Steijlen PM. Oral treatment of ichthyosis by the cytochrome P-450 inhibitor liarozole. Br J Dermatol 1997; 136:71–75.

33. Griffiths CEM, Finkel LJ, Tranfaglia MG, Hamilton TA, Voorhees JJ. An in-vivo experimental model for effects of topical retinoic acid in human skin. Br J Dermatol 1993; 129:389–394.
34. Fisher GJ, Esmann J, Griffiths CEM, Talwar HD, Duell EA, Hammerberg C, Elder JT, Finkel LJ, Karabin GD, Nickoloff BJ, Cooper KD, Voorhees JJ. Cellular, immunologic and biochemical characterization of topical retinoic acid-treated human skin. J Invest Dermatol 1991; 96:699–707.
35. Kang S, Duell EA, Fisher GJ, Datta SC, Wang ZQ, Reddy AP, Tavakkol A, Yi JY, Griffiths CEM, Elder JT, Voorhees JJ. Application of retinol to human skin in vivo induces epidermal hyperplasia and cellular retinoid binding proteins characteristic of retinoic acid but without measurable retinoic acid levels or irritation. J Invest Dermatol 1995; 105:549–556.
36. Kang S, Duell EA, Kim KJ, Voorhees JJ. Liarozole inhibits human epidermal retinoic acid 4-hydroxylase activity and differentially augments human skin responses to retinoic acid and retinol in vivo. J Invest Dermatol 1996; 107:183–187.
37. Kang S, Li XY, Voorhees JJ. Pharmacology and molecular action of retinoids and vitamin D in skin. J Invest Dermatol Symp Proc 1996; 15–21.

11
Chemistry and Pharmacology of Calcipotriol

Anne-Marie Kissmeyer, Martin J. Calverley, and Lise Binderup
Leo Pharmaceutical Products, Ballerup, Denmark

I. CHEMISTRY

Structural modification of a natural compound that has been found to have useful biological activity is most frequently desirable in order to create a therapeutic drug. The advantages of the resulting analog over the parent compound can include increased biological potency, improved pharmacological profile and/or pharmacokinetics, and decreased toxicity, together with pharmaceutical considerations like improved availability or stability of the bulk substance and patent protectability. In the case of calcitriol, which was already an established drug for treating bone disease at the time its potential in dermatology was discovered, the primary consideration was to see whether it was possible to select the beneficial potent effects on the modulation of cell growth and immune regulation from the undesired and potentially toxic influence on the systemic calcium homeostasis. The use of synthetic calcitriol itself (or its prodrug alphacalcidol) in bone disease, rather than an analog, is related to its administration in *physiological* quantities to correct a deficient endogenous production of this hormone. This is to be contrasted with the supraphysiological (i.e. *pharmacological*) concentrations of the hormone which are required for regulating keratinocyte dysfunction in psoriasis, a disease that has not been causatively associated with an endogenous calcitriol insufficiency (see Chapter 5).

A prerequisite to the rational design of analogs is an understanding of the biological processes involved and the mechanism of action of the natural substance with a view to interfering at a particular stage by chemical modification. At the time the vitamin D analog program at Leo Pharmaceutical Products was started in

1984, it was appreciated that the effects of calcitriol are hormonal and are receptor-mediated, relying upon the recognition of the molecule by the vitamin D receptor (VDR), for which calcitriol is the natural ligand. For an analog to function it must therefore at least fulfil the minimum requirements for binding to the VDR. At that time it was not, however, known whether activation of different VDR subtypes was responsible for eliciting effects in different cell types, so a possibility for achieving selectivity by structural modification was appreciated. It was also known that calcitriol was subject to further metabolic oxidation in the sterol side chain, producing metabolites with altered activity profiles. Sterols constitute a group of biologically important alcohols with a steroid nucleus and a long eight- to ten-carbon side chain. Vitamin D and its metabolites, including the hormone calcitriol [$1\alpha,25(OH)_2D_3$; Figure 1, left], are seco-sterols, wherein the 9,10-bond, and hence ring B, of the steroid nucleus is cleaved. Chemical methods for modifying the side chains of sterols were well established, and since it was known that the side chain hydroxyl (25-OH) of calcitriol is crucial for receptor binding and therefore hormonal activity, the side chain was an attractive region for investigation. Furthermore, it had already been shown that certain non-metabolic modifications around the 25-OH could be tolerated by the VDR. Some of these are indicated on the structure of calcitriol in Figure 1.

As a new idea, it was proposed to investigate the effect of incorporating the geminal methyl groups (C-26 and C-27) of calcitriol into a ring. This alter-

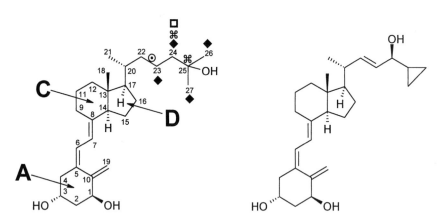

Figure 1   Left: Chemical structure of calcitriol showing the conventional steroid-derived ring nomenclature and carbon atom numbering system and indicating some of the modifications in the side chain tolerated by the VDR known prior to the discovery of calcipotriol. ⌘, transposition of 25-OH to 24-position; ◆, fluorine substitution around C-25; □, methyl substitution at C-24; ⊙, (*E*-) 22,23-double bond. Right: Chemical structure of calcipotriol.

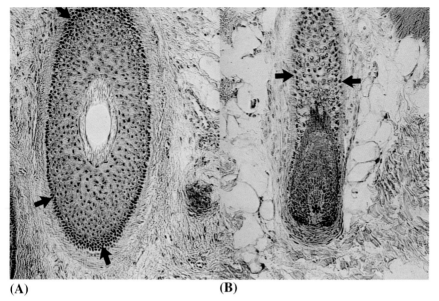

(A) **(B)**

Figure 6.1 Immunohistochemical detection of VDR (mAb 9A7γ 1 : 1500; streptavidin-peroxidase without counterstain) in the midportion of a human anagen hair follicle (**A**, horizontal section, original magnification x400) and a human proximal anagen VI follicle (**B**, longitudinal section, original magnification x400). Notice nuclear VDR immunoreactivity in hair follicle keratinocytes (arrows) and cells of the dermal papilla (asterisk).

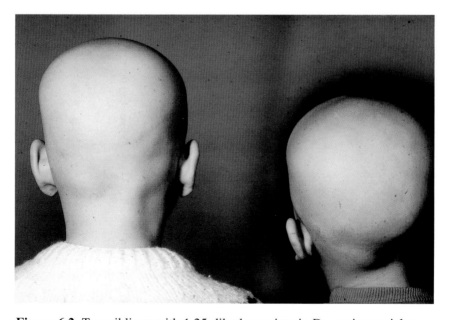

Figure 6.2 Two siblings with 1,25-dihydroxyvitamin D_3–resistant rickets type II. Note alopecia totalis, which developed during the first year of life and did not improve with oral calcitriol treatment.

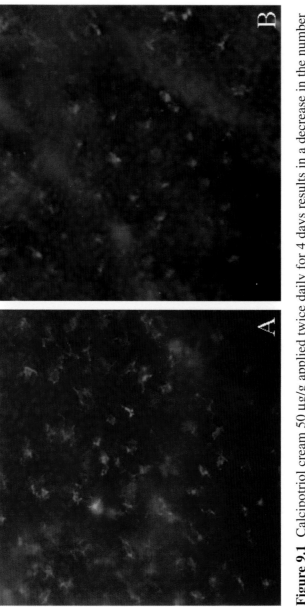

Figure 9.1 Calcipotriol cream 50 µg/g applied twice daily for 4 days results in a decrease in the number of CD1a⁺Langerhans cells and the number of dendrites per LC. Suction blisters were induced on the skin areas after treatment for 4 days. The blister roofs were incubated overnight at 4°C with anti-CD1a-FITC (green) and propidium iodide added to stain nuclei (red). CD1a⁺LC were studied using a laser scanning microscope (optical sectioning parallel to the epidermis). Computer-assisted image analysis of the images detected a 33% increase in average cell size after treatment. **A**, vehicle control; **B**, calcipotriol cream 50 µg/g. (From Ref. 41.)

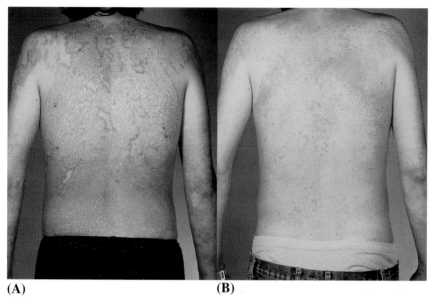

(A)   (B)

Figure 12.1 Patient with plaque-type psoriasis before (**A**) and after (**B**) topical application of calcipotriol ointment bid for 6 weeks.

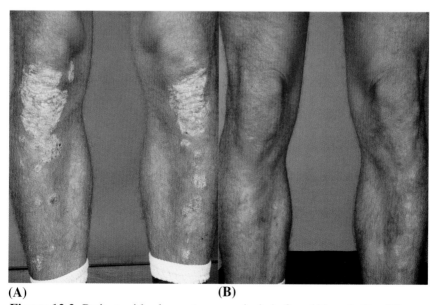

(A)   (B)

Figure 12.2 Patient with plaque-type psoriasis before (**A**) and after (**B**) topical application of calcipotriol ointment bid for 6 weeks.

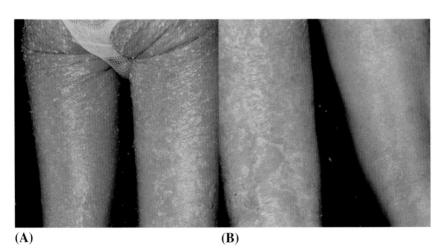

(A)   **(B)**

Figure 15.1 Calcipotriol-cyclosporine (right) versus vehicle-cyclosporine (left) in erythrodermic psoriasis: **A,** before treatment, **B,** after 1 week of treatment.

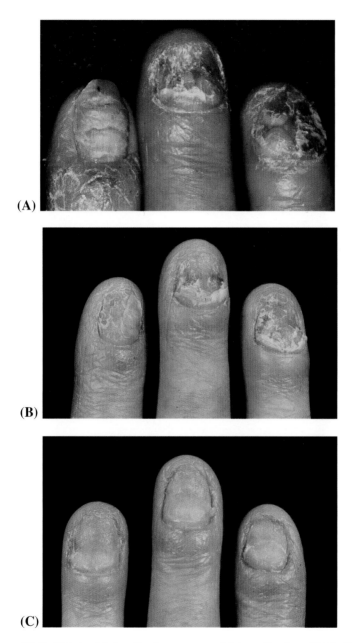

Figure 15.2 Calcipotriol-acitretin versus vehicle-acitretin: **(A)** before treatment; **(B)** after 1 month of treatment, calcipotriol-treated side; **(C)** after 1 month of treatment, vehicle-treated side.

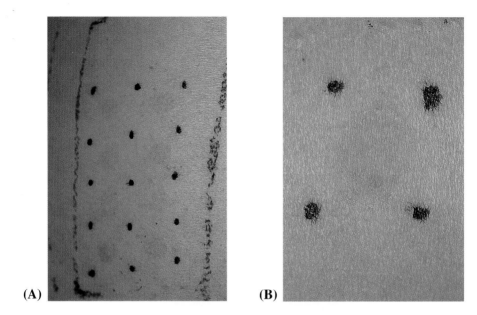

(A) (B)

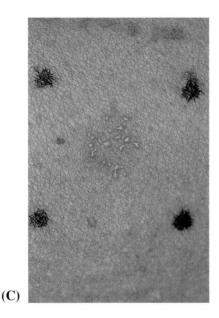

(C)

Figure 17.1 **A.** Typical 1+ patch test reaction to calcipotriol in alkaline-buffered isopropanol. The typical reaction is dominated by redness, but stronger reactions may show both edema and papules. The testee was a healthy volunteer. **B.** Typical 1+ patch test reaction in a healthy volunteer, closeup. **C.** A vesicular reaction to a patch test application of calcipotriol in alkaline-buffered isopropanol. Papules and vesicles were prominent. The testee was a healthy volunteer. (From Ref. 6.)

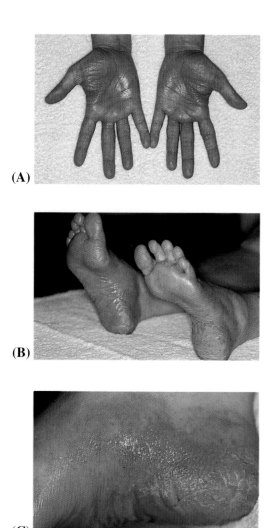

(A)

(B)

(C)

Figure 17.2 An alarming case of dermatitis in a patient with palmoplantar psoriasis about 5 weeks after start of treatment with calcipotriol ointment **(A, B, C).** 24-hour occlusive patch test with a dilution series of calcipotriol in alkaline buffered isopropanol (50/10/5/2 µg/L) was negative **(D).** A 7-day ROAT test on anticubital skin with application of calcipotriol ointment bid for 7 days was negative as well **(E).** Despite alarming symptoms, it was unlikely that the patient was allergic to calcipotriol. The case was concluded to be a probable case of cumulative irritant contact dermatitis. Calcipotriol treatment was stopped and not reinstituted because of the severity of the reaction, but the outcome of testing did not exclude its future use in a smaller dose or combined with a corticosteroid.

(D),(E) continued on next page

(D), (E) continued from **Figure 17.2**

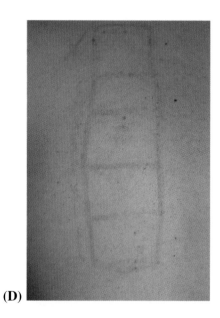

(D)

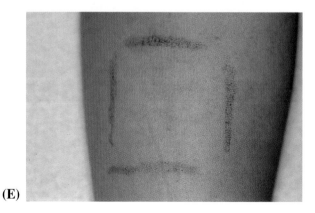

(E)

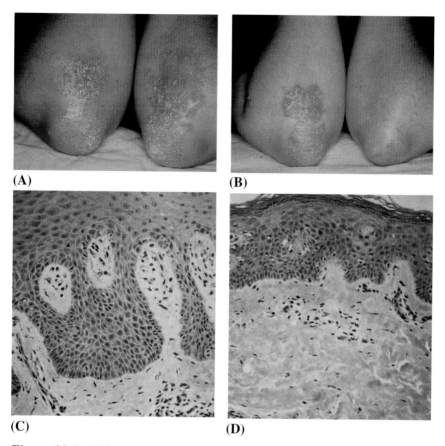

(A) **(B)**

(C) **(D)**

Figure 20.1 A 23-year-old woman with a 20-year history of psoriasis. **A** and **B**. The lesions on the patient's right and left forearms were treated with placebo petroleum jelly and calcitriol ointment, respectively. There is obvious improvement in the calcitriol-treated side. **C** and **D**. Photomicrograph (x20) of the biopsies stained with hematoxylin and eosin and toluidine blue. **C**. Right elbow (placebo). **D**. Left elbow (calcitriol). (From Ref. 10.)

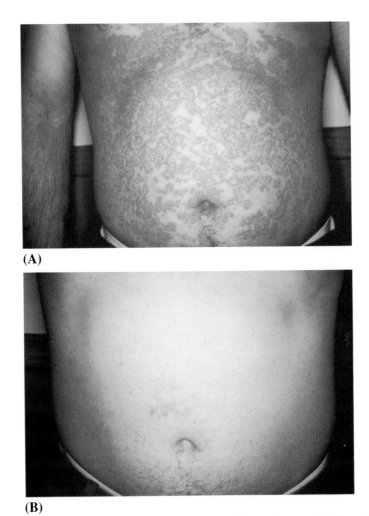

(A)

(B)
Figure 20.9 A 40-year-old male with psoriasis for 15 years. Before **(A)** and 6 months after 2 µg each night of oral calcitriol **(B)**. (From Ref. 13.)

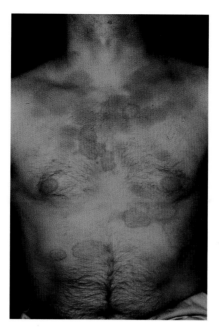

Figure 21.1 Erythema multiforme-like lesions in patients with plaque psoriasis treated topically with 15 µg/g calcitriol ointment twice daily.

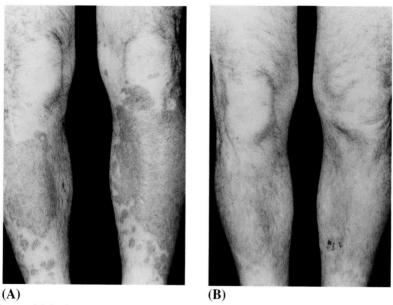

(A)   **(B)**

Figure 21.2 A. Patient before treatment with 3µg/g calcitriol ointment. **B.** Patient after successful treatment with 3 µg/g calcitriol ointment.

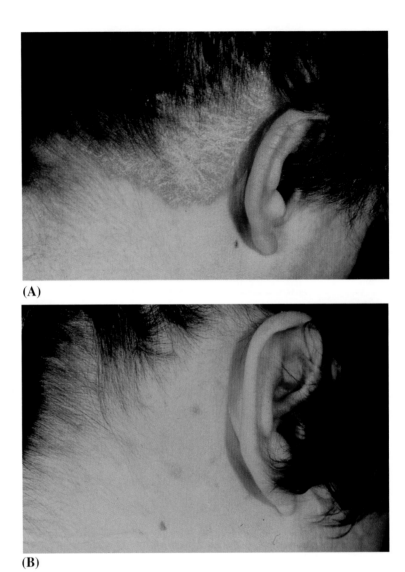

(A)

(B)

Figure 21.3 A. Patient with chronic plaque psoriasis on the scalp before treatment with 3 μg/g calcitriol ointment. **B.** Patient with chronic plaque psoriasis on the scalp after successful treatment with 3 μg/g calcitriol ointment (fast responder). No hyperpigmentation or acanthosis remained.

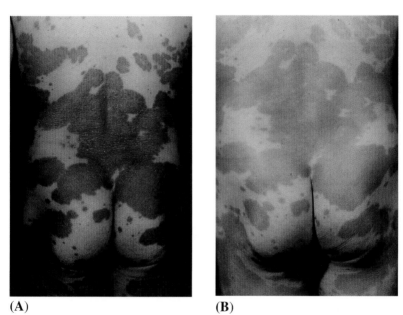

(A)   (B)

Figure 21.4 A. Patient with chronic plaque psoriasis on the trunk before treatment with 3 μg/g calcitriol ointment in a long-term study. **B.** Patient with chronic plaque psoriasis on the trunk after successful treatment with 3 μg/g calcitriol ointment in a long-term study (fast responder). Note pronounced hyperpigmentation but no acanthosis.

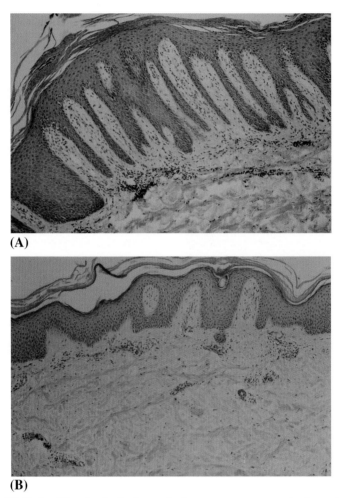

(A)

(B)

Figure 21.5 A. Histological picture before treatment—typical psoriasis. (H & E, low magnification.) **B.** Histological picture after 6 weeks of successful treatment with calcitriol. No signs of psoriasis despite the presence of infiltrates composed of PMNs in some papillae and around superficial blood vessels. (H & E, low magnification.)

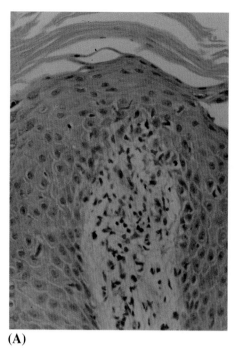

(A)

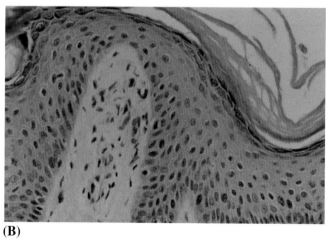

(B)

Figure 21.6 A. Histological picture before treatment—PMNs in papillae penetrating to the epidermis. (H & E, high magnification.) **B.** Histological picture after 6 weeks of successful treatment with calcitriol. PMNs are still present in papillae without penetration to the epidermis. (H & E, high magnification.)

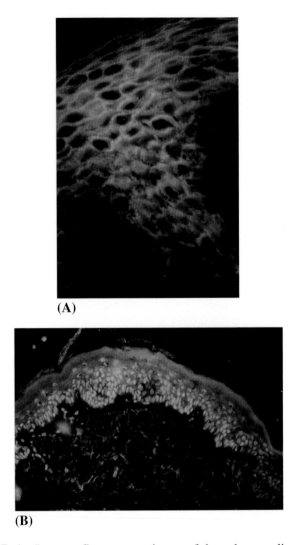

(A)

(B)

Figure 21.7 A. Immunofluorescent picture of thrombospondin staining before treatment with calcitriol ointment. **B.** Immunofluorescent picture of thrombospondin staining after successful treatment with calcitriol ointment.

ation could be anticipated to influence both receptor binding and further metabolism of the hormone. Among the compounds synthesized in 1985 was the compound with laboratory code MC 903 (Figure 1, right) [1], in which a cyclopropane ring occurs, at the same time as two of the other modifications already indicated in Figure 1, left were made—i.e., the transposition of the 25-OH to the 24 position, and the addition of a 22,23 double bond having the E configuration. Formally, the three-membered ring is the result of constituting a direct bond between carbons 26 and 27, and the carbon framework may be described as a 26,27-cyclo-vitamin D_3 derivative. MC 903 was found to have an ideal pharmacological profile, and a patent was applied for in the same year. Although early literature (1987 to 1992) may refer only to the laboratory code MC 903, the names *calcipotriol* [International Nonproprietary Name (INN)] and *calcipotriene* [U.S. Adopted Name (USAN)] are now universally recognized. Calcipotriol is a white crystalline powder (melting point: 166–168°C), although it is usually encountered in its formulated forms. It is manufactured by multistage synthesis from vitamin D_2, employing the intermediates described in the published synthesis outlined in Figure 2 [1]. Note that it is necessary to cleave off

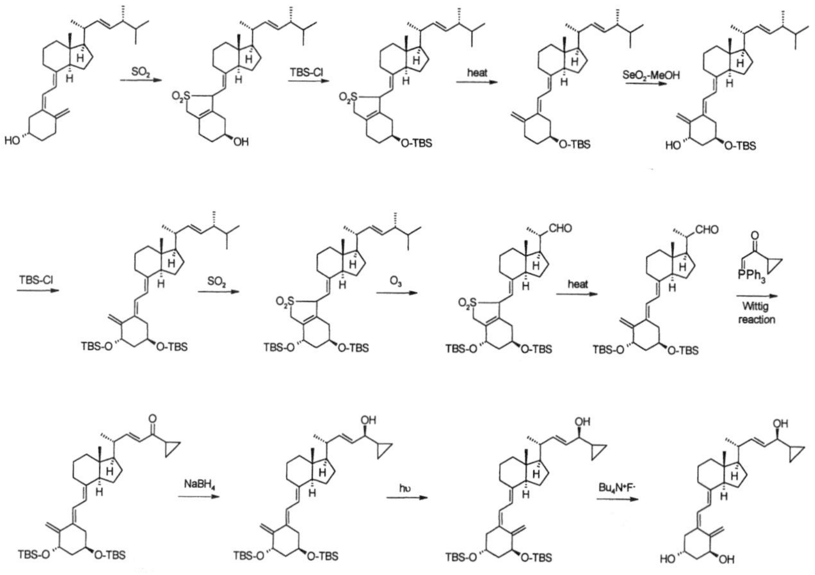

Figure 2 Chemical synthesis of calcipotriol from vitamin D_2 [1]. The initial steps are concerned with introducing the 1α-hydroxyl group into the seco-steroid ring system, while the later steps involve the replacement of the steroid side chain. TBS, tertiary-butyldimethylsilyl, an alcohol protective group.

the steroid side chain and replace it with the residue containing a prefabricated cyclopropane moiety. The chemical structure was confirmed by x-ray analysis ([2]; the systematic chemical name for calcipotriol is given in the title of this reference), and the conformations of the ring system and the side chain as found in the crystal are illustrated in Figure 3. The *S* configuration of the side chain hydroxyl at C-24 is an important feature of the molecule for preserving high VDR-binding affinity.

An account of the synthesis and effect of side-chain structure on the selective biological actions of congeners of calcipotriol is beyond the scope of this chapter but can be found in Ref. 3. Discussed are various analogs in which the ring size is changed or the ring is opened, that have chlorine or fluorine substitution at C-25, that are modified at C-24 or the 24-OH group, or that differ in the nature of the 22,23 bond (single or *Z* double). The analogs having the opposite configuration at C-20 (i.e., 20-epi) or a 22,23-triple bond (22-yne) have also been investigated [4,5]. It is important to note that not only the size of the side chain ring but also the combination of all three modifications relative to the structure of calcitriol found in calcipotriol is critical for the advantageous selectivity of activities. Radi-

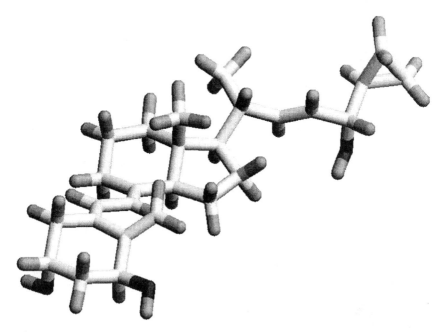

Figure 3 "Cylinder-model" representation of the crystal structure of calcipotriol, showing the conformations of the ring system and the side chain. The three darkest-shaded cylinders represent the oxygen atoms.

olabeled calcipotriol for pharmacokinetic and metabolic studies (see Sections III and IV of this chapter) was produced by a modified synthesis also described in Ref. 3. A tritium (^{3}H) label was employed and the labeling position is on the side chain at carbon 23.

II. PHARMACOLOGY

The effect of calcipotriol on cell-growth regulation has been investigated in various cells of human origin. Calcipotriol has been found to be a potent inducer of cell differentiation and to inhibit proliferation and DNA synthesis of cells possessing the receptor for calcitriol [6–8]. The most widely used cell line has been the human histiocytic lymphoma cell line U 937, which possesses well-characterized, high-affinity receptors for calcitriol [9]. Calcipotriol inhibits U 937 cell proliferation in concentrations from 10^{-8} M, with a potency comparable to that of calcitriol, and induces cell differentiation along the monocyte-macrophage pathway at slightly lower concentrations (Table 1) [6].

The antiproliferative and differentiation-inducing effects of calcipotriol have also been demonstrated in various cultured keratinocyte systems, in which calcipotriol displayed an activity similar to that of calcitriol. Cellular DNA content in primary human keratinocytes is significantly inhibited by calcipotriol and terminal differentiation is induced [10]. In HaCaT, a spontaneously immortal-

Table 1 Effect on Receptor Binding, Cell Proliferation, and Cell Differentiation[a]

Compound tested	Receptor binding 50% displacement of [^{3}H]1α,25(OH)$_2$D$_3$ (M)	Inhibition of cell proliferation IC$_{50}$ (M)	Induction of cell differentiation (M)
Calcipotriol	3.9×10^{-11}	1.4×10^{-8}	1.0×10^{-9}
Calcitriol	3.0×10^{-11}	2.8×10^{-8}	1.0×10^{-9}
MC 1046	9.5×10^{-9}	$>1.0 \times 10^{-7}$	1.0×10^{-7}
MC 1080	1.0×10^{-9}	$>1.0 \times 10^{-7}$	1.0×10^{-7}

[a] 1,25(OH)$_2$D$_3$ receptor protein from the intestinal epithelium of rachitic chicken was incubated with [^{3}H]1α,25(OH)$_2$D$_3$ and test compound. The concentration of the test compound resulting in 50% displacement of bound [^{3}H]1α,25(OH)$_2$D$_3$ was calculated. U 937 cells (1×10^5 cells/mL) were cultured at 37°C for 96 hr in presence of test compound. At the end of incubation, the cells were counted and the concentration of the compound resulting in 50% inhibition of cell proliferation was assessed (IC$_{50}$). The nonadherent cells were also collected and stained for the presence of nonspecific esterase activity as a marker of cell differentiation.

ized, nontumorigenic human skin keratinocyte cell line, the antiproliferative effect was accompanied by a change in the cytokeratin pattern of the skin cells as an indicator of a differentiating effect [11]. Besides the effects on cell growth regulation in cancer cells and keratinocytes, calcipotriol also exerts inhibitory effects on various cell types of the immune system [12,13]. Most of the biological effects observed with calcipotriol are suggested to be mediated via binding to the calcitriol receptor (VDR) [14]. The binding affinities for VDR of calcipotriol and of calcitriol were also found to be very similar (Table 1). In conclusion, the concentrations at which calcipotriol and calcitriol are active in vitro are generally the same. However, when administered in vivo, calcipotriol was found to be much less active than calcitriol with regard to its effects on calcium metabolism ([6]; Leo Pharmaceutical Products: toxicological studies of calcipotriol, 1986–1989). Studies have been performed in mice, rats, dogs, and minipigs. The most extensive studies have been performed in rats using oral, intraperitoneal, intravenous, and dermal administration. A comparative study of the calcemic effects of calcipotriol and calcitriol has been performed in rats and the urinary excretion of calcium after oral and intraperitoneal administration is shown in Figure 4. As it can be seen, calcipotriol is at least 100–200 times less active than calcitriol, and the same difference is seen with serum calcium values (data not shown).

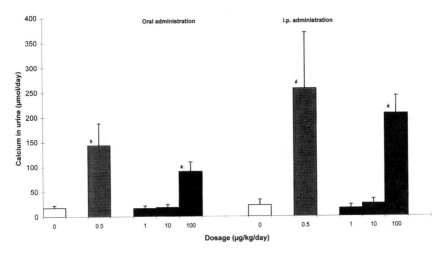

Figure 4   Calcium excretion in urine after administration of calcipotriol and calcitriol. Rats were treated orally or intraperitoneally daily for 7 days. Open box, control (vehicle); gray box, calcitriol; black box, calcipotriol. Urine was collected daily. Mean calcium excretion was calculated from days 3–7. In comparison with the control value, $*p < 0.05$.

III. PHARMACOKINETICS

One of the major advantages of calcipotriol in relation to calcitriol lies in its low calcemic activity in vivo; it is, of course, of obvious importance to elucidate the reasons for this difference in the mode of action of the two compounds. Since the biological potency of calcipotriol and that of calcitriol are, as described in Section II of this chapter, very similar in most in vitro systems, the selective action on the calcium metabolism of calcipotriol compared with that of calcitriol is most likely related to pharmacokinetic differences.

A. Analysis

The analysis of vitamin D analogs in blood presents a number of difficulties, as the blood levels reached after administration of pharmacological doses are very low and cannot be determined by using conventional high-performance liquid chromatography (HPLC) methodology. Consequently, it has been necessary to administer high doses and to use radiolabeled compound or an HPLC-radioreceptor assay in order to study the pharmacokinetics of calcipotriol [15–20]. However, the administration of high doses of any vitamin D analog is impossible in humans owing to the risk of calcemic side effects. The value of giving radioactive doses is also limited, as the amount of radioactivity that can be administered to humans is very small and therefore only little information can be extracted from such human studies. On the other hand, the HPLC-radioreceptor assay is very sensitive and does not require administration of high doses or administration of radiolabeled compounds. However, the assay is difficult and not very robust, as it involves a solid-phase extraction and an HPLC step for purification and isolation of the vitamin D analog before the assay is completed by performing a radioreceptor assay using a purified vitamin D receptor.

B. Animal Studies

In a single high-dose study in rats, the pharmacokinetics of calcipotriol and that of calcitriol were compared [15]. The serum half-life ($t_{1/2}$), the area under the serum level/time curve (AUC_{∞}), and the serum clearance were calculated from the serum concentrations determined by HPLC (Table 2). Calcitriol was still detectable 6 hr after intravenous dosing with either 10 or 50 μg/kg. The elimination of calcitriol could be separated into α and β phases with half-lives of 15 min and 2.3–3.8 hr, respectively. For calcipotriol only, an α phase was observed, with a half-life of approximately 4 min. Furthermore, calculation of the area under the serum level/time curve revealed that the value for calcitriol was more than 100 times higher than for calcipotriol. This correlates well with the effect on calcium metabolism found in vivo in normal and rachitic rats [6], where it was demonstrated that the antirachitic activity of calcipotriol was 100–200 times lower than

Table 2   Pharmacokinetic Profile of Calcipotriol and Calcitriol after

| Treatment | Dose (μg/kg) | 0 min | 5 min | Nanograms of unchanged compound per | | | |
				10 min	30 min	1 hr	2 hr
Calcitriol	10		130	99	83	40	38
Calcitriol	50	—	676	537	422	370	263
Calcipotriol	10	—	12	—	—	—	—
Calcipotriol	50	—	62	27	—	—	—

[a] The half-life is separated into an α-phase (0–10 min) and a β-phase (1–6 hr) after dosing. The serum concentrations were determined by HPLC [15].

that of calcitriol. These pharmacokinetic findings were further confirmed in an experiment where the effects on cell proliferation/differentiation in human histio-cytic lymphoma U 937 cells were evaluated after incubation for 4 days with serum from calcipotriol- or calcitriol-dosed rats [15]. As already stated, this cell line pos-sesses high-affinity receptors for calcitriol [9] and has been shown to be equally responsive to calcipotriol and to calcitriol at concentrations from 10^{-9} M (about 0.4 ng/mL) [6]. Figure 5 shows the effects on cell proliferation. The maximum in-

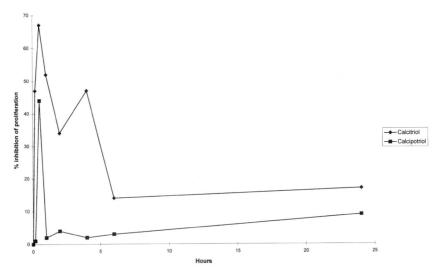

Figure 5   Effects of calcipotriol and calcitriol on cell proliferation. U937 (1×10^5 cells/mL) were cultured at 37°C for 96 hr in the presence of serum from calcipotriol- or cal-citriol-dosed rats (10 μg/kg). The sera were collected 0–24 hr following intravenous drug administration. At the end of the incubation, cell proliferation was determined by cell counting.

Intravenous Administration to Rats[a]

milliliter of serum			$t_{1/2}$ α-Phase (min)	β-Phase (hr)	AUC∞ (ng/mL $\times$ hr)	Cl (mL/hr)
4 hr	6 hr	24 hr				
23	17	—	13	3.8	309	6
165	78	—	15	2.3	1683	5
—	—	—	—	—	—	—
—	—	—	4	—	12	679

hibition of cell proliferation was observed with serum collected 30 min after dosing with either calcipotriol or calcitriol. This inhibitory effect could be observed with serum collected up to 4 hr after dosing with calcitriol, whereas no effect was observed with serum samples collected later than 30 min from rats dosed with calcipotriol. Figure 6 shows the effects on cell differentiation. Differentiation to cells with monocyte/macrophage characteristics was assessed using the appearance of α-naphthyl acetate esterase activity as a cell-differentiating marker. Cell cultures

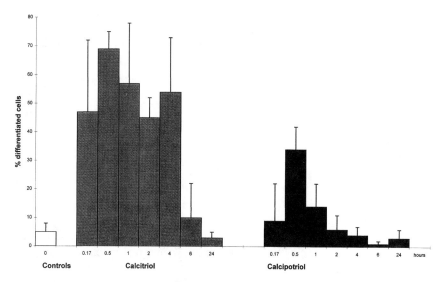

Figure 6 Effects of calcipotriol and calcitriol on cell differentiation. U937 (1 $\times$ 10^5 cells/mL) were cultured at 37°C for 96 hr in the presence of serum from calcipotriol- or calcitriol-dosed rats (10 μg/kg). The sera were collected 0–24 hr following intravenous drug administration. At the end of the incubation, samples of cells were stained for esterase activity as a marker for cell differentiation.

incubated with the 30-min samples had the highest effect on cell differentiation: 69% of the cells were differentiated by serum from the calcitriol-dosed rats and 34% of the cells by serum from the calcipotriol-dosed rats. Furthermore, serum samples collected at 1, 2, and 4 hr after dosing with calcitriol were able to differentiate about 50% of the cells, whereas the effect seen with the serum collected at 1 hr or later after dosing with calcipotriol rapidly disappeared. A similar rapid elimination of calcipotriol was also observed in other single-dose studies in rats performed at the much lower dose of 0.39 μg/kg intravenously [20] or 0.4–10 μg/kg subcutaneously [16]. Repeated subcutaneous administration of ^{3}H-calcipotriol to rats once daily for 21 days revealed an equally rapid elimination rate [18]. In contrast to this very rapid systemic biotransformation of calcipotriol, it has been reported that in the skin at the application site, the metabolic rate of calcipotriol is very low [17]. Thus, 40% of the radioactivity present 24 hr after application of ^{3}H-calcipotriol (5 μg/100 mg ointment per animal) to rats is recovered as intact calcipotriol. Moreover, the same study demonstrated that the major part of the total radioactivity was present in the skin and that the radioactivity in the skin declined very slowly; i.e., 50% of the maximal concentration of the radioactivity found in the skin was still present 48 hr after its application. A low metabolic rate at the application site and a very rapid metabolism as soon as calcipotriol reaches the systemic circulation ensure that the effects of calcipotriol in the target tissue are maximal and that the systemic side effects are minimal.

In addition to the pharmacokinetics in rats, a rapid elimination of calcipotriol was also found in minipigs. Thus, the plasma half-life of calcipotriol in minipigs after a single intravenous administration of calcipotriol was about 30 min (E. Eilertsen, personal communication, 1986). Finally, in the rats and minipigs, the major part of the biotransformed calcipotriol is excreted in the feces and only a minor part is excreted in the urine both after topical and systemic treatment [16–18] (M.K. Thomsen, personal communication, 1989).

C. Human Studies

The systemic exposure to calcipotriol in humans has mainly been determined indirectly by using serum calcium as a marker (see Chapter 19). This is due to analytical difficulties in measuring very low serum levels of calcipotriol after dermal application. The in vitro half-life of calcipotriol and that of calcitriol in the postmitochondrial liver fraction from rats, minipigs, and humans were investigated (Table 3) [21]. These results have shown that a similar rapid metabolism of calcipotriol is found in vitro in rats, minipigs, and humans and that the metabolism of calcitriol in the three species is much slower than that of calcipotriol. The rapid metabolism of calcipotriol found in vitro in rats and minipigs was also observed in vivo, as described in Section IIIB above, but a similar in vitro/in vivo comparison in humans cannot be performed, as no such in vivo data have been generated.

Table 3 The Half-Life ($t_{1/2}$) of Calcipotriol and Calcitriol In Vitro (in Postmitochondrial Liver Fraction)[a]

	Rats (hr)	Minipigs (hr)	Humans (hr)
Calcipotriol	0.3	0.2	0.2
Calcitriol	3.1	2.9	2.0

[a] The in vitro system consisted of 100 μL postmitochondrial liver fraction per milliliter in 8 mM MgCl$_2$, 33 mM KCl, 5 mM glucose-6-phosphate, 4 mM NADP, and 0.1 M phosphate buffer. The test compound was added to a final concentration of 4×10^{-6} M. The incubations were performed at 37°C, and samples were collected at 0–6 hr. The concentration of test compound was determined by HPLC [22].

Furthermore, the percutaneous absorption of ^{3}H-calcipotriol ointment (50 μg/g) has been investigated after a single application to five healthy volunteers, after a single application on the psoriatic plaques of four patients and after a single dose on the psoriatic plaques of four patients following multiple-dose treatment with nonradiolabeled calcipotriol ointment (50 μg/g) for 2 weeks [23]. Based on the excretion of radioactivity in urine and feces, the percutaneous absorption was calculated to be approximately 6% (range, 2.4–12.1%) both after a single application to normal skin in healthy subjects and after single and repeated application on psoriatic plaques in psoriatic patients. In these studies, it was not possible to detect any calcipotriol or metabolites in the blood. A rapid metabolism of ^{3}H-calcipotriol was indirectly indicated by the rapid formation of ^{3}H$_2$O, which was already found 4 hr after the application of ^{3}H-calcipotriol. Altogether, both the in vitro and in vivo studies in humans indicate that the systemic exposure to intact calcipotriol is low, which minimizes the risk of calcemic side effects after dermal application of calcipotriol.

IV. METABOLISM

The very rapid elimination of calcipotriol is associated with the formation of a number of metabolites. Many of these have been identified and a metabolic pathway for calcipotriol has been proposed. The biological activity of the major metabolites formed early in the degradation was tested and was found to be reduced.

A. In Vitro Metabolism

The in vitro systems that have been used to study the metabolism of calcipotriol include both broken cells (subcellular fractions) and intact cell systems. The liver-based models have been used to study the general catabolism, which is the process that deactivates the drug. Using the postmitochondrial fraction from livers obtained from rats, minipigs, and humans, the rapidly formed major metabolites of calcipotriol, MC 1046 and MC 1080, were identified (Figure 7) [24]. These two major metabolites were also formed in human hepatoma cell lines (Hep 3B and G2) [25].

The target cell metabolism has been studied in order to contribute to an understanding of the pharmacological effects of the drug. Thus, the metabolism has been studied in the keratinocyte cell lines HPK1A and HPK1A-*ras,* the osteosarcoma cell lines UMR 106 and ROS 17/2, and the kidney cell line LLC-PK1 [25]. The metabolism of calcipotriol was most extensively investigated in the immortalized, nontumorigenic HPK1A cell line and the malignant HPK1A-*ras* cell line. The rate of metabolism was different in the two cell lines. The metabolism was slowest in the HPK1A cells, which are most similar to normal basal keratinocytes, whereas the metabolism was more rapid in the HPK1A-*ras* cells, which are more similar to cancer cells. Thus, the slower metabolism in the HPK1A cells correlates well with the findings in vivo in rat skin [17]. It was furthermore revealed that MC 1046 and MC 1080 are not the terminal metabolites of calcipotriol, as several other metabolites were identified from the keratinocyte incubations. Based on these findings, a metabolic pathway of calcipotriol has been proposed (Figure 7) [25]. The metabolism of calcipotriol to MC 1046 and MC 1080 involves oxidation at carbon 24 in the side chain, similar to the C-24 oxidation pathway of metabolism of calcitriol and a reduction of the double bond between carbons 22 and 23. These two initial steps are suggested to be carried out by nonspecific enzymes [21,25], whereas the subsequent steps are similar to the catabolism of calcitriol. Hence, 23-hydroxylation and side chain cleavage followed by oxidation leads to calcitroic acid [26], and these steps are likely to be carried out by the same enzymes that catabolize calcitriol.

Finally, the biological activity of the two major metabolites, MC 1046 and MC 1080, has been demonstrated to be very low both on cell proliferation and cell differentiation in vitro (Table 1) [15]. This low biological activity of the two metabolites can be explained by their decreased ability to bind to the calcitriol receptor.

B. In Vivo Metabolism

The metabolic pathway of calcipotriol has also been investigated after administration of radiolabeled calcipotriol to rats, dogs, and minipigs. In a single-dose dermal study in rats (5 μg/100 mg ointment per animal), it was seen that the major part of the radioactivity was present in the skin within the observation period— i.e., 4–168 hr after application [17]. In the skin at the application site, the metabolic rate of calcipotriol was, as described in Section IIIB above, very low, and 40% of the radioactivity present 24 hr after dosing was intact calcipotriol. The

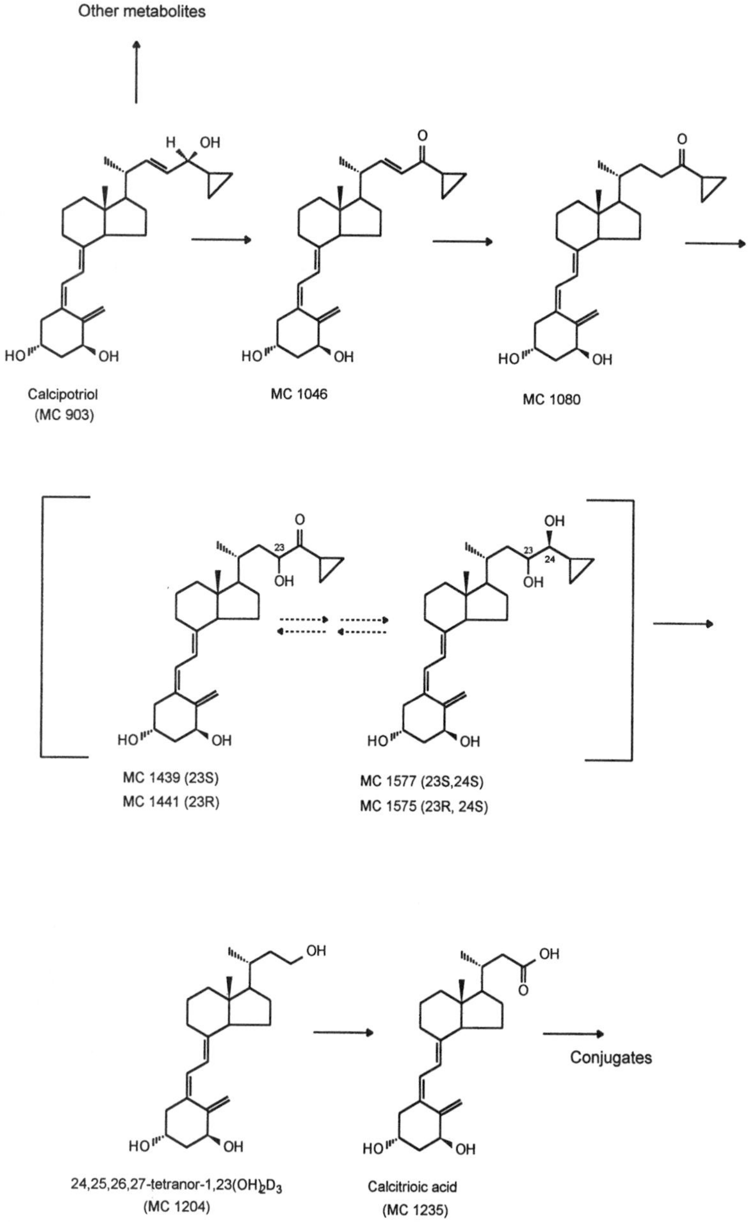

Figure 7 Proposed metabolic pathway of calcipotriol.

remaining part of the radioactivity was present as several metabolites, including MC 1046, MC 1080, and calcitroic acid. Among many other tissues investigated, the liver was found to contain the second highest level of radioactivity, which was only about 1% of that found in the skin, thus explaining why it is difficult to study the metabolic profile of calcipotriol after dermal application in most tissues with the exception of the application site. This also explains why the other in vivo metabolism studies were conducted after systemic administration of calcipotriol. Thus, single and repeated subcutaneous administration of calcipotriol to rats have revealed that only 6–12% of the radioactivity found in plasma and kidney was present as intact calcipotriol 1 hr after administration, and that although the concentration of radioactivity in the liver was high, only the metabolites of calcipotriol and not calcipotriol itself could be detected [16,18]. The major metabolite observed in plasma, liver, and kidney were, in order of magnitude, MC 1080 and an unidentified metabolite; MC 1046 and calcitroic acid were also present among several other minor metabolites detected. The major metabolites observed in feces collected 0–24 hr after dosing was calcitroic acid and the major unknown metabolite found in plasma, kidney, and liver; but several other minor metabolites were also observed, including known metabolites. In urine collected 0–24 hr after dosing, none of the known metabolites was observed, but several unknown metabolites were found. Several metabolites were also excreted in the bile 0–24 hr after dosing. Two of the major metabolites were glucuronide conjugates, one of calcitroic acid and one of the major unknown metabolite found in plasma, liver, kidney, and feces. In dogs, a similar metabolic profile of calcipotriol was observed, although the metabolic rate was lower in dogs than in rats [19]. Thus, the major metabolite in plasma was MC 1080, and in feces almost the same profile was observed as in the rat feces. In dog urine, one of the major metabolites was a glucuronide of calcitroic acid, which was not found in rat urine. A study in minipigs showed that MC 1080 was the major metabolite in serum (M. K. Thomsen, personal communication, 1989). Taken together, more or less the same metabolic pathway of calcipotriol has been observed in vivo in rats and dogs as in vitro in various cell systems. The proposed metabolic pathway as shown in Figure 7 fits very well with the in vivo findings, as major metabolites as well as minor metabolites are found also in vivo. However, other minor pathways cannot be excluded due to the observation of many minor unidentified metabolites.

V. CONCLUSIONS

Calcipotriol is a synthetic vitamin D analog, differing from calcitriol only in the structure of the side chain, most characteristically by the incorporation of a cyclopropane ring. Calcipotriol and calcitriol have similar effects on cell growth regulation in vitro in keratinocytes, cancer cells, and cells from the immune system.

However, in vivo calcipotriol has 100–200 times less effect on calcium metabolism. This low calcemic activity is associated with a rapid systemic rate of metabolism, which has been demonstrated both in vitro and in vivo in several species. In contrast, calcipotriol is only slowly metabolized in keratinocytes and in the skin after dermal application to rats. Consequently, the effect of calcipotriol in the target tissue is maximal and the systemic side effects are minimal.

REFERENCES

1. Calverley MJ. Synthesis of MC 903, a biologically active vitamin D metabolite analogue. Tetrahedron 1987; 43:4609–4619.
2. Larsen S, Hansen ET, Hoffmeyer L, Rastrup-Andersen N. Structure and absolute configuration of a monohydrate of calcipotriol ($1\alpha,3\beta,5Z,7E,22E,24S$)-24-cyclopropyl-9,10-secochola -5,7,10(19),22-tetraene-1,3,24-triol. Acta Cryst 1993; C49:618–621 and 2184 (erratum).
3. Calverley MJ. Novel vitamin D analogues in the calcipotriol (MC 903) series: Synthesis and effect of side chain structure on the selective biological actions. In: Sarel S, Mechoulam R, Agranat I, eds. Trends in Medicinal Chemistry '90. Oxford, UK: Blackwell, 1992:299–306.
4. Calverley MJ, Binderup E, Binderup L. The 20-epi modification in the vitamin D series: selective enhancement of "non-classical" receptor mediated effects. In: Norman AW, Bouillon R, Thomasset M, eds. Vitamin D: Gene Regulation, Structure-Function Analysis and Clinical Application. Berlin: de Gruyter, 1991:163–164.
5. Calverley MJ, Bretting CAS. $1\alpha,24S$-dihydroxy-26,27-cyclo-22-yne-vitamin-D_3—the side chain triple bond analogue of MC 903 (calcipotriol). BioMed Chem Lett 1993; 3:1841–1844.
6. Binderup L, Bramm E. Effects of a novel vitamin D analogue MC 903 on cell proliferation and differentiation in vitro and on calcium metabolism in vivo. Biochem Pharmacol 1988; 37:889–895.
7. Binderup L. MC 903—A novel vitamin D analogue with potent effects on cell proliferation and cell differentiation. In: Norman AW, Schaefer K, Grigoleit HG, Herrath DV, eds. Vitamin D Molecular, Cellular and Clinical Endocrinology. Berlin: de Gruyter, 1988:300–309.
8. Kragballe K, Wildfang IL. Effects of calcipotriol (MC 903), novel vitamin D_3 analogue, on human keratinocyte differentiation and on psoriasis. Skin Pharmacol 1989; 2:44–45.
9. Mezzetti G, Bagnara G, Monti MG, Bonsi L, Brunelli MA, Barbiroli B. $1\alpha,25$-dihydroxycholecalciferol and human histiocytic lymphoma cell line (U 937): The presence of receptor and inhibition of proliferation. Life Sci 1984; 34:2185–2191.
10. Kragballe K, Wildfang IL. Calcipotriol (MC 903), a novel vitamin D_3 analogue stimulates terminal differentiation and inhibits proliferation of cultured human keratinocytes. Arch Dermatol Res 1990; 282:164–167.
11. Hansen CM, Mathiasen IS, Binderup L. The anti-proliferative and differentiation-inducing effects of vitamin D analogs are not determined by the binding affinity for the vitamin D receptor alone. J Invest Dermatol Symp Proc 1996; 1:44–48.

12. Binderup L. Immunological properties of vitamin D analogues and metabolites. Biochem Pharmacol 1992; 43:1885–1892.

13. Hustmyer FG, Benninger L, Manolagas SC. Comparison of the effects of 22-oxa-1,25(OH)$_2$D$_3$ and MC 903 on the production of IL-6, γ-IFN and lymphocyte proliferation in peripheral blood mononuclear cells. J Bone Min Res 1991; 6:S292.

14. Morrison NA, Eisman JA. Nonhypercalcemic 1,25(OH)$_2$D$_3$ analogs potently induce the human osteocalcin gene promoter stably transfected into rat osteosarcoma cells (ROSCO-2). J Bone Min Res 1991; 6:893–899.

15. Kissmeyer A-M, Binderup L. Calcipotriol (MC 903): Pharmacokinetics in rats and biological activities of metabolites. Biochem Pharmacol 1991; 41:1601–1606.

16. Tomida M, Shirakawa K, Masaki K, Konishi R, Esumi Y, Ninomiya S, Inaba A, Mashiko T. Metabolic fate of MC903 (1): Absorption, distribution, metabolism, excretion, transfer into fetus and milk of MC 903 after single subcutaneous administration in rats. Xenob Metab Disp 1996; 11:57–80.

17. Tomida M, Shirikawa K, Masaki K, Konishi R, Esumi Y, Ninomiya S, Inaba A, Mashiko T. Metabolic fate of MC903 (2): Absorption, distribution, metabolism and excretion after single dermal application in rats. Xenob Metab Disp 1996; 11:81–92.

18. Tomida M, Shirakawa K, Masaki K, Konishi R, Esumi Y, Ninomiya S, Inaba A, Mashiko T. Metabolic fate of MC903 (3): Absorption, distribution, metabolism, excretion and effect on drug metabolizing enzymes after multiple dermal application and subcutaneous administration in rats. Xenob Metab Disp 1996; 11:93–105.

19. Tomida M, Shirakawa K, Masaki K, Konishi R, Esumi Y, Ninomiya S, et al. Metabolic fate of MC903 (4): Absorption, metabolism and excretion after dermal application and subcutaneous administration in dogs. Xenob Metab Disp 1996; 11:106–118.

20. Levan LW, Knutson JC, Valliere CR, Bishop CW. Low-dose pharmacokinetics of calcipotriol in rats after oral and intravenous administration. J Invest Dermatol Symp Proc 1996; 1:111.

21. Kissmeyer A-M, Binderup L. The in vitro metabolism of calcipotriol, 1,24(OH)$_2$D$_3$ and 1,25(OH)$_2$D$_3$. In: Norman AW, Bouillon R, Thomasset M, eds. Vitamin D A Pluripotent Steroid Hormone: Structural Studies, Molecular Endocrinology and Clinical Applications. Berlin: de Gruyter, 1994:178–179.

22. Kissmeyer A-M, Mathiasen IS, Latini S, Binderup L. Pharmacokinetic studies of vitamin D analogues: relationship to vitamin D binding protein (DBP). Endocrine 1995; 3:263–266.

23. Delaney C, Liao W, Cohen M, Fancher M, Kripalani K, Uderman H, Stoltz R, Siskin SB. Percutaneous absorption of calcipotriene (calcipotriol) in normal volunteers and psoriatic patients after a single dose of ^{3}H-calcipotriene and in psoriatic patients after a single dose of ^{3}H-calcipotriene following multiple dose treatment with non-radiolabeled calcipotriene 0.005% ointment. J Invest Dermatol Symp Proc 1996; 1:112.

24. Sorensen H, Binderup L, Calverley MJ, Hoffmeyer L, Andersen NR. In vitro metabolism of calcipotriol (MC 903), a vitamin D analogue. Biochem Pharmacol 1990; 39:391–393.

25. Masuda S, Strugnell S, Calverley MJ, Makin HLJ, Kremer R, Jones G. In vitro metabolism of the anti-psoriatic vitamin D analog, calcipotriol, in two cultured human keratinocyte models. J Biol Chem 1994; 269:4794–4803.

26. Makin G, Lohnes D, Byford V, Ray R, Jones G. Target cell metabolism of 1,25-dihydroxyvitamin D$_3$ to calcitroic acid. Biochem J 1989; 262:173–180.

12
Monotherapy—Including Long-Term Therapy with Calcipotriol

Karsten Fogh and Knud Kragballe
Marselisborg Hospital, University of Aarhus, Aarhus, Denmark

I. INTRODUCTION

Psoriasis is a common, chronically relapsing inflammatory skin disease occurring in about 1.5–2% of the population in many Western countries. Affected skin areas are characterized by guttate, nummular, and plaque lesions. Individual lesions are erythematous infiltrations covered by scales located primarily at the knees and elbows. In severe cases, the whole skin area may be affected. Impaired differentiation and increased proliferation of epidermal keratinocytes are key features in psoriatic lesions, together with a local activation of T lymphocytes. Treatments for psoriasis include topical preparations (corticosteroids, tar, dithranol), phototherapy (ultraviolet B [UVB]), photochemotherapy (psoralen plus ultraviolet A [PUVA]) and systemic drugs (methotrexate, retinoids, cyclosporin A). Topical corticosteroids are used extensively for psoriasis. However, topical corticosteroids can induce skin atrophy and may result in the development of tachyphylaxis. Furthermore, topical corticosteroids may have systemic effects when applied to widespread, thin lesions. Therefore new, effective, and nontoxic drugs are needed.

As mentioned in previous chapters, the active form of vitamin D_3 [1,25-dihydroxyvitamin D_3, $1,25(OH)_2D_3$] is known to play an important role in the regulation of intestinal calcium absorption, bone mineralization, and prevention of rickets. In addition to these mechanisms, $1,25(OH)_2D_3$ has several additional biological effects, including stimulation of cellular differentiation, inhibition of proliferation [1,2] and immunomodulation [3,4]. These biological actions make $1,25(OH)_2D_3$ a potential candidate for treatment of psoriasis [5–7]. Improvement of psoriasis has been demonstrated in one patient with osteoporosis, who received oral 1-d-OH-D$_3$, a prodrug of 1,25(OH)$_2$D$_3$, at 0.75 μg/day and had a dramatic improvement of her severe psoriasis [8]. This observation, together with evidence that the bioactive form of 1,25(OH)$_2$D$_3$ inhibits keratinocyte proliferation and promotes keratinocyte differentiation [9], prompted further investigation of the role of 1,25(OH)$_2$D$_3$ and its analogs in psoriasis.

1,25(OH)$_2$D$_3$ itself may not be suitable for treatment of psoriasis due to its hypercalcemic effects. As a consequence, several more selective vitamin D$_3$ analogs with potent biological effects on the cellular level have been developed [10]. One of these analogs, calcipotriol, has been extensively investigated and is now available for topical treatment of psoriasis in most countries. This chapter deals with monotherapy and long-term therapy with topical calcipotriol in psoriasis.

II. BIOLOGICAL ACTIONS OF CALCIPOTRIOL IN THE SKIN

The in vitro effects of calcipotriol on keratinocytes and on the immunocompetent cells are similar to those of 1,25(OH)$_2$D$_3$ both quantitatively and qualitatively. Calcipotriol binds to the vitamin D receptor (VDR) with the same affinity as 1,25(OH)$_2$D$_3$ in a number of different cell types. Calcipotriol inhibits cell proliferation and induces cell differentiation at concentrations similar to those of 1,25(OH)$_2$D$_3$ in the human histiocytic lymphoma cell line U937 [11] and in cultured human keratinocytes [2,12]. In addition, calcipotriol induces VDR-mediated gene transcription in transfected cultures of human keratinocytes [13]. Furthermore, topical application of calcipotriol twice daily for 4 days suppresses the number of Langerhans cells, the antigen-presenting cells (APCs) of the epidermis, as well as their accessory cell function [14]. Compared with 1,25(OH)$_2$D$_3$, calcipotriol has much lower calcemic potency in mice, rats, dogs, and guinea pigs. After oral and intraperitoneal administration, it was found that calcipotriol was 100–200 times weaker than 1,25(OH)$_2$D$_3$ with respect to serum calcium and calcium excretion [11]. Calcipotriol is a 1,25(OH)$_2$D$_3$ analog containing a double-bond and a ring structure in the side chain. As a consequence of this modification of the side chain, it is rapidly transformed into inactive metabolites [10]. Therefore, calcipotriol is about 200 times less potent than 1,25(OH)$_2$D$_3$ in producing hypercalcemia and hypercalciuria after oral and intraperitoneal administration in rats. In contrast, calcipotriol and 1,25(OH)$_2$D$_3$ are equipotent in their affinity for the VDR and in their in vitro effects [10].

III. MODE OF ACTION OF VITAMIN D$_3$ IN PSORIASIS

Together with epidermal hyperproliferation and incomplete terminal differentiation, activated immunocytes are key features of the psoriatic lesion. Treatment with vitamin D_3 analogs has been shown to modulate each of these processes. It is, however, unclear which of these actions are most important for the antipsoriatic effect of vitamin D_3 and its analogs.

In hematoxylin and eosin–stained skin biopsies, treatment with topical $1,25(OH)_2D_3$ results in reappearance of the granular layer, regression of acanthosis and parakeratosis, and resumption of the orthokeratotic horny layer. Also, the infiltrating leukocytes disappear from epidermis but may still be detected around superficial blood vessels and in the papillary dermis [15]. Immunohistopathological evaluation shows normalization of the epidermal staining with the monoclonal antibodies CD15, CD16, CD36, CD1a, and Ki67 during $1,25(OH)_2D_3$ therapy. These and later results suggest that treatment with $1,25(OH)_2D_3$ has an essential effect on epidermal proliferation and differentiation in psoriasis.

During treatment with topical calcipotriol, the keratin levels have been assessed by electrophoretic and immunehistochemical analysis of skin biopsies. Improvement of the psoriatic lesions is accompanied by a reduction in the amount of keratins 5, 16, and 18 (markers of basal and hyperproliferating keratinocytes) and an increase in keratins 1, 2, and 10 (markers of differentiating keratinocytes) [16–22]. The changes of these markers of epidermal growth correlate with the degree of clinical improvement. The changes in levels of markers of differentiation during calcipotriol therapy are similar to those observed in patients treated with photochemotherapy—i.e., small changes in keratin 1 levels and large increases in keratin 2 levels—but contrast with those observed during retinoid therapy, where a large increase in keratin 1 levels with no increase in keratin 2 levels is seen [23].

Calcipotriol treatment also produces a profound effect on immunocytes in psoriatic epidermis and dermis. The number of T lymphocytes is reduced, relatively more for T4+ cells than for T8+ cells [20,21]. In contrast, the epidermal T6+ cells (Langerhans cells) may increase during treatment, although clinical resolution is accompanied by a decrease in T6+ cells [20]. The biphasic effect on T6+ cells has also been reported with PUVA and cyclosporin A treatment. Using elastase activity as a marker of neutrophil infiltration, there is a significant decrease in neutrophils during calcipotriol treatment. These changes are already detectable after treatment for 1 week and may precede the decrease of T lymphocytes [19]. Recently, it has been shown that calcipotriol-induced improvement of psoriasis is associated with reduced interleukin-8 and increased interleukin-10 levels in lesional skin, further supporting the idea that calcipotriol affects the immunological processes in the psoriatic skin [24].

Topical treatment of normal human skin with calcipotriol is accompanied by an increase in the VDR expression in epidermis, as revealed by Western blot analysis [25]. A similar increase of VDR protein and message has been found in cultured human keratinocytes after $1,25(OH)_2D_3$ treatment [26]. Because the in vitro responsiveness to vitamin D_3 correlates with the VDR levels, it is of interest that the induction of VDR mRNA expression in psoriatic plaques correlates with the clinical response to $1,25(OH)_2D_3$ [27].

Taken together, these results indicate that treatment with vitamin D_3 analogs has effects on the proliferation and differentiation of keratinocytes as well as on the infiltration and activation of neutrophils and immunocytes in psoriatic skin lesions. From the existing data, it is controversial whether the effect on epidermal keratinocytes precedes or is more marked than the effect on the cellular infiltrate. A primary target cell has not been identified, and it is likely that topical treatment with vitamin D_3 analogs has multiple target points in psoriatic skin.

IV. USE OF CALCIPOTRIOL AS MONOTHERAPY IN PSORIASIS

Within the past decade the effect of topical calcipotriol in psoriasis has been documented in a number of clinical trials involving several thousands of patients. Calcipotriol ointment 50 μg/g is marketed for the treatment of plaque-type psoriasis vulgaris under the trade names Daivonex®, Dovonex®, and Psorcutan®. A calcipotriol cream [28–30] and solution [31,32] have also been found to be effective. Table 1 summarizes clinical trials conducted with topical calcipotriol in psoriasis.

Table 1 Comparative Studies with Topical Calcipotriol in Psoriasis

Calcipotriol	Comparison	Outcome	References
Ointment 50 μg/g	Vehicle, calcipotriol 25 μg/g and 100 μg/g	50 μ/g better than vehicle and 25 μg/g but equal to 100 μg/g	5, 33
Ointment 50 μg/g	Betamethasone 17-valerate	Calcipotriol better than corticosteroid	35,49
	Betamethasone dipropionate		37
	Fluocinonide		38
Cream 10–100 μg/g	Vehicle	Calcipotriol better than vehicle	28, 29, 30
Cream 50 μg/g	Betamethasone 17-valerate	Calcipotriol equal to corticosteroid	36
Ointment 50 μg/g	Anthralin	Calcipotriol better than anthralin	41, 42
Ointment 50 μg/g	Tar	Calcipotriol better than tar	43, 44, 45

Figures 12.1 and 12.2 (see color insert) show psoriatic patients before and after topical applications of calcipotriol bid for 6 weeks.

A. Comparison with Placebo

In a dose-finding, randomized, double-blind, right-left comparative study, calcipotriol ointment (25, 50, and 100 μg/g) and vehicle were compared in 50 patients with psoriasis vulgaris [5]. After treatment for 8 weeks, calcipotriol 50 μg/g had a significantly greater antipsoriatic effect than vehicle. Calcipotriol 50 μg/g was more effective than calcipotriol 25 μg/g ointment, whereas no difference was found between calcipotriol 50 and 100 μg/g. From this study it was concluded that a calcipotriol concentration of 50 μg/g in an ointment is optimal for the treatment of psoriasis. Treatment with this calcipotriol concentration induces a significant improvement after only 1 week, and a marked improvement is observed in about two-thirds of patients after 8 weeks. The efficacy and safety of calcipotriol ointment 50 μg/g was later confirmed in a multicenter, double-blind, placebo-controlled, right-left study including 66 psoriatic patients [33]. When calcipotriol was used as a twice-daily treatment, the mean psoriasis is area and severity index (PASI) score fell in 4 weeks from 14.2 to 6.3 with calcipotriol and from 14.1 to 9.2 with placebo [33]. However, calcipotriol has also been investigated as a once-daily regimen in a double-blind multicenter, placebo-controlled study including 245 psoriatics evaluated over an 8-week period [34]. It was found that calcipotriol was effective and well tolerated and that it was significantly better in terms of efficacy than its vehicle as early as the first week of treatment. This difference was maintained throughout the study [34]. A once-daily regimen produces better patient compliance than the twice-daily regimens.

Other formulations of calcipotriol have been investigated. In a double-blind study [28], it was found that calcipotriol cream resulted in a statistically significant decrease in erythema, thickness, and scaling of psoriatic lesions compared with cream base alone. Calcipotriol was investigated at three different concentrations: 10 μg/g, 33 μg/g, and 100 μg/g. After 6 weeks, moderate or excellent improvement was found in 2 of 9 patients treated with 10 μg/g, 5 of 9 patients treated with 33 μg/g, and 7 of 9 patients treated with 100 μg/g of calcipotriol [28]. In another study [29], 10 inpatients with chronic plaque psoriasis, the antipsoriatic effect of calcipotriol was evaluated. In each patient two symmetrically located psoriatic plaques were selected for the study. Topical treatment with calcipotriol cream containing 1200 μg calcipotriol per gram of cream was compared with placebo cream in a double-blind, controlled, left-right, randomized way during 6 weeks of therapy. Compared with baseline, the clinical (erythema, scaling, and infiltration) improvement was significant after 1 week of therapy with calcipotriol cream, while lateral comparison showed calcipotriol cream significantly better than cream base after 4 weeks of therapy. From these studies it was concluded that calcipotriol cream is also useful in the treatment of psoriasis, although calcipotriol cream appears to be less effective than ointment.

Calcipotriol has also been investigated as a solution for scalp psoriasis (see Chapter 16). The efficacy and safety of calcipotriol solution in the treatment of scalp psoriasis were compared with those of placebo (vehicle solution) in a multicenter, double-blind, randomized, parallel-group study of 49 adult patients [31]. Calcipotriol solution (50 μg/mL) or placebo was applied twice daily over a 4-week period. At the end of the study period, 60% of patients on calcipotriol showed clearance or marked improvement of their psoriasis compared with 17% on placebo. Overall assessment of treatment response showed that calcipotriol was superior to placebo, and the solution was generally well tolerated [31]. The use of calcipotriol for scalp psoriasis was investigated in a multicenter, prospective, randomized, double-blind, parallel group study [32]. A total of 474 patients with scalp psoriasis were investigated in a twice-daily regimen and treatment was compared with betamethasone 17-valerate solution (1 mg/mL) over a 4-week treatment period. The decrease in total sign score (sum of scores for erythema, thickness, and scaliness) at the end of treatment was statistically significantly greater in the betamethasone group (61%) than the calcipotriol group (45%). Adverse events (lesional or perilesional irritation) were reported more frequently in the calcipotriol group (87 patients) than in the betamethasone group (31 patients).

From these studies it can be concluded that calcipotriol is significantly better that its vehicle. Although the two were not directly compared, it is the general impression that the ointment formulation is better than the cream and solution formulations. Furthermore, it is the impression that the effect of calcipotriol is more pronounced on lesional infiltration and scaling and less pronounced on redness.

B. Comparison with Topical Corticosteriod

The efficacy of calcipotriol has been compared with that of a number of topical corticosteroids. Calcipotriol ointment 50 μg/g has been compared with betamethasone 17-valerate ointment 0.1% in a multicenter, randomized, double-blind, right-left comparison [35]. A total of 345 patients with symmetrical stable plaque-type psoriasis were randomized to treatment for 6 weeks. Both treatments produced a time-dependent improvement, and after 6 weeks the PASI was reduced by 68.8% with calcipotriol and 61.4% with betamethasone. Recently, calcipotriol cream 50 μg/g (210 patients) was compared with betamethasone 17-valerate cream, 1 mg/g (211 patients) in a multicenter, double-blind, parallel group study [36]. It was found that both substances induced a significant reduction in PASI after 8 weeks of 47.8 and 45.4%, respectively. However, no difference was observed between the two groups. These results suggest that the efficacy of calcipotriol ointment is superior to that of the cream formulation. Calcipotriol ointment was also shown to be more effective than the potent corticosteroids betamethasone dipropionate plus salicylic acid [37] and fluocinonide [38]. In the later study, calcipotriol was compared with fluocinonide in a randomized, double-blind, parallel-group, active-controlled trial. Treatments were applied twice daily for 6 weeks. Mean scores for signs of scaling and plaque elevation in calcipotriol-treated subjects were significantly lower by week 2 than in the fluocinonide-treated subjects. These scores continued to be significantly lower than those with fluocinonide through week 6, and it was concluded that calcipotriol was superior to fluocinonide in the treatment of plaque psoriasis.

Calcipotriol monotherapy has also been compared with combination therapy calcipotriol/corticosteriods [39,40]. It was found that a combination of calcipotriol/corticosteroid was better than monotherapy alone. These results are dealt with elsewhere in this review.

Taken together, these comparative studies document that treatment with calcipotriol ointment and creme 50 μg/g is efficacious for psoriasis, with a potency comparable to that of potent topical corticosteriods.

C. Comparison with Dithranol and Tar

Calcipotriol ointment 50 μg/g has been compared with anthralin (Dithrocreme®) used either as short-contact therapy in outpatients [41] or as conventional overnight inpatient therapy [42]. In a multicenter, open, randomized, parallel-group comparison, patients were treated for 8 weeks with either calcipotriol 50 μg/g ointment applied twice daily or anthralin applied once daily for 30 min according to a short-contact regimen [41]. Both the percentages and absolute reductions of in PASI scores were significantly greater in the calcipotriol group (58.1%) than in the anthralin group (41.6%) at the end of treatment. In a study using a left-right comparative design, 10 patients hospitalized with refractory psoriasis showed a better therapeutic response to calcipotriol ointment 50 μg/g than to anthralin after 2 weeks [42]. Despite the low number of patients and the lack of follow-up, these results challenge one of the "gold standards" of antipsoriatic therapy.

Calcipotriol therapy has also been compared with tar treatment in a prospective, right/left randomized, investigator-blinded controlled study [43]. Calcipotriol 50 μg/g was applied to one-half of the body and compared with a tar solution applied to the opposite side of the body. A total of 27 patients were evaluated and it was found that a decrease in PASI score occurred on both sides at 2, 4, and 6 weeks. However, improvement was significantly better on the calcipotriol-treated side. High-dose calcipotriol (usage of an average of 377 g of calcipotriol ointment for body lesions and 100 mL solution for scalp psoriasis per week) has also been compared with topical tar/anthralin in a 4-week multicenter, prospective, randomized, open parallel-group study [44]. It was found that PASI decreased significantly more in the calcipotriol group (58.4%) than the tar/anthralin group (35.6%). Recently, calcipotriol ointment 50 μg/g was compared with a cream containing 5% coal tar/2% allantoin/0.5% hydrocortisone applied twice daily in a multicenter, randomized, controlled study [45]. A total of 122 patients participated in the study, and it was found that calcipotriol was significantly better than 5% coal tar/2% allantoin/0.5% hydrocortisone.

D. Occlusion

The therapeutic response to calcipotriol ointment can be increased by occlusion under a polyethylene film [46] or a hydrocolloid dressing [47]. Forty-eight patients with symmetrical chronic plaque psoriasis affecting the limbs were recruited for a single-blind right/left within-patient study to assess the effect of combining hydrocolloid occlusion with topical calcipotriol [47]. The combination of calcipotriol plus occlusion was significantly better than calcipotriol alone. The results indicate that occlusion improves the response to calcipotriol by enhancing its penetration. Indices of calcium metabolism remained unchanged throughout the study.

The beneficial effect of occlusion is mainly due to greater penetration and delivery of calcipotriol. Because of the risk of increased systemic absorption of calcipotriol, calcipotriol ointment should be occluded only in small areas. In particular, very thick plaques benefit from occlusive therapy.

E. Long-Term Therapy

Because psoriasis is a chronic and relapsing disease, it becomes important to determine whether the beneficial effect of calcipotriol seen in the short-term studies can be maintained when patients are treated on a long-term basis. This question has been assessed in two prospective noncomparative open studies. Included were patients who had a good clinical response to calcipotriol previously. In the first study, 15 patients from a single center were treated with calcipotriol 50 μg/g ointment twice daily (maximally 100 g ointment per week) for at least 6 months [48]. Assessment of efficacy at the end of therapy showed at least a moderate improvement in 80% of the treated patients.

These results have been confirmed and extended in a multicenter study including 167 patients [49]. In most patients, the beneficial effect seen in short-term trials was maintained over the course of 1 year. Although approximately 10% of the patients had to be withdrawn because of insufficient effect of calcipotriol, the dose required to maintain efficacy did not to have be increased with time. Thus, the mean quantity of ointment used fell from 35 g/week to 23 g/week during the last 6 months of therapy [49]. Therefore, there was no suggestion of the development of a pharmacological tolerance to calcipotriol. The major advantage of calcipotriol over corticosteroids may be that it does not induce skin atrophy during long-term treatment [49].

In a third study, the long-term safety and effectiveness of calcipotriol 0.005% ointment was evaluated in the treatment of 397 patients with stable plaque psoriasis [50]. In this multicenter open-label clinical investigation, the psoriasis characteristics of scaling, erythema, and plaque elevation and overall disease severity were evaluated periodically. At the end of the study, 235 subjects were considered assessable. Psoriatic plaques were cleared by week 8 in 25% of the subjects. The median time to initial clearing was between 16 and 17 weeks. This study showed that calcipotriol 0.005% ointment is safe and effective for long-term use in the treatment of plaque psoriasis [50].

V. CONCLUSION

Topical calcipotriol is an efficacious and safe drug for topical treatment of chronic plaque psoriasis and should be regarded as the first-line topical drug for this condition. The effects are well documented in several clinical trials. However, few reports indicate that calcipotriol can be used in other clinical presentations of the disease, such as generalized pustular psoriasis [51] and erythrodermic psoriasis [52,53].

Calcipotriol can be used on all locations of the body and is available as an ointment, a cream, and a scalp solution. The ointment formulation has been found to be the most efficacious of the three formulations. The effect of calcipotriol begins within the first week of treatment and a marked improvement occurs in most patients after 8 weeks. It is recommended that calcipotriol usage is limited to a maximum of 100 g of ointment/cream per week. In general, the average remission time after stopping calcipotriol therapy is rather short. This means that patients may require repeated treatment courses. From the long-term studies, there was no evidence of pharmacological tolerance, and no evidence of skin atrophy was observed. Furthermore, it is important to notice that calcipotriol treatment can be stopped without a resulting exacerbation of psoriasis.

REFERENCES

1. Smith EL, Walworth NC, Holick MF. Effect of 1,25-dihydroxyvitamin D_3 on the morphologic and biochemical differentiation of cultured human epidermal keratinocytes grown in serum-free conditions. J Invest Dermatol 1986; 86:706–716.
2. Kragballe K, Wildfang IL. Calcipotriol (MC903), a novel vitamin D_3 analogue stimulates terminal differentiation and inhibits proliferation of cultured human keratinocytes. Arch Dermatol Res 1990; 282:164–167.
3. Bhalla, AK, Amento EP, Clemens TL. Specific high-affinity receptors for 1,25-dihydroxy-vitamin D_3 in human peripheral blood mononuclear cells: Presence in mono-

cytes and induction in T-lymphocytes following activation. J Clin Endocrinol Metab 1983; 57:1308–1310.

4. Müller K, Bendtzen K. 1,25-Dihydroxyvitamin D_3 as a natural regulator of human immune functions. J Invest Dermatol Symp Proc 1996; 1:68–71.

5. Kragballe K. Treatment of psoriasis by the topical application of the novel cholecalciferol analogue calcipotriol (MC903). Arch Dermatol 1989; 125:1647–1652.

6. Kragballe K, Iversen L. Calcipotriol (MC903): A new topical antipsoriatic. Dermatol Clin 1993; 11:137–141.

7. Green C, Ganpule M, Harris D, Kavanagh G, Kennedy C, Mallett R, Rustin M, Downes N. Comparative effects of calcipotriol (MC903) solution and placebo (vehicle of MC903) in the treatment of psoriasis of the scalp. Br J Dermatol 1994; 130:483–487.

8. Morimoto S, Kumahara Y. A patient with psoriasis cured by 1-d-hydroxyvitamin D_3. Med J Osaka Univ 1985; 35:51.

9. Hosomi J, Hosoi J, Abe E, Suda T, Kuroki T. Regulation of terminal differentiation of mouse cultured epidermal cells by 1,25-dihydroxyvitamin D_3. Endocrinology 1983; 113:1950–1957.

10. Binderup L, Kragballe K. Origin of the use of calcipotriol in psoriasis treatment. Rev Contemp Pharmacother 1992; 23:401–409.

11. Binderup L, Bramm E. Effects of a novel vitamin D analogue MC903 on cell proliferation and differentiation in vitro and on calcium metabolism in vivo. Biochem Pharmacol 1988; 37:889–895.

12. Binderup L, Carlberg C, Kissmeyer A, Latini S, Mathiasen IS, Hansen CM. In: Norman AW, Bouillon R, Thomasset M, eds. Vitamin D. New York: de Gruyter, 1994:55–63.

13. Henriksen LØ, Kragballe K, Jensen TG, Fogh K. Transcriptional activation by 1,25-dihydroxyvitamin D_3 and synthetic vitamin D_3 analogues in transfected cultures of human keratinocytes. Skin Pharmacol 1997; 10:10–20.

14. Dam TN, Møller B, Hindkjær J, Kragballe K. The vitamin D analog calcipotriol suppresses the number and antigen-presenting function of Langerhans celle in normal human skin. J Invest Dermatol Symp Proc 1996; 1:72–77.

15. Matsouka LY, Wortsman J, Haddad J, Hollis B. Cutaneous formation of vitamin D_3 in psoriasis. Arch Dermatol 1990; 126:1107–1108.

16. Langner A, Verjans H, Stapor V, Mol M, Fraczykowska M. 1-d 25 dihydroxyvitamin D_3 ointment in psoriasis J Dermatol Treat 1992; 3:177–180.

17. Holland DB, Roberts SG, Russell A, Wood EJ, Cunliffe WJ. Changes of epidermal keratin levels during treatment of psoriasis with topical Vitamin D_3 analogue MC 903. Br J Dermatol 1990; 122:284.

18. De Mare S, De Jong EGJM, van de Kerkhof PCM. DNA content and Ks 8.12 binding of the psoriatic lesions during treatment with the vitamin D_3 analogue MC 903 and betamethasone. Br J Dermatol 1990; 123:291–295.

19. Mallett RB, Coulson IH, Purkis PE. An immunohistochemical analysis of the changes in the immune infiltrate and keratin expression in psoriasis treated with calcipotriol compared with betamethasone ointment. Br J Dermatol 1990; 123:837.

20. De Jong EMGJ, van de Kerkhof PCM. Simultaneous assessment of inflammation and epidermal proliferation plaques during long-term treatment with the vitamin D_3 analogue MC 903: Modulations and interrelations. Br J Dermatol 1991; 124:221–229.

21. Berth-Jones J, Fletcher A, Hutchinson PE. Epidermal cytokine and immunocyte responses during treatment of psoriasis with calcipotriol and betamethasone valerate. Br J Dermatol 1992; 126:356–361.

22. Nieboer C, Verburgh CA. Psoriasis treatment with vitamin D_3 analogue MC 903. Br J Dermatol 1992; 126:302–303.

23. Holland DB, Wood EJ, Cunliffe WJ, Turner DM. Keratin gene expression during the resolution of psoriatic plaques: Effect of dithranol, PUVA, etretinate and hydroxyurea regimes. Br J Dermatol 1989; 120:9–19.

24. Kang S, Yi S, Griffiths CEM, Fancher L, Hamilton TA, Choi JH. Calcipotriene-induced improvement in psoriasis is associated with reduced interleukin-8 and increased interleukin-10 levels within lesions. Br J Dermatol 1998; 138:77–83.

25. Sølvsten H, Svendsen ML, Fogh K, Kragballe K. Upregulation of vitamin D receptor levels by 1,25 dihydroxyvitamin D_3 in cultured human keratinocytes Arch Dermatol Res 1997; 289:367–372.

26. Jensen TJ, Sørensen S, Sølvsten H, Kragballe K. The vitamin D_3 receptor and retinoid X receptors in psoriatic skin: the receptor levels correlate with receptor binding. Br J Dermatol 1998; 138:225–228.

27. Chen ML, Perez A, Sanan DK, Heinrich G, Chen TC, Holick M. Induction of vitamin D receptor mRNA expression in psoriatic plaques correlates with clinical response to 1,25-dihydroxyvitamin D_3. J Invest Dermatol 1996; 106:637–641.

28. Kragballe K, Beck HI, Søgaard H. Improvement of psoriasis by a topical vitamin D_3 analogue (MC903) in a double-blind study. Br J Dermatol 1988; 119:223–230.

29. Staberg B, Roed-Petersen J, Menne T. Efficacy of topical treatment in psoriasis with MC 903: A new vitamin D analogue. Acta Derm Venereol (Stockh) 1989; 69: 147–150.

30. Harrington CI, Goldin D, Lovell CR, van de Kerkhof P, Nieboer C, Austad J, Molin L, Clareus BW, Rask-Petersen E. Comparative effects of two different calcipotriol (MC903) cream formulations versus placebo in psoriasis vulgaris: A randomized, double-blind, placebo-controlled, parallel group multi-centre study. J Eur Acad Dermatol Venereol 1996; 6:152–158.

31. Green C, Ganpule M, Harris D, Kavanagh G, Kennedy C, Mallett R, Rustin M, Downes N. Comparative effects of calcipotriol (MC 903) solution and placebo (vehicle of MC 903) in the treatment of psoriasis of the scalp. Br J Dermatol 1994; 130:483–487.

32. Klaber MR, Hutchinson PE, Pedvis-Leftick, Kragballe K, Reunala TL, van de Kerkhof PCM, Johnsson MK, Molin L, Corbett MS, Downes N. Comparative effects of calcipotriol solution (50 $\mu g/ml$) and betamethasone 17-valerate solution (1 mg/ml) in the treatment of scalp psoriasis. Br J Dermatol 1994; 131:678–683.

33. Dubertret L, Wallach D, Souteyrand P, Perussel M, Kalis B, Meyaadier J, Chevrant-Breton J, Beylot E, Bazex JA, Jürgensen HJ. Efficacy and safety of calcipotriol (MC903) ointment in psoriasis vulgaris. J Am Acad Dermatol 1992; 27:983–988.

34. Pariser MD, Pariser RJ, Breneman D, Lebwohl M, Kalb R, Moore J, Moss, H, Parker C, Fiedler V. Calcipotriene ointment applied once a day for psoriasis: A double-blind multicenter placebo-controlled study (letter). Arch Dermatol 1996; 132:1527.

35. Kragballe K, Gjertsen BT, De Hoop D, Karlsmark T, van de Kerkhof PCM, Larkö O, Nieboer C, Roed-Petersen J, Strand A, Tikjøb G. Double-blind, right-left comparison

of calcipotriol and betamethasone valerate in treatment of psoriasis vulgaris. Lancet 1991; 337:193–196.

36. Molin L, Cutler TP, Helander I, Nyfors B, Downes N. Comparative efficacy of calcipotriol (MC903) cream and betamethasone 17-valerate cream in the treatment of chronic plaque psoriasis: A randomized, double-blind, parallel group multicentre study. Br J Dermatol 1997; 136:89–93.

37. Scarpa C. Calcipotriol: Clinical trial versus betamethasone dipropionate + salicylic acid. Acta Derm Venereol Suppl (Stockh) 1994; 186:47.

38. Bruce S, Epinette WW, Funicella T, Ison A, Jones EL, Loss R Jr, McPhee ME, Whitmore C. Comparative study of calcipotriene (MC 903) ointment and fluocinonide ointment in the treatment of psoriasis. J Am Acad Dermatol 1994; 31:755–759.

39. Lebwohl M, Siskin SB, Epinette W. A multicenter trial of calcipotriene ointment and halobetasol ointment compared with either agent alone for the treatment of psoriasis. J Am Acad Dermatol 1996; 35:268–269.

40. Ruzicka T, Lorenz B. Comparison of calcipotriol monotherapy and a combination of calcipotriol and betamethasone valerate after 2 weeks' treatment with calcipotriol in the topical therapy of psoriasis vulgaris: A multicentre, double-blind, randomized study. Br J Dermatol 1998; 138:254–258.

41. Berth-Jones J, Chu AC, Dodd WAH, Ganpule M, Griffths WAD, Haydey RO, Klaber MR, Murray SJ, Rogers S, Jürgensen HJ. A multicentre parallel-group comparison of calcipotriol ointment and short-contact dithranol therapy in chronic plaque psoriasis. Br J Dermatol 1992; 127:266–271.

42. Van der Vleuten CJM, de Jong EMGJ, Ruto EHFC, Gertsen M-J P, van der Kerkhof PCM. In-patient treatment with calcipotriol versus dithranol in refractory psoriasis. Eur J Dermatol 1995; 5:676–679.

43. Tham SN, Lun KC, Cheong WK. A comparative study of calcipotriol ointment and tar in chronic plaque psoriasis. Br J Dermatol 1994; 131:673–677.

44. Van de Kerkhof PCM. Topical use of high dose calcipotriol in psoriasis does not affect bone turnover or calcium metabolic profile. 56th Annual Meeting of the American Academy of Dermatology, 1998 (abstract).

45. Pinheiro N. Comparative effects of calcipotriol ointment (50 micrograms/g) and 5% coal tar/2% allantoin/0.5% hydrocortisone cream in treating plaque psoriasis Br J Clin Pract 1997; 51:16–19.

46. Bourke JF, Berth-Jones J, Hutchinson PE. Occlusion enhances the efficacy of topical calcipotriol in the treatment of psoriasis vulgaris. Clin Exp Dermatol 1993; 18:504–506.

47. Nielsen PG. Calcipotriol or clobetasol propionate occluded with a hydrocolloid dressing for treatment of nummular psoriasis. Acta Dermatol Venereol (Stockh) 1993; 73:394.

48. Kragballe K, Fogh K, Søgaard H. Long-term efficacy and tolerability of topical calcipotriol in psoriasis. Acta Dermatol Venereol 1991; 71:475–478.

49. Ramsay CA, Berth-Jones J, Brundin G, Cunliff WJ, Dubertret L, van de Kerkhof PCM, Menné T, Wegmann E. Long-term use of topical calcipotriol in chronic plaque-type psoriasis. Dermatology 1994; 189:260–264.

50. Cullen SI. Long-term effectiveness and safety of topical calcipotriene for psoriasis. South Med J 1996; 89:1053–1056.

51. Berth-Jones J, Bourke J, Bailey K, Graham-Brown RA, Hutchinson PE. Generalized pustular psoriasis: Response to topical calcipotriol. BMJ 1992; 305:868–869.

52. Dwyer C, Chapman RS. Calcipotriol and hypercalcaemia. Lancet 1991; 338:764–765.

53. Russell S, Young MJ. Hypercalcaemia during treatment of psoriasis with calcipotriol. Br J Dermatol 1994; 130:795–796.

13
Combination Therapy: Calcipotriol and Corticosteroids

Mark Lebwohl and David J. Hecker
Mount Sinai Medical Center, New York, New York

I. RATIONALE

Superpotent topical corticosteroids have been used for many years as first-line therapy in the treatment of psoriasis. However, problems with their long-term use include the development of tachyphylaxis and such adverse effects as cutaneous atrophy, perioral dermatitis, exacerbation of rosacea, telangiectasia, striae, and hypopigmentation. If overuse of topical corticosteroids occurs either through increased frequency of application or use of occlusion, systemic effects such as suppression of the hypothalamic-pituitary-adrenal axis may be seen. In order to avoid this problem, regulatory agencies such as the U.S. Food and Drug Administration have limited the use of superpotent corticosteroids to twice daily application for 2 weeks only, followed by application on weekends only. While minimizing adverse effects, this regimen is often insufficient to maintain optimal responses in patients with chronic plaque psoriasis.

The vitamin D_3 analog calcipotriol has recently been developed as an alternative and/or adjunct topical medication in the treatment of psoriasis. At the molecular level, calcipotriol induces differentiation of keratinocytes with very little effect on calcium metabolism systemically [1,2]. In clinical trials, calcipotriol 0.005% ointment has been shown to be more effective than betamethasone valerate 0.1% ointment [3], fluocinonide 0.05% ointment [4], and short-contact anthralin therapy [5]. In direct comparison to superpotent corticosteroids, calcipotriol 0.005% ointment has been shown to be less effective than halobetasol ointment in decreasing plaque thickness after 2 weeks of application [6]. However, none of the adverse effects associated with long-term use of topical corticosteroids have been seen with calcipotriol. The main adverse effect seen with calcipotriol is local irritation, particularly when the medication is applied to the face or intertriginous areas.

Given the anti-inflammatory effect of corticosteroids, one would hope that these agents could be used to suppress irritation caused by calcipotriol. Conversely, calcipotriol could be used as a corticosteroid-sparing agent, thus preventing cutaneous atrophy, formation of telangiectasia and striae, and other undesired effects such as tachyphylaxis.

II. EFFECT OF CALCIPOTRIOL ON SKIN THICKNESS

These expectations were supported by an early study by Levy et al. who compared the effects of calcipotriol, prednicarbate, and clobetasol 17-propionate on skin thickness (epidermis plus dermis) using ultrasound [7]. Calcipotriol 50 μg/g, calcipotriol placebo ointment, clobetasol propionate ointment 0.5 mg/g, and prednicarbate ointment 2.5 mg/g were applied to the volar aspect of the forearm three times per week for 6 weeks. A fifth site was occluded without treatment. Skin thickness was measured with 20 MHz ultrasound equipment. Of 12 volunteers, 4 had to discontinue application of clobetasol because of severe signs of atrophy and telangiectasia. Clobetasol and prednicarbate resulted in dermal atrophy as measured by ultrasonography after 3 weeks. Both agents caused equivalent degrees of atrophy. Nine patients showed clinical manifestations of atrophy such as telangiectasia and blanching of the two test sites. Calcipotriol, on the other hand, resulted in an increase in skin thickness, which peaked at 3 weeks and stayed at a plateau thereafter. The increase in skin thickness seen with calcipotriol may have been due to an inflammatory infiltrate and/or edema. Ten of the volunteers has erythema and two had a papular reaction at the calcipotriol-treated site, a finding that should be expected when calcipotriol is occluded. One week after treatment, nearly all calcipotriol- and corticosteroid-induced changes normalized.

III. CLINICAL STUDIES COMBINING CALCIPOTRIOL AND
CORTICOSTEROIDS

The demonstration that calcipotriol does not thin the dermis naturally suggests that a regimen using both calcipotriol and corticosteroids is logical for the treatment of psoriasis. The steroid-sparing effect of calcipotriol might be expected to prevent or reverse any atrophy induced by corticosteroids. Conversely, the anti-inflammatory effect of corticosteroids might be expected to inhibit or reverse the cutaneous irritation that is a side effect of calcipotriol. Most importantly, because the two agents work in different ways, their effects might be additive or synergistic. In fact, Ortonne studied a regimen of calcipotriol ointment and betamethasone dipropionate ointment and found that the application of calcipotriol ointment in the morning and betamethasone dipropionate ointment in the evening was more effective than applying calcipotriol ointment alone [8].

Based on the above findings, a multicenter trial was conducted to compare the combination therapy of calcipotriol ointment and halobetasol ointment with either agent alone [6]. One hundred twenty-seven psoriatic patients were evenly divided into three treatment groups: those receiving calcipotriol ointment each morning and halobetasol ointment at night, those receiving calcipotriol ointment twice daily, and those receiving halobetasol ointment twice daily. At the end of the 2-week study, mean overall severity of psoriasis was significantly lower with combination therapy than with either agent alone. In addition, plaque thickness, erythema, and scaling were each more improved by the combination therapy than with either agent alone. In regard to local adverse effects, findings again favored the combination therapy. Of 42 patients, 3 complained of local side effects, versus 11 of 42 and 6 of 43 within the calcipotriol and halobetasol groups, respectively.

Lebwohl et al. further examined the long-term efficacy of the use of calcipotriol ointment in combination with halobetasol ointment for the treatment of psoriasis [9]. In this double-blind placebo-controlled parallel-group study, 44 patients received calcipotriol ointment in the morning and halobetasol ointment in the evening for 2 weeks. The 40 patients who achieved at least 75% improvement were subsequently divided into two treatment groups: (1) those receiving halobetasol ointment twice daily on weekends and calcipotriol ointment twice daily on weekdays and (2) those receiving halobetasol ointment twice daily on weekends and placebo ointment twice daily on weekdays. Of the patients continuing combination therapy, 76% maintained improvement of at least 75% for 6 months. Some increased their improvement further during 6 months of follow-up. Of patients applying halobetasol ointment on weekends and placebo on weekdays, only 40% maintained marked improvement, defined as 75% improved or better, for 6 months. There were significant differences between the two groups in degree of scaling, plaque thickness, and overall severity in favor of those who were maintained with calcipotriol and halobetasol ointments as compared with halobetasol ointment alone. Physician global assessments also favored weekday calcipotriol ointment and weekend halobetasol ointment over weekday placebo ointment and weekend halobetasol ointment. Differences in erythema were not significant but also favored halobetasol and calcipotriol ointments over halobetasol and placebo ointments (Figure 1A–E). None of the patients exhibited cutaneous atrophy throughout the study. In addition, only 4 of the 20 patients receiving combination therapy reported mild local irritation.

Ruzicka and Lorenz studied 169 patients in a double-blind trial in which all patients were treated twice daily for 2 weeks with calcipotriol. Thereafter, patients were randomized into two groups. In one group, 87 patients continued calcipotriol

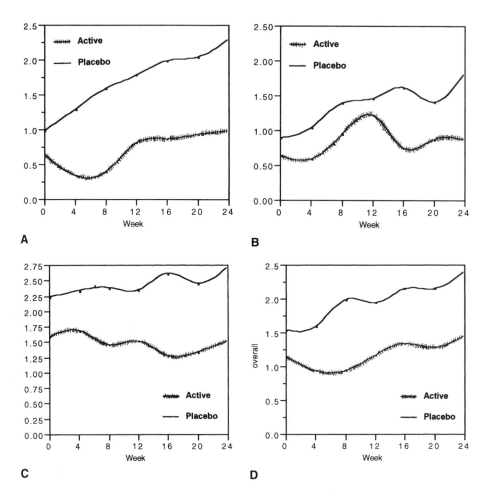

Figure 1   Following 2 weeks of therapy with halobetasol 0.05% ointment in the morning and calcipotriol 0.005% ointment in the evening, subjects were randomized into two groups. Both groups applied halobetasol 0.05% ointment twice daily on weekends only. One group (active) applied calcipotriol 0.005% ointment twice daily on weekdays, and the second group (placebo) applied vehicle twice daily on weekdays. Plaque thickness (A), scaling (B), erythema (C), overall severity (D), and global evaluations (E) were rated on a 0–3 scale. An absence of signs of psoriasis is indicated by 0; 1 indicates mild, 2 moderate, and 3 severe clinical findings.

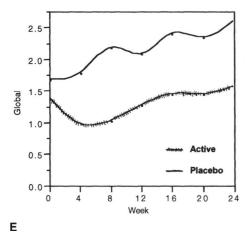

E

Figure 1 *(Continued)*

monotherapy for 4 weeks, and in the second group calcipotriol and betamethasone valerate were used for 4 weeks. Patients were followed for 8 weeks and psoriasis area severity index (PASI) scoring was used to assess the two treatments. The combination of calcipotriol and betamethasone was superior to calcipotriol monotherapy. In particular, patients who did not respond adequately to two weeks of calcipotriol monotherapy improved when the combination treatment was instituted. The authors therefore recommend that calcipotriol be combined with topical corticosteroids in patients who do not show an adequate response after 2 weeks of calcipotriol alone. The authors also pointed out an observation that has been made in many studies in which calcipotriol is combined with corticosteroids: long-term side effects of corticosteroids, including atrophy and rebound, are reduced by adding calcipotriol, and calcipotriol-induced irritation is less common when the combination therapy is used [10].

IV. MIXING CALCIPOTRIOL WITH CORTICOSTEROIDS

In both of the studies examining the use of halobetasol and calcipotriol ointments, the two drugs were applied separately, one in the morning and one in the evening. There was concern that calcipotriol, a relatively unstable chemical, would be broken down by ingredients in halobetasol. Patel et al. subsequently studied various combinations of topical preparations [11]. These investigators mixed calcipotriol 0.005% ointment with equal quantities of each of five products: 12% ammonium lactate lotion, hydrocortisone-17-valerate 0.2% ointment, halobetasol propionate 0.05% ointment, halobetasol propionate 0.05% cream, and a 5% tar gel. Salicylic acid was also added to calcipotriol to reach a concentration of 6%. Calcipotriol concentration was measured by reversed-phase high-performance liquid chromatography (HPLC) with ultraviolet detection at 265 nm. Viability of lactic acid was measured by ion-exchange HPLC using an ion-exchange column and ultraviolet detection at 214 nm. Reversed-phase HPLC with ultraviolet detection at 254 nm was used to measure hydrocortisone-17-valerate and halobetasol propionate. The mixtures were assayed at baseline and regular intervals up to 336 hr following mixing.

When mixed with hydrocortisone valerate 0.2% ointment, calcipotriol was degraded over a period of hours, with less than 50% present at 20 hr. Hydrocortisone-17-valerate was not affected for at least 72 hr. Combining calcipotriol ointment with 6% salicylic acid resulted in immediate degradation of the calcipotriol. Even after raising the pH of that mixture by adding sodium hydroxide, a combination of salicylic acid and calcipotriol was stable for only a few hours. Likewise, ammonium lactate lotion inactivated nearly a third of calcipotriol immediately upon mixing, with subsequent gradual loss of calcipotriol over the ensuing 24 hr. The concentration of lactic acid was not affected for at least 24 hr. In contrast, calcipotriol was stable when mixed with halobetasol cream or ointment for up to 13 days. Similarly, the halobetasol propionate was not affected. A 6% tar formulation (Estar®) did not degrade calcipotriol for up to 13 days as well. Future regimens will thus likely combine halobetasol ointment and calcipotriol ointment, so that each agent could be applied twice daily without any loss of effect.

V. TREATMENT OF FACE AND INTERTRIGINOUS SITES

The combination of corticosteroids and calcipotriol can play an important role in the management of psoriasis of the face and intertriginous sites. The face and intertriginous sites are particularly susceptible to corticosteroid side effects. Telangiectasia and perioral dermatitis are common occurrences in patients who use corticosteroids on the face. These are particularly common with strong corticosteroids but also occur with prolonged use of weak topical corticosteroids. Since psoriasis is a chronic condition, most therapies are used for long periods, so that the benefit of corticosteroid-sparing agents such as calcipotriol is apparent. Unfortunately, the cutaneous irritation associated with calcipotriol is more common on the face and intertriginous sites, precisely those areas where it is important to minimize use of topical corticosteroids.

In published studies, 20% of patients who use calcipotriol experience irritation on the face and the intertriginous sites. Nevertheless, some investigators have developed regimens to minimize irritation, so that calcipotriol can be used on intertriginous sites. John Koo, for example, advocates combining calcipotriol with petrolatum to reduce the cutaneous irritation that results from calcipotriol ointment alone [12]. Kienbaum et al. studied the use of calcipotriol for intertriginous psoriasis [13]. He and his colleagues studied 12 psoriasis patients in an open, uncontrolled trial of calcipotriol 0.005% ointment twice daily for 6 weeks in intertriginous sites. Five patients responded within 3 weeks or less and five responded more slowly over the 6 weeks of treatment. Of the 12 patients, 2 did not respond to this regimen. Burning occurred in one patient and irritation in five. It should not be surprising that calcipotriol treatment of intertriginous sites results in faster improvement than treatment of sites on the elbows, knees, and trunk, as similar findings have been reported with corticosteroids [14]. It should also not be surprising that cutaneous irritation is more likely to develop in these treatment-sensitive sites.

Anecdotally, we have treated 10 patients with a combination of both 0.1% mometasone furoate ointment daily and calcipotriol ointment at night for 1 week, followed by daily calcipotriol ointment application and use of mometasone furoate ointment once a day on weekends only. Marked improvement occurred in all patients within 1 week, and improvement was maintained without side effects for at least 4 weeks of follow-up thereafter. The rapid response of patients to this regimen can be attributed to the mometasone furoate, as previous studies have demonstrated that the face and intertriginous sites respond more quickly than other body sites [14].

VI. CONCLUSION

In conclusion, studies have shown that a combination regimen of calcipotriol ointment and halobetasol ointment (a superpotent topical corticosteroid) is more efficacious than either agent used alone in the treatment of chronic plaque-type psoriasis vulgaris. Further investigation regarding the use of other topical corticosteroids in combination with calcipotriol is warranted. When using corticosteroids that have not been shown to be compatible with calcipotriol, it is important that the medications are applied at different times until studies have shown that the particular topical corticosteroid used does not inactivate calcipotriol [15]. Regimens using calcipotriol and corticosteroids may be particularly useful for intertriginous sites, which are more easily irritated by calcipotriol and more susceptible to corticosteroid-related side effects. Patients who are not responsive to monotherapy with either agent alone and those who have developed tachyphylaxis in the past benefit from regimens using both calcipotriol and topical corticosteroids. These regimens may also be useful for long-term maintenance and to induce remission of psoriasis.

REFERENCES

1. Kragballe K, Wildfang IL. Calcipotriol (MC903), a novel vitamin D$_3$ analogue, stimulates terminal differentiation and inhibits proliferation of cultured human keratinocytes. Arch Dermatol Res 1990; 228:164–167.
2. Binderup L, Bramm E. Effects of a novel vitamin D analogue MC903 on cell proliferation and differentiation in vitro and on calcium metabolism in vivo. Biochem Pharmacol 1988; 37:889–895.
3. Cunliffe WJ, Berth-Jones J, Fairiss G, Goldin D, Gratton D, Henderson CA, Holden CA, Maddin WS, Ortonne JP, Young M. Comparative study of calcipotriol (MC903) ointment and betamethasone 17-valerate ointment in patients with psoriasis vulgaris. J Am Acad Dermatol 1992; 26:736–743.
4. Bruce S, Epinette WW, Funicella T, Ison A, Jones EL, Loss R Jr, McPhee ME, Whitmore C. Comparative study of calcipotriene (MC903) ointment and fluocinonide ointment in the treatment of psoriasis. J Am Acad Dermatol 1994; 31(part 1):755–759.
5. Berth-Jones J, Chu AC, Dodd WAH, Ganpule M, Griiffiths WAD, Haydey RP, Klaber MR, Murray SJ, Rogers S, Jurgensen HJ. A multicentre, parallel group comparison of calcipotriol ointment and short contact dithranol therapy in chronic plaque psoriasis. Br J Dermatol 1992; 127:266–271.
6. Lebwohl M, Siskin S, Epinette W, Breneman D, Funicella T, Kalb R, Moore J. A multicenter trial of calcipotriene ointment and halobetasol ointment compared to either agent alone for the treatment of psoriasis. J Am Acad Dermatol 1996; 35:268–269.
7. Levy J, Gassmuller J, Schroder G, Audring H, Sonnichsen N. Comparison of the effects of calcipotriol, prednicarbate and clobetasol 17-propionate on normal skin assessed by ultrasound measurement of skin thickness. Skin Pharmacol 1994; 7:231–236.
8. Ortonne JP. Psoriasis: Nouvelle modalite therapeutique par le calcipotriol plus le dipropionate de betamethasone. Nouv Dermatol 1994; 13:746–751.
9. Lebwohl M, Yoles A, Lombardi K, Lou W. A regimen of calcipotriene ointment and halobetasol ointment in the long-term treatment of psoriasis: Effects on the duration of improvement. J Am Acad Dermatol 1998; 39:447–450.
10. Ruzicka T, Lorenz B. Comparison of calcipotriol monotherapy and a combination of calcipotriol and betamethasone valerate after 2 weeks' treatment with calcipotriol in the topical therapy of psoriasis vulgaris: A multicentre, double-blind, randomized study. Br J Dermatol 1998; 138:254–258.
11. Patel B, Siskin S, Lebwohl M. Compatibility of calcipotriene with other topical medications. J Am Acad Dermatol 1998; 38:1010–1011.
12. Koo J. Diluting Dovonex. Psoriasis Forum 1995; 1(2):6.
13. Kienbaum S, Lehmann P, Ruzicka T. Topical calcipotriol in the treatment of intertriginous psoriasis. Br J Dermatol 1996; 135:647–650.
14. Lebwohl M, Peets E, Chen V. Limited application of mometasone furoate on the face and intertriginous areas: Analysis of safety and efficacy. 1993; Intl J Dermatol 32:830–831.
15. Lebwohl M. Topical application of calcipotriene and corticosteroids: combination regimens. J Am Acad Dermatol 1997; 37(3 suppl):S55–S58.

14

Calcipotriol/Calcipotriene (Dovonex/Daivonex) in Combination with Phototherapy

John Koo and Jack Maloney
University of California–San Francisco Medical Center, San Francisco, California

In the treatment of psoriasis, the use of combination therapy is common. Even if the patient is using only topical therapy, several different agents are often used simultaneously. The use of combination therapy is even more prevalent in patients who are receiving phototherapy or systemic agents. Therefore, it is not surprising that calcipotriol ointment became an adjunct to phototherapy almost as soon as it became available. The published data regarding the safety and efficacy of the use of calcipotriol with ultraviolet light are reviewed.

I. CALCIPOTRIOL WITH UVB PHOTOTHERAPY

Kragballe conducted a bilateral comparison study of 20 patients with bilateral, symmetrical psoriatic lesions [1]. One side received calcipotriol ointment twice daily, while the other side received calcipotriol ointment twice daily and UVB phototherapy three times per week. After 8 weeks, 39% of the sides treated with the combination cleared, compared with 17% of the sides treated with calcipotriol ointment alone. Owing to the small number of patients involved, the results were not statistically significant. The side effects included only a facial dermatitis in two patients.

The second report came from a study in Germany in which a Philips TL 01 narrow-band ultraviolet B (UVB) machine was used [2,3]. In this right/left bilateral comparison, calcipotriol ointment was applied on both sides daily. Only one side received UVB (at 311 nm) 5 times per week. Although the treatment period was just 2 weeks, the mean psoriasis area and severity index (PASI) reduction for the combination side was 68%, whereas the reduction with calcipotriol alone was 35% ($p < 0.001$). No significant adverse effects occurred in this study.

The third evaluation of calcipotriol with UVB was a multicenter study in Sweden, the Netherlands, and Norway [4]. A total of 101 patients were involved in an 8-week study, during which UVB phototherapy was given three times per week. By week 4, the mean reduction in PASI was 70% for the sites treated with UVB and calcipotriol and 52% in the areas treated with calcipotriol alone. By the end of the study, the combination treatment produced a mean reduction of 82%, while the areas treated with calcipotriol alone had a 70% reduction in PASI. During the follow-up period, it was noted that new psoriatic lesions occurred sooner on the sides treated with calcipotriol alone than on those treated with calcipotriol and UVB. The only side effects were mild to moderate skin irritation, which occurred equally on both sides.

The fourth study is an Italian one with a different design from those previously mentioned [5]. In this bilateral comparison study, UVB therapy was given on both sides by means of a suberythemogenic regimen three times per week. One side also received calcipotriol ointment twice per day except in the morning, when UVB radiation was given. No placebo was used on the side treated with UVB alone. Of 19 patients, 17 (89%) showed greater improvement with combination therapy than with UVB alone. Because of the small number of patients, no statistical analysis was performed. No side effects were observed during the study.

It should be noted that in all of these studies, patients were instructed to apply calcipotriol after phototherapy. This precaution probably helped to minimize any adverse interactions between the UVB and calcipotriol [6].

A Canadian multicenter study involving 164 patients with psoriasis was recently completed; this study investigated the use of calcipotriol cream plus twice-weekly UVB phototherapy versus vehicle cream plus UVB phototherapy three times weekly [7]. The UVB equipment was standardized and calibrated prior to the study, and initial UVB dosing was based on the subject's minimal erythema dose (MED). Over the treatment period of 12 weeks, the reduction in PASI was similar in the two groups, but fewer exposures were required for the group receiving calcipotriol plus twice-weekly UVB to achieve an 80% reduction in PASI score from baseline versus the comparative group (12 versus 19) as well as to achieve total clearance. Thus, in terms of cumulative UVB dosage, the patients treated with calcipotriol received a median of 1570 mJ/cm^2, compared with 5430 mJ/cm^2 in the placebo group ($p < 0.001$). Furthermore, the patients who received the twice-weekly UVB experienced significantly fewer adverse events than those who received UVB three times per week. Therefore this study demonstrates that using calcipotriol in combination with UVB phototherapy results in a decreased number of UVB exposures and lower energy density requirements.

II. CALCIPOTRIOL WITH PUVA PHOTOTHERAPY

The first and largest study of this kind was performed in France and Belgium [8]. A total of 103 patients were evaluated in a randomized, double-blind, vehicle-controlled, parallel-group study. The patients received pretreatment with either calcipotriol or vehicle for 2 weeks. For the next 10 weeks, psoralen plus ultraviolet A (PUVA) therapy was administered three times per week while the patients continued to be treated with either calcipotriol or vehicle. At the end of the treatment period, the mean reduction in PASI from baseline was 91.4% in those treated with the combination of calcipotriol and PUVA and 75.7% for those treated with vehicle and PUVA ($p = 0.013$). Of 46 patients in the combination group 40 had a PASI reduction of greater than 75%, whereas only 29 of 46 patients in the group receiving PUVA with vehicle experienced a similar degree of improvement. The mean duration of treatment required to achieve a PASI reduction $\geq 75\%$ was 22 days for those in the combination therapy group and 34 days for the patients in the other group. The cumulative UVA dose for the combination group was 30 J/cm^2 (10 irradiations), whereas for those who received PUVA and vehicle, it was 57 J/cm^2 (15 irradiations). All of these differences were statistically significant.

The second study, by Speight and Farr [9], involved 13 patients in a bilateral comparison, placebo-controlled design in which PUVA therapy was administered on both sides twice weekly; only one side received calcipotriol. After 6 weeks, the lesions treated with PUVA and calcipotriol cleared sooner than the PUVA-and-placebo sides in 7 of 11 patients. Also, the combination of PUVA and calcipotriol had a median reduction in UVA dose of 26.5%.

The third study, from Brazil, was a parallel group design, in which patients received either PUVA alone or calcipotriol with PUVA. After 8 weeks, it was once again demonstrated that the improvement in patients treated with the combination appeared to be greater than in those treated with PUVA phototherapy alone. No increase in adverse effects was noted with the combination. Owing to the small number of patients, statistical analysis was not conducted.

Finally, Lebwohl et al. [10] found that when calcipotriol was exposed to UVA or UVB radiation, there was a consistent and significant drop in the concentration of calcipotriol in the ointment after UVA irradiation but not after UVB irradiation. The UVB doses ranged from 100–150 mJ/cm^2, so there is a possibility that higher levels of UVB might decrease the concentration of calcipotriol. Also, they observed that after a thick application of calcipotriol ointment, the average MED for UVB phototherapy increased from 22.6–55.4 mJ/cm^2, whereas the amount of UVA required for immediate pigment darkening increased from 20.2–24.5 J/cm^2.

III. CONCLUSION

Both UVB and PUVA phototherapy can be enhanced by the use of calcipotriol. However, it is important to instruct patients to apply the calcipotriol after phototherapy for three reasons. First, this precaution will ensure that the calcipotriol does not impede the transmission of UV light. Second, applying calcipotriol after phototherapy will prevent the destruction of calcipotriol by the ultraviolet light. Third, it will minimize the possibility of burning sensations, which may occur in a minority of patients—especially if calcipotriol is applied just before phototherapy. The following list contains recommendations for combining calcipotriol/calcipotriene (Dovonex/Daivonex) with UV therapy:

- Calcipotriol should be applied *after* the application of UVB or UVA (for PUVA therapy), and should never be applied immediately before the application of UV light.
- If the patient applies calcipotriol more than 2 hr before the application of UV light but yet complains of burning sensations or irritation, the patient should be advised to skip the application of calcipotriol the morning before the UV light is administered.
- Since there is a limitation on how much calcipotriol can be used per week, it may be most useful to combine the treatment of calcipotriol with UV light for the more recalcitrant plaques, such as those on the shins or other parts of the lower legs.

REFERENCES

1. Kragballe K. Combination of topical calcipotriol (MC 903) and UVB radiation for psoriasis vulgaris. Dermatologica 1990; 181:211–214.
2. Kerscher M, Plewig G, Lehmann P. Kombinationstherapie der Psoriasis vulgaris mit einem Schmalspektrum UB-B-Strahler (Philips TL 01,311 nm) und Calcipotriol. Akt Dermatol 1994; 20:151–154.
3. Kerscher M, Plewig G, Lehmann P. Combination therapy of psoriasis with calcipotriol and narrow-band UVB. Lancet 1993; 342:923.
4. Molin L. Combined therapy better for psoriasis than just calcipotriol. Dermatol Times 1994; 15:3.
5. Kokelj F, Lavaroni G, Guadagnini A. UVB versus UVB plus calcipotriol (MC 903) therapy for psoriasis vulgaris. Acta Derm Venereol (Stockh) 1995; 75:386–387.
6. McKenna KE, Stern RS. Photosensitivity associated with combined UVB and calcipotriene therapy. Arch Dermatol 1995; 131:1305–1307.
7. Ramsay CA, Schwartz BE, Lowson D, Papp K, Bolduc A, Gilbert M. Calcipotriol cream combined with twice weekly broad band UVB phototherapy: a safe, effective and UVB-sparing anti-psoriatic combination treatment. Dermatology (in press).

8. Frappaz A, Thivolet J. Calcipotriol in combination with PUVA: A randomized double-blind placebo study in severe psoriasis. Eur J Dermatol 1993; 3:351–354.
9. Speight EL, Farr PM. Calcipotriol improves the response of psoriasis to PUVA. Br J Dermatol 1994; 130:79–82.
10. Lebwohl M, Hecker D, Martinez J, Sapadin A, Patel B. Interactions between calcipotriene and ultraviolet light. J Am Acad Dermatol 1997; 37:93–95.

15

Combination of Calcipotriol with Systemic Antipsoriatic Treatments

Peter C. M. van de Kerkhof
University Hospital Nijmegen, Nijmegen, The Netherlands

I. INTRODUCTION

Combination treatment is a common principle in the treatment of psoriasis [1]. Several useful combinations have been shown to have a beneficial effect. Perhaps the most time-honored approaches are ultraviolet therapy in combination with tar [2] and ultraviolet therapy in combination with anthralin [3].

This chapter focuses on combination treatment with calcipotriol and systemic treatments, in particular cyclosporine and acitretin.

II. RATIONALE FOR COMBINATION TREATMENT WITH CALCIPOTRIOL

The mode of action of calcipotriol has already been presented in Chapters 5–10. In vitro, calcipotriol affects epidermal proliferation, keratinization, and inflammation in several respects [4]. In vivo, however, the most marked effect is on epidermal proliferation and keratinization [4]. Indeed, the residual redness after successful treatment with calcipotriol is a well-known feature. Therefore, it is likely that combination treatment with calcipotriol and immunosuppressive treatments such as cyclosporine, photo(chemo)therapy, methotrexate, and topical corticosteroids is promising. Within the immunomodulatory effects of treatment, an important synergism has been demonstrated. Calcitriol was shown to augment the immunosuppressive effect of cyclosporin on interleukin-2 secretion [5]. Calcipotriol has been shown to potentiate the immunosuppressive effects of cy-

closporine in human allogeneic mixed lymphocyte and mixed epidermal cell reactions [6].

Vitamin D_3 analogs belongs to the nuclear receptor superfamily. This principle is presented in Chapter 7. Interactions of vitamin D_3 with other ligands of the
nuclear receptor superfamily have been described previously [7]. The vitamin D_3
receptor binds with the retinoid X receptor (RXR). Via this principle, vitamin D_3
interacts with retinoids having RXR as a receptor. However, the molecular actions
of retinoids and vitamin D_3 are not always understood; for example the receptor
for acitretin, the standard retinoid for psoriasis, is not yet understood. Therefore,
combination treatment with calcipotriol and acitretin is a challenge.

From a clinical point of view, combination treatment might be useful to enhance efficacy but also to minimize side effects [1]. Indeed, if the duration of treatments can be restricted or the dosages used can be reduced, the potential cumulative toxicity of the treatment is reduced. With respect to the combination of
calcipotriol with systemic treatments, the combination with cyclosporine and acitretin has been studied and experimental data are available. With respect to the
combination with methotrexate, our information is restricted to clinical experience, although an ongoing study will inform us in the near future.

III. COMBINATION OF CALCIPOTRIOL AND
CYCLOSPORINE

Cyclosporine is a highly effective treatment for patients with severe psoriasis [8].
The usual dosage of cyclosporine treatment in psoriasis is 3–5 mg/kg body weight
per day. However, side effects restrict the use of cyclosporine to severe psoriasis,
and prolonged treatment is for this reason prohibited. In particular, impairment of
kidney function implies that maintenance therapy with cyclosporine should be
avoided.

A multicenter study was carried out to evaluate the efficacy and safety of the
combination of 2 mg/kg/day of cyclosporin with calcipotriol ointment (50 μg/g
with a maximum of 125 g/week) in the treatment of severe plaque psoriasis [9].
The relatively low dosage of cyclosporine was selected in order to find out to what
extent the addition of calcipotriol might enhance the efficacy of this relatively safe
low-dose approach.

In total, 69 patients with severe plaque psoriasis were included in this double blind, multicenter investigation. One group of patients ($n = 35$) were treated
with cyclosporine in combination with calcipotriol ointment and a second group
($n = 34$) were treated with the vehicle ointment only in combination with cyclosporine. The duration of psoriasis varied between 14 and 396 months and the
psoriasis area and severity index (PASI) ranged between 6.2 and 39.6. Both
groups were comparable with respect to duration and severity of psoriasis. The

comparison—using the multicenter, prospective, randomized, double-blind parallel group approach—was made over a 6-week treatment period with a 4-week period of washout of all systemic psoriasis treatments and a 2-week period of washout of all topical antipsoriatic treatments. Patients were evaluated 1–2 weeks before randomization, at randomization, and after 2, 4, and 6 weeks of treatment. At these investigations, parameters for efficacy and safety were evaluated.

Successful treatment, defined as clearing of plaques or 90% improvement of the PASI was observed in 50% of the patients receiving the combination of calcipotriol/cyclosporine and 11.8% of the patients receiving the combination of vehicle and cyclosporine ($p = 0.0019$). Also, both groups were different, in favor of the calcipotriol cyclosporine group, with respect to the global assessment of efficacy by the patients themselves ($p = 0.005$).

Side effects were reported in 18 patients in the calcipotriol/cyclosporine group and 19 patients in the vehicle/cyclosporine group. Lesional and perilesional irritation was recorded in 22.9% of the patients treated with calcipotriol/cyclosporine and 17.6% of those treated with vehicle/cyclosporine. No patient discontinued treatment for reason of irritation. Other side effects were facial irritation, cutaneous infections, hypertrichosis, fatigue, digestive problems, and general infections. No increases in mean serum calcium were observed in either group and four patients had to decrease the dosage of cyclosporine in view of side effects.

This multicenter investigation clearly demonstrated that combination treatment of calcipotriol/cyclosporine can enhance the response to treatment. In particular, the combination treatment permits the use of a lower dose of cyclosporine and hence improves the risk/benefit ratio beyond cyclosporine monotherapy.

The combination of cyclosporine/calcipotriol can be a highly effective principle in therapeutically recalcitrant psoriasis. Recently a case was presented to illustrate the therapeutic strength of the combination (Figure 15.1, see color insert) [10]. An 83-year-old erythrodermic man was admitted to our inpatient department. The patient had had psoriasis vulgaris for 5 years. However, 6 months before the admission, his skin condition had advanced to erythrodemic psoriasis. Previous treatment for the patient with acitretin, methotrexate, oral corticosteroids, cyclosporine and the combination of cyclosporine and acitretin had not been effective. The patient then was treated with calcipotriol on the right side and the vehicle only on the controlateral side while continuing treatment with cyclosporine at a dosage of 5 mg/kg/day.

The calcipotriol-treated side showed a marked improvement as compared with the side receiving vehicle alone. After 1 week the patients entire body was treated with calcipotriol ointment twice daily on alternate days. Using this approach, the skin condition was markedly improved with up to 100 g ointment per week.

The combination of calcipotriol and cyclosporine is a useful combination with enhanced efficacy as compared with each of the monotherapies, permitting a low-dose approach of 2 mg/kg/day for cyclosporine.

IV. COMBINATION OF CALCIPOTRIOL AND ACITRETIN

Acitretin is a highly effective treatment for patients with severe psoriasis. Patients with pustular and erythrodermic psoriasis respond well to acitretin monotherapy [11–13]. Patients with chronic plaque psoriasis prove to be relatively resistant to acitretin monotherapy; only 50–60% of them showed an improvement and 30% showed an unsatisfactory response [11–13]. Therefore, acitretin is mainly used in combination with other treatments, such as ultraviolet B (UVB) phototherapy and psoralen plus ultraviolet A (PUVA) [14,15]. These combinations are well-established, highly effective principles. Although calcipotriol and acitretin both belong to the nuclear receptor superfamily, until recently no data were available on the clinical outcome of the combination as compared with monotherapy.

A multicenter, parallel group, randomized, double-blind, placebo-controlled study on safety and efficacy of calcipotriol in combination with acitretin as compared to the vehicle and acitretin was undertaken [16]. After a washout and qualification phase of 2 weeks, a double-blind phase of combined treatment followed for 12 weeks. Patients with severe psoriasis were included who had had no systemic treatment or photo(chemo)therapy for 2 weeks (12 weeks for etretinate or acitretin). A maximum of 120 g of calcipotriol ointment (50 μg/g) was permitted per week. Acitretin was started at a dose of 20 mg once daily.

The dose was increased every 2 weeks in steps of 10 mg as required until the maximum dose (70 mg/day or, in patients weighing below 60 kg, 1 mg/kg per day) was reached. Between 1 and 2 weeks before randomization, at randomization, and at 2-weekly intervals, the patients came in for investigation.

In total, 76 patients were treated with calcipotriol/acitretin and 59 patients with vehicle/acitretin. In both groups the mean duration of psoriasis was 18 years and the mean PASI before treatment was 17. As females of childbearing age were excluded in this investigation, only 35 females participated versus 100 males.

Clearance or marked improvement was reached by 67% of the calcipotriol acitretin–treated group and 41% of the patients treated with vehicle/acitretin. At the end of the treatment there was a highly significant difference between the two groups, favoring the calcipotriol/acitretin–treated patients ($p = 0.006$). The mean change in PASI in the calcipotriol/acitretin–treated group was -13.2 and in the vehicle/acitretin treated group -8.8 ($p < 0.007$). The patients' overall assessments revealed that, in comparing the two treatment groups at the end of treatment, there was a trend which appeared to favor calcipotriol therapy ($p = 0.05$).

Within the group of patients treated with the combination, the median total dose of ointment to reach clearance or marked improvement was 660.8 g calcipotriol ointment versus 1195.4 g vehicle only in the other group ($p = 0.01$). The median total dose of acitretin to reach clearing or marked improvement was 1680 mg in the calcipotriol acitretin group versus 2100 mg in the other group ($p = 0.01$).

The most frequent side effect was dryness of the skin without any difference between the two treatment groups. In total, 12% of the patients in the calcipotriol acitretin group and 22% of the patients in the vehicle-acitretin group were withdrawn due to adverse events, which was not a statistically significant difference. No significant differences were observed between the two groups with respect to any of the safety parameters.

The combination of calcipotriol acitretin has been described to be of benefit in a severe manifestation of pustular psoriasis: acrodermatitis continua Hallopeau [17].

A 73-year-old woman with a 3-year history of acrodermatitis continua Hallopeau had been treated with topical corticosteroids, crude coal tar, UVB, UVB in combination with anthralin and calcipotriol without a significant effect. Acitretin was initiated at a dosage of 35 mg/day (0.5 mg/kg). One hand and foot were treated with the vehicle only. After 1 month of combined treatment, a substantial improvement of the lesions at the vehicle-treated sites was present (Figure 15.2, see color insert). However, the calcipotriol-treated site was far more improved (Figure 15.2): pustulation had disappeared completely and only slight erythema and desquamation remained.

Combination treatment of calcipotriol-acitretin proved to be a highly effective principle, which permits a reduction of the dosage of acitretin.

V. CONCLUSION

Calcipotriol-cyclosporine and calcipotriol-acitretin are highly effective and safe combinations indicated in patients with severe psoriasis.

REFERENCES

1. Van de Kerkhof PCM. Combinations and comparisons. In: Van de Kerkhof PCM, ed. The Management of Psoriasis. Clin Dermatol 1997; 15:831–844.
2. Goëckerman WH. The treatment of psoriasis. Northwest Med 1925; 24:229–242.
3. Ingram JT. The approach to psoriasis. BMJ 1953; 2:591–594.
4. Kerkhof van de PCM. Biological activity of vitamin D analogues in the skin, with special reference to antipsoriatic mechanisms. Br J Dermatol 1995; 132:675–682.
5. Gupta S, Fass D, Shimuzi M. Potentiation of immunosuppressive effects of cyclosporin A by 1 alpha, 25-dihydroxyvitamin D_3. Cell Immunol 1989; 121:290–297.
6. Bagot M, Charve D, Pamphile R. Calcipotriol potentiates the immunosuppressive effects of cyclosporin A in allogeneic reactions. J Invest Dermatol 1991; 96:1023.
7. Carlberg K. The vitamin D_3 receptor in the context of the nuclear receptor superfamily. Endocrine 1996; 4:91–105.
8. DeRie MA, Bos JD. Cyclosporin and immunotherapy. In: Van de Kerkhof PCM, ed. Textbook of Psoriasis. Cambridge, MA: Blackwell Science, 1999:257–274.

9. Grossman RM, Thivolet J, Cloudy A, Soutegrand P, Guilhou JJ, Thomas P, Amblard P, Belaich S, Belilovsky C, de la Brassine M, Martinet C, Bazex JA, Beylet C, Combemale P, Iambert D, Ostojic A, Denouex JP, Lauret Ph, Vaillant L, Weber M, Pamphile R, Dubertret L. A novel therapeutic approach to psoriasis with combination calcipotriol ointment and very low-dose cyclosporine: Results of a multicenter placebo-controlled study. J Am Acad Dermatol 1994; 31:68–74.

10. Vleuten van der CJM, Gerritsen MJP, Steijlen PM, de Jong EMGJ, van de Kerkhof PCM. A therapeutic approach to erythrodermic psoriasis: Report of a case and a discussion of therapeutic options. Acta Derm Venereol 1996; 76:65–67.

11. Saurat JH. Side effects of systemic retinoids and their clinical management. J Am Acad Dermatol 1992; 27:23–28.

12. Gollnick H, Bauer R, Brindley C. Acitretin versus etretinate in psoriasis. J Am Acad Dermatol 1988; 19:458–469.

13. Kragballe K, Jansen CT, Geiger JM. A double blind comparison of acitretin and etretinate in the treatment of severe psoriasis. Acta Derm Venereol 1989; 69:35–40.

14. Saurat JH, Geiger JM, Amblard P. Randomized double blind multicenter study comparing acitretin-PUVA, etretinate-PUVA and placebo-PUVA in the treatment of severe psoriasis. Dermatologica 1988; 177:218–224.

15. Orfanos CE, Steigleder GK, Pullman H. Oral retinoid and UVB radiation. Acta Derm Venereol (Stockh) 1979; 59:241–244.

16. Kerkhof van de PCM, Cambazard F, Huchinson PE, Haneke E, Wong E, Souteyrand P, Damstra RJ, Combemale P, Neumann MHAM, Cholmers RJJ, Olsen L, Revuz J. The effect of addition of calcipotriol ointment (50 μg/g) to acitretin therapy in psoriasis. Br J Dermatol 1998; 138:84–89.

17. Kuijpers ALA, van Dooren-Greebe RJ, van de Kerkhof PCM. Acrodermatitis continua Hallopeau: response to combined treatment with acitretin and calcipotriol ointment. Dermatology 1996; 192:357–359.

16

Treatment of Scalp, Face, and Skin Folds with Calcipotriol

Michael R. Klaber
Royal London Hospital, London, England

I. INTRODUCTION

Psoriasis commonly affects the extensor surfaces of the skin and also the scalp. Involvement of the face is uncommon, while the flexures are usually spared except in the so-called inverse psoriasis. These three areas—the scalp, face, and flexures—constitute the "difficult areas" in psoriasis management. They are difficult to manage because the various antipsoriatic drugs have drawbacks regarding efficacy, tolerability, and/or safety.

Coal tar may be acceptable as a shampoo: as an ointment, however, it is less tolerable. This applies especially to the flexures, where coal tar ointment cannot be used because of irritancy and the risk of causing folliculitis. A cream preparation containing 10% coal tar may be used on the face without significant side effects. In the scalp, however, the severest forms of plaque psoriasis justify the use of unpleasant tar preparations such as coal tar and salicylic acid ointment.

Anthralin is even more unsuitable for the difficult areas because it causes both burning and staining. Some dermatologists still use it in the scalp—though it does stain both scalp and hair. Its use is absolutely contraindicated on the face and in the flexures.

What about topical corticosteroids? They have, after all, been the most widely used treatment for psoriasis, especially by general practitioners. Four different levels of potency are recognized: mild, moderately potent, potent, and very potent. Unfortunately, mild topical corticosteroids such as 1% hydrocortisone, although safe and well tolerated, have little or no efficacy in the treatment of psoriasis. Potent and especially very potent topical steroids, though effective in the

219

short term, are quite unsafe for use on the face, where they will cause prominent side effects including "steroid face." In the flexures, too, the degree of occlusion that the anatomy dictates means that absorption is enhanced and side effects result. The use of potent steroids on the scalp is common and is discussed below.

This leaves only the group of moderately potent corticosteroids such as clobetasone butyrate 0.05% (Eumovate (U.K.)), which may be suitable short-term treatment of flexural or facial psoriasis. However, it must be noted that these preparations cannot be considered entirely safe and must be closely monitored in these circumstances.

II. USE OF TOPICAL CALCIPOTRIOL ON THE DIFFICULT AREAS OF PSORIASIS

A. Scalp

A solution containing calcipotriol (50 μg/mL) is both safe and effective in the treatment of scalp psoriasis [1,2]. It has been compared with Betamethasone 17-valerate solution (1 mg/mL), which is the most frequently prescribed topical treatment for scalp psoriasis, and also with a shampoo containing tar, salicylic acid, and coconut oil (Capasal (U.K.)). There has also been a small trial using calcipotriol ointment on the scalp under occlusion for 5 or 10 days [3].

1. Comparative Effects of Calcipotriol Solution (50 μg/mL) and Betamethasone 17-Valerate Solution (1 mg/mL) in the Treatment of Scalp Psoriasis

A multicenter, prospective, randomized, double-blind, parallel-group study was carried out in Canada and six European countries [1]. A total of 474 patients with scalp psoriasis were enrolled and, following a 2-week washout period, were randomized to receive either calcipotriol solution or betamethasone twice daily for 4 weeks. Calcipotriol-treated patients were offered 6 weeks of further treatment if they relapsed during the 4-week observation period.

The two groups were well matched at baseline. At the end of 4 weeks, 75% of the betamethasone group were rated "clear" or "markedly improved," compared with 58% of the calcipotriol group ($p < 0.001$). Moreover, the decrease in total sign score (the sum of scores for erythema, thickness, and scaliness) was also statistically significantly greater in the betamethasone group (61%) than in the calcipotriol group (45%) ($p < 0.001$).

Adverse events—mainly lesional or perilesional irritation—occurred in 26% of calcipotriol-treated patients but in only 8% on betamethasone ($p < 0.001$). A total of 6% of the calcipotriol group and 1% of the betamethasone group withdrew from the study because of adverse events or a poor response to treatment. The serum total calcium did not change significantly in either group. The subsequent relapse rate was the same for each group; of the 69 calcipotriol-treated patients who relapsed and were retreated with calcipotriol for 6 weeks, 82% reported "a marked improvement" or "clearance."

It might appear that these results were unimpressive, since betamethasone outperformed calcipotriol, which is not only less effective but also less well tolerated. To put this in perspective, it needs to be borne in mind that most patients with psoriasis have scalp involvement—either continuously or intermittently [3]. All currently available treatments have significant drawbacks, which makes them far from ideal. They are either messy and malodorous, like tar; stain and burn, like anthralin; or produce typical corticosteroid side effects, like betamethasone. None of these drawbacks apply to calcipotriol, which is pleasant to use. Any facial irritation may be related to the solution running onto the face; care should be taken to prevent this.

2. Calcipotriol Scalp Solution Versus a Tar, Salicylic Acid, and Coconut Oil–Based Shampoo (Capasal) in Patients with Scalp Psoriasis

In this trial, 475 patients with scalp psoriasis entered an 8-week, randomized open-label study comparing calcipotriol scalp solution with a tar/salicylic acid/coconut oil shampoo [2]. Patients treated with calcipotriol scalp solution also used calcipotriol ointment for body psoriasis, while the shampoo group used a cream containing tar and hydrocortisone. At 8 weeks, 46% of the calcipotriol-treated patients had moderate improvement or better, compared with only 30% of the shampoo-treated subjects ($p < 0.001$). One hundred calcipotriol treated patients were followed up while continuing treatment for a total of 24 weeks; the reduction in total sign score was maintained throughout the follow-up. Irritation tended to occur early in the course of treatment with calcipotriol solution and to resolve or lessen subsequently during long term treatment. Calcium homeostasis was unaffected [2].

3. Five and Ten Days of Occlusive Treatment with Calcipotriol Ointment in Scalp Psoriasis

In this small open trial [4], calcipotriol ointment was applied to the scalp under occlusion overnight for either 5 or 10 days and washed out every morning. "Marked improvement" or "clearance" of scalp psoriasis was found in 85% of the 5-day group and 92% of the 10-day group. Some 12.5% experienced a degree of irritation; the serum calcium did not change. The author concluded that 5 days of occlusion with calcipotriol ointment was a suitable treatment for scalp psoriasis.

4. The Hair Root Pattern After Calcipotriol Treatment for Scalp Psoriasis

There is some evidence that hair loss may occur in scalp psoriasis [5]. Since calcipotriol is both a potent regulator of cell differentiation and an inhibitor of cell proliferation [6], it might be expected to produce hair loss. A study from the Netherlands [7] demonstrated no difference in telogen counts between patients using Calcipotriol scalp application and those on placebo. Moreoever there was no correlation between the efficacy of treatment and any change in telogen count.

B. Calcipotriol in the Treatment of Inverse (Flexural) Psoriasis

The flexures are difficult areas to treat because the degree of occlusion results in increased absorption of applied medicaments. This renders the use of potent topical corticosteroids unsafe. Topical calcipotriol causes some irritation [8] and might, therefore, be thought unsuitable for use in the flexures.

A small open German study [9] in 12 patients showed a good response using calcipotriol ointment for psoriasis in intertriginous areas. Eighty-three percent showed a significant reduction in induration and scaling after 3 weeks; by 6 weeks, there was also a significant reduction in erythema and in the area of involvement. The authors were impressed by the apparent lack of serious adverse reactions.

However, ointment bases are far from ideal in the flexures and creams are to be preferred. Another German group [10] used calcipotriol cream successfully in a number of patients who had either flexural psoriasis or sebopsoriasis.

C. Calcipotriol on the Face

Psoriasis on the face, while not common, is a cause of considerable psychological distress when present and remains a major therapeutic dilemma. Effective treatments have been unsafe or intolerable: acceptable preparations are often ineffective. At present, the data sheet advises against the use of calcipotriol on the face and warns that hands must be washed after application so as to diminish the risk of transferring calcipotriol onto the face and producing irritation.

Because of the urgent need for treatment of facial psoriasis, trials of calcipotriol have been carried out. A cream formulation has been used to treat facial psoriasis for up to 6 weeks. A mean reduction of over 50% was observed in the total sign score for redness, thickness, and scaliness. In each case the reduction was significantly greater than that observed with the cream vehicle. Both patients and investigators judged over 50% of patients to have been "cleared" or "markedly improved." Tolerance was acceptable, the most frequently reported adverse event being lesional or perilesional irritation (Leo Pharmaceuticals, personal communication).

In conclusion, calcipotriol cream, ointment, and scalp solution are the treatments of choice for psoriasis involving the difficult areas of face, scalp, or flexures. Their therapeutic ratio is high, with considerable efficacy and acceptable side effects.

REFERENCES

1. Klaber MR, Hutchinson PE, Pedvis-Leftick A, Kragballe K, Reunala TL, Van de Kerkhof PCM, Johnsson MK, Molin L, Corbett MS, Downess N. Comparative effects of calcipotriol solution (50 μg/ml) and betamethasone 17 valerate solution (1 mg/ml) in the treatment of scalp psoriasis. Br J Dermatol 1994; 131:678–683.
2. Klaber MR for the UK Study Group. Calcipotriol scalp solution (Daivonex/Dovonex) vs a tar, salicylic acid and coconut oil based shampoo (Capasal) in patients with scalp psoriasis (abstract). J Eur Acad Dermatol Venereol 1996; 6(suppl 1).
3. Green C, Ganpule M, Harris D, Kavanagh G, Kennedy C, Mallet R, Rustin M, Downes N. Comparative effects of calcipotriol (MC903) solution and placebo (vehicle of MC903) in the treatment of psoriasis of the scalp. Br J Dermatol 1994; 130:483–487.
4. Köse O. 5 and 10 days occlusive treatment with calcipotriol ointment in scalp psoriasis. J Eur Acad Dermatol Venereol 1995; 5(suppl 1):S148.
5. Shuster S. Psoriatic alopecia. Br J Dermatol 1972; 87:73–77.
6. Kragballe K. MC 903, a non-calciotropic vitamin D analogue stimulates differentiation and inhibits proliferation of cultured human keratinocytes (abstract). J Invest Dermatol 1988; 91:383.
7. Kuijpers ALA, Van Baar HMJ, Van Gasselt MW, Van de Kerkhof PCM. The hair root pattern after calcipotriol treatment for scalp psoriasis. Acta Derm Venereol (Stockh) 1995; 75:388–390.
8. Kragballe K. Treatment of psoriasis with calcipotriol and other vitamin D analogues. J Am Acad Dermatol 1992; 27:1001–1008.
9. Kienbaum S, Lehmann P, Ruzicka T. Topical calcipotriol in the treatment of intertriginous psoriasis. Br J Dermatol 1996; 135:647–650.
10. Schlehaider UK, Kowalzick L. Cream based calcipotriol for the treatment of "inverse" psoriasis and seborrhoeic dermatitis. Akt Dermatol 1996; 22:345–348.

17
Skin Tolerability of Calcipotriol

Jørgen Serup
Leo Pharmaceutical Products, Ballerup, Denmark

I. INTRODUCTION

This chapter primarily addresses calcipotriol (USAN: calcipotriene, MC903) because much knowledge has accumulated on this analog owing to its widespread use and status as an international reference drug. However, both the genuine vitamin D hormone (1,25-dihydroxy vitamin D_3), calcipotriol, tacalcitol, and a number of other analogs all seem to elicit clinically and experimentally similar skin adverse reactions, and it is likely that experience obtained with the genuine hormone and calcipotriol may be extrapolated to cover other analogs as well, although some quantitative differences may exist. The safety of calcipotriol and skin irritation with vitamin D (irritant contact dermatitis) were recently reviewed; the reader is referred to these sources of general information [1,2] and to the detailed reports on calcipotriol irritation studied in humans and in animals [3–9].

This chapter primarily addresses diagnostic assessment of the problem case showing an adverse drug reaction during calcipotriol therapy. A primer of diagnostic assessment is proposed and the pros and cons of such assessment are outlined.

II. CLINICAL MANIFESTATIONS OF CUTANEOUS ADVERSE REACTIONS TO CALCIPOTRIOL

The dominating manifestation is irritant contact dermatitis of the cumulative type with a debut 4–6 weeks after initiation of the treatment. The dermatitis may be lesional, confined to the psoriatic plaque treated, and/or perilesional in which case the normal-appearing skin around the plaque is also involved. A scaly demarcation line toward unaffected skin is characteristic. The face is especially sensitive to irritation. Skin irritation (in some studies reported as total number of local adverse events) was recorded in 4–25% of patients in 11 studies performed from 1989–1995 [10], but only a few dropped out because of irritation.

Registrational studies operating with a fixed protocol, however, do not directly reflect clinical practice. A German postmarketing surveillance study among 1664 patients and 339 dermatologists showed only 4.7% drug-related local adverse events during calcipotriol treatment [11]. This is probably closer to a general figure during practical use of calcipotriol. Nevertheless, even if irritant contact dermatitis to calcipotriol is relatively uncommon, occasional cases of alarming irritant skin reactions are expected to occur with a drug such as calcipotriol, used by millions of patients worldwide. Such very special cases are typically those where the dermatologist suspects allergic sensitization and wishes to conduct diagnostic testing in his or her professional search for clarification of the case as a prerequisite for a proper future treatment strategy or for the purpose of academic interest.

III. MECHANISM OF ADVERSE REACTIONS

Cumulative irritant contact dermatitis is, as mentioned, dominating and by far commonest. The mechanism is believed to be a direct effect on the epidermis and the vasculature in the rete papillae with no specific involvement of the immune system. Irritant reactions are characterized by redness followed by some edema, papules, and possibly vesicles (Figure 17.1, see color insert). Clinical manifestations due to irritation cannot be distinguished from manifestations expected to occur in allergic reactions. The fact that an adverse reaction is alarming; appears after 4–6 weeks of treatment (normally needed for primary allergic sensitization to take place, but also for cumulative irritation to escalate); and shows redness, papules, and vesicles is in itself no proof of allergy (Figure 17.2, see color insert). It is more likely to represent irritation with progressive skin barrier disruption due to abrupt and direct exposure of deeper skin layers to the irritant drug.

Calcipotriol is not primarily a corrosive irritant [4,5,7]. Transepidermal water loss (TEWL) is increased only as a secondary event in protracted or advanced reactions [8]. Initial reactions are red with increased a* by colorimetry and with increased blood flow.

Constitutional and environmental factors (i.e., the inbuilt tolerance toward a vitamin D substance, season of the year, mental stress and other typical predisposing factors in irritant contact dermatitis) are also expected to modulate adverse reactions to calcipotriol, although this has not been shown directly.

Interestingly, it was recently shown that irritation to calcipotriol in the scalp is less when patients receive simultaneous treatment with the antifungal itraconazole. Thus, *Pityrosporum ovale* overgrowth may play a role in D-vitamin irritation on the scalp (Leo data, to be published).

There is no known easy predictor of a vitamin D–sensitive person especially prone to irritation, although special persons with such special constitution and increased risk are likely to exist. Testing should aim to identify such individuals with delicate skin.

The irritation potential of various vitamin D analogs (about 90 studied) does not correlate with vitamin D receptor affinity or in vitro effects on cell proliferation (Leo, data on file). The genuine vitamin D hormone, calcipotriol, and tacalcitol are concluded to be equally irritant when tested in similar dose, and initial claims that tacalcitol was less irritant were not confirmed [5]. A clinical study with open application indicated that tacalcitol in a low dose may be more irritant than calcipotriol in a higher dose [12]. In patch testing with the three substances, cross-irritation is foreseeable [5].

A few reports on allergic reactions or possibly allergic contact dermatitis due to calcipotriol and tacalcitol have appeared in the literature [13–24], based on the testing of selected cases with alarming symptoms. With today's knowledge about pitfalls in patch testing with vitamin D, no case of verified allergic sensitization has been reported. A case of calcipotriol-induced dermatitis claimed to be "unequivocal" allergy was published recently [24a]. However, patch test reactions to calcipotriol lower than 2 μg/ml were 0 or ?+ (compare with Figures 3 and 4). Although allergy may appear likely, irritant reactions in a person with especially delicate skin remain to be excluded.

The allergy patch test described by Jadassohn in 1896 remains a crude experiment and not a real test with acceptable predictive values of positive and negative findings, albeit in the hands of qualified dermatologists it is a helpful adjunct to other sources of diagnostic information. Calcipotriol and D vitamins in general may not be suited for patch testing at all because of their well-known irritant effect on skin, with reactions that easily mimic allergic manifestations. Thus, a statement that a patient with adverse reaction to calcipotriol, tacalcitol, or some other analog of vitamin D by the use of patch testing is concluded an "unequivocal case of allergy" is not justified and not academically correct simply because no validated test of vitamin D allergy exists and since such allergy testing of known irritant substances is from the beginning controversial. Only inconclusive statements such as "doubtful," "possible," or "likely allergic sensitization" are academically acceptable.

In order to establish a diagnosis of "likely allergic sensitization" to any substance, the classical premises should be fulfilled: a relevant past and present exposure, manifestations in conformity with expected manifestations of allergy, hyperreactivity to low exposure normally tolerated by healthy individuals (availability of a proper control series of healthy individuals), specificity of this hyperreactive mode of reaction, in principle lifelong memory of that specific hyperreactivity or at least a demonstration that the abnormal hyperreactivity is reproducible after a certain time lapse—for example, of some months. These prerequisites are surrogates of a specific activation of the immune system involving T cells that is difficult or impossible to measure directly and reliably.

Thus, for practical reasons and as key information, the threshold of nonirritation in healthy individuals both need to exist and to be known (and such a threshold may show geographical, climate, seasonal, racial, etc., variation). Reproducibility of findings on repeated testing should also be documented. Such essential basic knowledge is crucial for the patch-test procedure to be a valid test and is not available with regard to calcipotriol and other D vitamins, although the contour of the dose-irritation curve of healthy skin is outlined (see below).

In a recent study of patch testing with a dilution series of calcipotriol, 179 healthy individuals never exposed to calcipotriol before and therefore known *not* to be allergic to this test compound were studied [6]. Irritant patch-test reactions showed similar findings, with redness, papules, and even vesicles, as known from allergic patch-test reactions (Figure 17.1). Reactions declined between a 48- and 72-hr reading. Readings of 1+ and doubtful reactions were common (Figure 3) and not convincingly related to the dose applied, with 1+ reactions observed even at very low exposure. Reactions of 2+ were few and observed only at a dose over 2 μg/ml, but such strong reactions might easily occur at a lower concentration if the study population had been bigger, since 1+ reactions were noted at very low exposure. Measurement of erythema by colorimetry and cutaneous blood flow by laser Doppler flowmetry, however, both demonstrated a dose irritation relationship, and a test dose of 2 μg or less may represent some threshold toward baseline reactivity (Figure 4). Nevertheless, it was not possible to define a distinct threshold of nonreactivity despite the use of advanced bioengineering techniques. Similar observations were made in a previous study of 30 healthy Japanese persons, indicating no racial difference in spontaneous reactivity [25]. A patch-test study from Spain with the ointment product (published papers says cream, later corrected) showing very low irritancy remains unexplained [26].

An allergy patch experiment with calcipotriol will always carry a high risk of false-positive readings and erroneous conclusions and the test will not be able clearly to distinguish between individuals who were truly allergic and individuals who were uniquely delicate cases, with possibly alarming clinical symptoms of irritant contact dermatitis, appearing as selected cases among the very many patients treated with this first-line antipsoriatic drug. In patch testing of special cases with alarming symptoms, a control group of only some 10–20 healthy individuals will never be adequate to support any conclusion for simple epidemiological and statistical reasons. A large control sample is required because the case with alarming dermatitis is a highly selected individual, a psoriasis sufferer with an abnormal threshold.

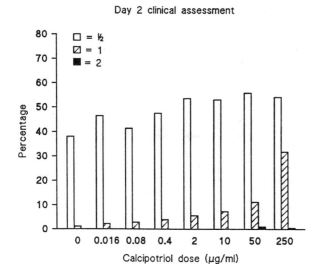

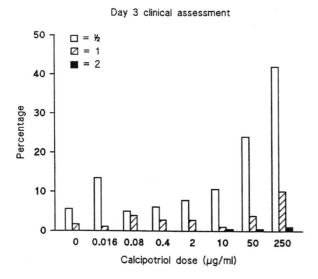

Figure 3 Clinical reading of irritant patch-test reactions in 179 healthy volunteers not previously exposed to calcipotriol and therefore not allergic, studied with 24 hr occlusive application of a dilution series of calcipotriol in alkaline-buffered isopropanol. (From Ref. 6.)

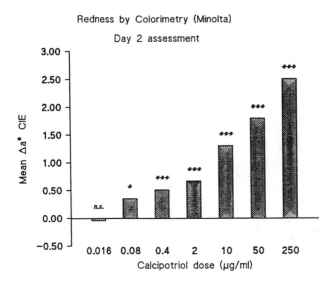

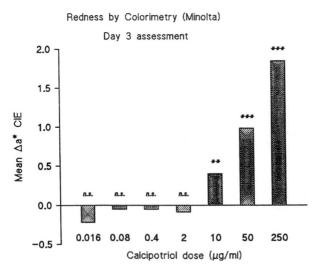

Figure 4 Same study as in Figure 4. Measurement of redness with a Minolta Chromameter. Measurement of cutaneous blood flow with laser Doppler flowmetry shows similar results. (From Ref. 6.)

IV. A TENTATIVE PRIMER TO DIAGNOSTIC EVALUATION IN ADVERSE DERMATITIS WHERE ALLERGY TO CALCIPOTRIOL IS SUSPECTED

Diagnostic evaluation may be conducted to answer the practical question of whether the patient, irrespective the mechanism of dermatitis, can or cannot use calcipotriol in the future for his or her psoriasis and/or to envisage the academic question about allergic sensitization as a possible or likely cause of dermatitis.

Initially it should be ensured that

1. The past and present exposure to calcipotriol is relevant.
2. Simple irritant contact dermatitis is unlikely albeit possible, and further clarification of the case is needed in order to decide whether the patient shall stop or continue the treatment, and if the patient stops if the drug can or cannot be given again on some later occasion, or maybe combined with other therapy.
3. The history should indicate that there is an abnormal hyperreactivity state—i.e., relative to the doctor's general experience with calcipotriol (which is relevant, based on treatment of other psoriasis sufferers and not on treatment of healthy individuals).
4. If additional testing is decided primarily a repeated open application test (ROAT test) should be performed on antecubital skin with two applications of the calcipotriol final product (the formulation actually used by the patient) daily for 7 days or alternatively 5 days, and reading on day 7 and 5, respectively [27]. The contralateral side may be treated the same way with the vehicle obtained from the manufacturer. If positive (1 + reactions or more) the test indicates intolerance to the product and it may be decided, depending on a contralateral vehicle experiment, if this intolerance is related to calcipotriol or to its vehicle. The ROAT experiment even conducted without a placebo control may help the doctor to decide if the patient can continue with calcipotriol, if the patient has to stop with calcipotriol, or if the patient perhaps should stop with calcipotriol for a limited time only and the treatment could be supplemented with or combined with a topical corticosteriod. The ROAT test will *not* allow the doctor to draw a conclusion as to whether intolerance is of allergic or irritant nature, although a very strong reaction might be indicative of the former. In this case additional patch testing may be decided on.
5. An occlusive patch experiment with a dilution series of calcipotriol 50–0.016 μg/ml in alkaline buffered isopropanol may be performed on the back using standard occlusion chambers such as the Finn chamber and paper disks, left for 24 hr. and read after 72 hr. Test so-

lutions may be requested from the manufacturer. Doubtful and 1+ readings are of no importance, since calcipotriol is an irritant that often induce such reactions in healthy volunteers (see Figure 3). Reactions of 2+ at 2 μg/ml or lower would demonstrate that the patient is hyperreacting to calcipotriol, and the patient should probably not be treated with calcipotriol in the future but considered an especially vulnerable individual. Although 2+ or 3+ reactivity at very low concentration might speak in favor of an allergic sensitization, the individual is still more likely to be a case especially sensitive to calcipotriol as an irritant.

6. Any testing where allergy is in question should be repeated after a minimum of 3 months to demonstrate reproducibility and "memory" of reactivity.

The test procedure above would allow the dermatologist to conclude whether the patient is or is not hyperreactive to calcipotriol and to decide about the future use of calcipotriol and the treatment strategy for that particular patient. Moreover, the test procedure might give the dermatologist some evidence as to whether allergic sensitization is possible or even likely, upon summing up and evaluating all the information the dermatologist can obtain about the problem case, which is then carefully and professionally analyzed.

A. The Lymphocyte Transformation Test

This in vitro test depends on the proliferative response measured by thymidine incorporation of lymphocytes exposed to the suspected antigen, but since the D vitamins may both down- and upregulate cell proliferation, depending on culture conditions [28–30], and since the test despite 20 years of use, is not validated either generally for contact allergy diagnosis or specifically with respect to calcipotriol, results of this test are easily misleading. The test should be used only with much reservation. The test laboratory should conduct the proper validation experiments and conclude the test to be valid prior to any conclusive statement. Hitherto lymphocyte transformation control experiments with allergic patients and healthy controls have included five or fewer individuals in the study groups—too few for any conclusion.

V. INTOLERANCE TO THE VEHICLE

In the registrational studies, adverse irritant contact dermatitis to the placebo ointment, placebo cream, and placebo solution were registered [10]. There are in such studies certain levels of "background noise" in the reporting; however, it is likely that at least some cases may not tolerate the vehicle well. Ingredients of the calcipotriol vehicles are given in Table 1. The ingredients are traditional. It was shown at least for the ointment vehicle that when applied under occlusion, this vehicle acts as a mild, corrosive irritant [3]. Mild corrosiveness of vehicles may be desirable to enhance the penetration of the drug into the skin. Propylene glycol as

Table 1 Composition of Calcipotriol Ointment, Cream, and Solution

Calcipotriol ointment
Calcipotriol 50 μ/g
Sodium dihydrogen phosphate
Liquid paraffin
Polyoxyethylene stearyl ether (Brij 72)
Propylene glycol[a]
Sodium edetate
DL-α-tocopherol
Water, purified
White soft paraffin
Calcipotriol cream
Calcipotriol 50 μg/g
Cetomacrogol 1000
Cetostearyl alcohol
Disodium hydrogen phosphate
Germall II + Myacide SP (preservatives)*
Glycerol
Disodium edetate
Liquid paraffin
White soft paraffin
Water, purified
Calcipotriol scalp solution
Calcipotriol 50 μg/ml
Hydroxypropylcellulose
Isopropanol[b]
Menthol
Sodium citrate
Propylene glycol[c]
Water, purified

[a] 10%.
[b] 40%.
[c] 4%.
*In the United States. Preservative in Europe: Dorvicil 200 (only).

solvent and enhancer is commonly used in pharmaceutical vehicles; it is a well-known irritant and allergen and has also been described as a reason for dermatitis during calcipotriol ointment treatment [31]. Also isopropanol contained in the solution vehicle may be a reason for alcohol-induced irritation, dominated by dryness and fissuring.

Irritant properties of a vehicle can sometimes be related to just one component—for example, propylene glycol, the alcohol solvent as mentioned above, or the emulsifier. Testing of problem cases with individual vehicle ingredients has resulted in positive readings with propylene glycol, the emulsifier, and even paraffin oil (Leo, data on file). No single component that could explain the majority of the vehicle adverse reactions has been identified.

Probably vehicle adverse reactions are typically not related to a single ingredient but rather to the formulation as a whole or a few ingredients working together. For example, studies in hairless mice and humans have indicated that the enhancers propylene glycol and isopropyl myristate may be tolerated well when applied undiluted on the skin, while they may cause irritation in alcoholic dilution even using a low concentration of the enhancer (Leo, data on file). Enhancers do not selectively enhance the penetration of the active substance, but they may easily enhance constituents of the vehicle as well, exaggerating the damaging effect of such constituents.

Testing adverse reactions to a vehicle is complicated. A test with application of the complete vehicle, either as a 48-hr or 24-hr occlusive patch may be practiceable; or a chamber scarification test; or a 3-week cumulative open application. Testing of single ingredients may easily be misleading. It is an open question which test concentration and which solvent to use. There is no "gold standard" for the testing of vehicle ingredients with respect to irritancy and allergy, although some guidance may be found in the literature and in the monographs of Bandman and Dohn and of de Groot [32,33].

The relevant question in the clinic of whether a problem case is intolerant to calcipotriol or to the vehicle can normally be solved simply by testing the complete placebo vehicle in parallel with testing of the final product with the active substance included. The testing can be performed in parallel with occlusive application of a calcipotriol dilution series and/or the final product as described above, and in parallel to the ROAT testing of the final product on the antecubital skin, with vehicle on the contralateral side.

A relevant testing to identify problem ingredients is probably a stepwise elimination of single vehicle ingredients one by one, maintaining the basic formulation and its hydrophilic and lipophilic phases as far as possible. Such stepwise procedure for testing of ingredients of the ointment has been used; see Table 2 (can be requested from the manufacturer).

A schematic review of test procedures is given in Table 3.

Table 2 Stepwise Testing of the Calcipotriol Ointment Vehicle[a]

Sample 1:	Vaseline + paraffin oil
Sample 2:	Vaseline + paraffin oil + Brij72 (emulsifier)
Sample 3:	Ointment vehicle with propylene glycol avoided
Sample 4:	Ointment vehicle with the phosphate buffer avoided
Sample 5:	Ointment vehicle with any component included
Product:	Ointment vehicle with calcipotriol 50 μg/g included

[a] Samples for patch testing of the calcipotriol ointment vehicle with the single ingredients avoided one by one.

VI. NOTIFICATION OF ADVERSE REACTIONS

Adverse reactions should be reported to national health authorities and to the manufacturer.

The manufacturer is obliged to conduct postmarketing surveillance and to have an updated register on adverse reactions to the product. Manufacturers are always interested in knowing about the performance of their product and to implement necessary refinements.

Table 3 Schematic Review of Diagnostic Procedures in the Assessement of Patients with Adverse Dermatitis During Calcipotriol Treatment with Ointment or Cream Formulations[a]

1. *Check patient's history* and past and present exposure to the product and exclude other reasons for dermatitis.
2. Conduct a 7- (or 5-) day *repeated open application test* (*ROAT*) with the commercial product used by the patient, twice daily, antecubital skin, reading day 7 (or 5). If possible conduct simultaneouosly a ROAT on the contralateral side with the calcipotriol placebo.

Decide future treatment of the patient, and proceed with optional testing only if necessary.

3. *Optional, calcipotriol suspected to be causative: occlusive 24-hr patch experiment on the back* with a dilution series of calcipotriol (50–0.016/0 μg/ml) in alkaline buffered isopropanol. If possible also apply patches with the calcipotriol ointment product, the ointment placebo, the calcipotriol cream product, and the cream placebo. Reading after 72 hr. Reference for reading see Fig. 3. Readings ?+ and 1+ are of no importance, and only 2+ and 3+ readings may indicate hyperreactivity.
4. *Optional, vehicle suspected to be causative.* Test selected ingredients under occlusion only if special suspicion arise. *Such test is individual.* A stepwise testing of the ointment vehicle is proposed (Table 2).

[a] For interpretation of test results, see text. Testing should always be repeated after a minimum of 3 months if allergy is in question.

REFERENCES

1. Serup J. Safety of and skin irritation with vitamin D. In: Roenigk HH, Maibach HI, eds. Psoriasis. New York: Marcel Dekker, 1998: 519–526.
2. Serup J. The spectrum of irritancy and applications of bioengineering techniques. In: Elsner P, Maibach HI, eds. Irritant Dermatitis: New Clinical and Experimental Aspects. Vol 23. Basel: Karger, 1995:131–143.
3. Fullerton A, Avnstorp C, Agner T, Dahl JC, Olsen LO, Serup J. Patch test study with calcipotriol ointment in different patient groups, including psoriatic patients with and without adverse dermatitis. Acta Derm Venereol (Stockh) 1996; 76:194–202.
4. Fullerton A, Serup J: Characterization of irritant patch test reactions to topical D vitamins and all-trans retinoic acid in comparison with sodium lauryl sulphate: Evaluation by clinical scoring and multiparametric non-invasive measuring techniques. Br J Dermatol 1997; 137:234–240.
5. Fullerton A, Serup J: Topical D-vitamins: Multiparametric comparison of the irritant potential of calcipotriol, tacalcitol and calcitriol in a hairless guinea pig model. Contact Dermatitis 1997; 36:184–190.
6. Fullerton A, Vejlstrup E, Roed Petersen J, Birk Jensen S, Serup J. The calcipotriol dose-irritation relationship: 48 hour occlusive testing in healthy volunteers using Finn chambers. Br J Dermatol 1998; 138:259–265.
7. Arafat SM, Turner RJ, Marks R: The irritant effect of topically applied vitamin D_3 analogue (calcipotriol), a placebo controlled, double blind, randomised study. Br J Dermatol 1995; 133(suppl 45):36.
8. von Brenken S, Proksch E. Calcipotriol and 1,25dihydroxyvitamin D_3 impair barrier function in normal mouse skin and in normal human skin. Arch Dermatol Res 1994; 286:157
9. Thieroff-Ekerdt R, Gerhard D, Hartung A, Krause A, Wiesinger H. Erythema induction by calcipotriol: A vitamin D receptor-mediated effect? Arch Dermatol Res 1994; 286(3/4):159.
10. Berth-Jones J: Calcipotriol in dermatology: A review and supplement. Br J Clin Pract 1996; 83(suppl):1–32.
11. Friedmann D, Schnitker J, Schroeder G. Efficacy and tolerability of calcipotriol ointment, proven in the course of a drug monitoring in 1664 patients. ESDR Symposium: Vitamin D, Actions and Applications in Dermatology, Århus, Denmark, 1995; April 27–29 (abstract).
12. Veien NK, Bjerke JR, Rossmann-Ringdahl I, Jakobsen HB. Once daily treatment of psoriasis with tacalcitol compared with twice daily treatment with calcipotriol: A double-blind trial. Br J Dermatol 1997; 137:581–586.
13. Yip J, Goodfield M. Contact dermatitis from MC903, a topical vitamin D_3 analogue. Contact Dermatitis 1991; 25:139.
14. Bruynzeel DP, Hol CW, Nierboer C. Allergic contact dermatitis to calcipotriol. Br J Dermatol 1992; 127:66.
15. de Groot AC. Contact allergy to calcipotriol. Contact Dermatitis 1994; 30:242–243.
16. Steinkjaer B. Contact dermatitis from calcipotriol. Contact Dermatitis 1994; 31:122.
17. Schmid P. Allergisches Kontaktekzem auf calcipotriol. Akt Dermatol 1995; 21:401–402.

18. Garrigue JL, Nicolas JL, Demidem A, Bour H, Viac J, Thivolet J, Schmitt D. Contact sensitivity in mice: Differential effect of vitamin D_3 derivative (calcipotriol) and corticosteroids. Clin Immunol Immunopathol 1993; 67:137–142.

19. Kimura K, Katayama I, Nishioka K. Allergic contact dermatitis from tacalcitol. Contact Dermatitis 1995; 33:441–442.

20. Molin L. Contact dermatitis after calcipotriol and patch test evaluation. Acta Derm Venereol (Stockh) 1996; 76:163–164.

21. Giordano-Labadie F, Laplanche G, Bazex J. Eczéma de contact au calcipotriol. Ann Dermatol Venereol 1996; 123:196–197.

22. Garcia-Bravo B, Camacho F. Two cases of contact dermatitis caused by calcipotriol cream. Am J Contact Dermatitis 1996; 7:118–119.

23. Zollner TM, Ochsendorf FR, Hensel O, Thasi D, Diehl S, Kalveram CM, Boehncke W-H, Wolter M, Kaufmann R. Delayed-type reactivity to calcipotriol without cross-sensitization to tacalcitol. Contact Dermatitis 1997; 37:251.

24. Fleming CJ, Burden DA. Contact allergy in psoriasis. Contact Dermatitis 1997; 36:274–276.

24a. Frosch PJ, Rüstemeyer T. Contact allergy to calcipotriol does exist: report of an unequivocal case and review of the literature. Contact Dermatitis 1999;40:66–71.

25. Mayakawa R, Ukei C, Suzuki M, Ogino Y, Fujimoto Y. Results of a dermal safety study of MC903 ointment incorporated with an active vitamin D_3 analogue. Skin Res 1993; 35:108–116.

26. Vilaplana J, Mascaro J, Lecha M, Romaguera C. Low irritancy of 2-day occlusive patch test with calcipotriol. Contact Dermatitis 1994; 30:45.

27. Hannuksela M, Salo H. The repeated open application test (ROAT). Contact Dermatitis 1986; 14:221–227.

28. Gniadecki R. Vitamin D—A modulator of cell proliferation. Retinoids 1997; 13:55–59.

29. Gniadecki R. Activation of faf-mitogen-activated protein kinase signaling pathway by 1,25-dihydroxyvitamin D_3 in normal human keratinocytes. J Invest Dermatol 1996; 106:1212–1217.

30. Gniadecki R. Bidirectional regulation of keratinocyte growth by 1,25-dihydroxyvitamin D_3: Stimulation and inhibition of growth dependent on the degree of cell differentiation. J Invest Dermatol 1996; 106:510–516.

31. Fisher DA. Allergic contact dermatitis to propylene glycol in calcipotriene ointment. Cutis 1997; 60:43–44.

32. Bandmann H-J, Dohn W. Die Epicutantestung. Munich: Verlag Bergmann, 1967.

33. De Groot AC. Patch Testing, Test Concentrations and Vehicles for 3700 Chemicals, 2d ed. New York: Elsevier, 1994.

18
Safety of Calcipotriol

John F. Bourke
South Infirmary–Victoria Hospital and University College Cork, Cork, Ireland

I. INTRODUCTION

The principal concern about the toxicity of calcipotriol is the potential for vitamin D toxicity. Calcipotriol was developed as an analog of 1,25dihydroxyvitamin D_3 (calcitriol), with much weaker effects on systemic calcium homeostasis. Although it binds to the vitamin D receptor as avidly as calcitriol, it was found in animal studies to have a 100- to 200-fold weaker effect on systemic calcium homeostasis [1]. This feature is presumed to hold true in humans, although human comparative studies have not been carried out. Other potential problems include local adverse effects (Chapter 17), teratogenicity, differential effects on any aspect of calcium homeostasis, and interaction with other treatment modalities.

Data on the safety of calcipotriol derive from three sources; in vitro studies, animal studies, and studies in humans.

II. IN VITRO STUDIES

A. Calcium Homeostasis and Cell Differentiation

Calcipotriol was first synthesised by Calverley [2] in 1987, while Leo laboratories were searching for a suitable alternative to calcitriol with less effect on systemic calcium homeostasis. It is a synthetic analog of vitamin D characterized by a terminal cyclopropyl ring and a 24- rather than a 25-hydroxyl group. The mode of action and potency of calcipotriol appear to be identical to those of 1,25-dihydroxyvitamin D_3. It combines with the vitamin D receptor in the same manner as calcitriol and binds as avidly as calcitriol in vitro [3]. It has also been shown in vitro to be equipotent to calcitriol in many respects.

Calcipotriol is a potent inhibitor of proliferation and promoter of differentiation of U937 lymphoma cells [1]. It has also been shown to promote differentiation and to inhibit proliferation of mouse and human keratinocytes [4]. Calcipotriol has been found to inhibit osteoblast-like cell proliferation [5], increase osteocalcin and alkaline phosphatase activity [6], and stimulate osteoclast-like cell formation in human bone marrow cultures [7] in a similar manner to 1,25-dihydroxyvitamin D_3.

Only two groups have demonstrated any differences in vitro between 1,25-dihydroxyvitamin D_3 and calcipotriol. Norman et al. [8] found that calcipotriol had a much weaker effect than 1,25-dihydroxyvitamin D_3 on acute gastrointestinal calcium absorption in vitro. Using an isolated loop of chick intestine, this group assessed the effects of a variety of vitamin D analogs and metabolites on the early phase of intestinal calcium absorption, which they have suggested is a process independent of the vitamin D receptor. Calcipotriol, which is referred to as BT in their work, was found to be weaker than 1,25-dihydroxyvitamin D_3. What this means in vivo is uncertain, but it could conceivably lead to an imbalance of vitamin D activity with increased resorption of calcium from bone without the associated increase intestinal absorption of calcium.

The second paper to demonstrate a differential effect on some aspects of vitamin D activities was that by Naveh-Many et al. [9]. This group reported a differential suppressive effect of calcipotriol on PTH mRNA production in vitro by bovine parathyroid cells. They found that calcipotriol was less effective by a factor of approximately 10 as compared to both 1,25-dihydroxyvitamin D_3 and oxacalcitriol. The clinical significance of this finding is also uncertain.

B. Carcinogenicity

Reverse mutation and chromosome abberation studies on calcipotriol in vitro have shown no evidence of mutagenicity [10].

C. Summary

In summary, most in vitro studies of calcipotriol have shown it to be very similar to 1,25-dihydroxyvitamin D_3 in range and potency of effects. Two studies have demonstrated a weaker effect in some areas of calcium homeostasis that might have clinical significance.

III. ANIMAL STUDIES

A. Calcium Homeostasis

Calcipotriol has been shown to have a much weaker effect on systemic calcium homeostasis in animals. Oral, intravenous, and intraperitoneal injection of calcipotriol in rats has a 100- to 200-fold weaker effect on systemic calcium home-ostasis than injection calcitriol [1]. This has been confirmed by further studies comparing the effects of calcipotriol with that of a variety of vitamin D metabo-lites and analog [11]. Topical administration to rats revealed a similar reduction in toxicity in comparison with other vitamin D analog [12].

The weaker effect on systemic calcium homeostasis in animals has been shown to be due to more rapid metabolism [1]. Calcipotriol was shown to have reduced effects on calcium mobilization from bone, which would fit in with the more rapid metabolism of the drug [1]. Bouillon et al. [13] found that cal-cipotriol did not bind as avidly to serum vitamin D–binding protein as calcitriol, putting this forward as a possible explanation for the more rapid metabolism of calcipotriol. However, a subsequent study involving a number of vitamin D analogs failed to demonstrate a relationship between $t1/2$ (time to reduction in serum concentration by a factor of 2) and affinity for serum vitamin D–binding protein for a variety of vitamin D analogs [14]. This suggests that other factors may contribute to the differential effect of calcipotriol on systemic calcium homeostasis.

Two principal metabolites of calcipotriol—MC 1080 and MC 1046—have been identified. Calcipotriol is metabolized to these two inactive products by rat and human hepatocytes in vitro by oxidation at the 24 position [15,16].

B. Calcipotriol in Pregnancy

Studies carried out in rats [17–19] and rabbits [20] indicate no evidence of terato-genicity of calcipotriol in animals. However, as vitamin D is known to be poten-tially teratogenic in humans, calcipotriol is contraindicated in pregnancy.

C. Summary

In summary, animal studies have shown calcipotriol to have weaker effects than 1,25-dihydroxyvitamin D_3 in animals. This reduced effect has been shown to be due to more rapid metabolism. The reason for this more rapid metabolism is uncertain but may involve weaker binding to vitamin D–binding protein in serum.

IV. STUDIES IN HUMANS

A. Pharmacokinetics

There have been two studies investigating the metabolism of calcipotriol. In the first, carried out in healthy human volunteers, approximately 1% of radiolabeled topical calcipotriol was absorbed and all of the calcipotriol was excreted within 48 hr, as judged by radioactivity levels [21]. In the second, three groups were investigated; healthy human volunteers, psoriatics after a single dose, and psoriatics after treatment for 2 weeks [22]. Between 2.6 and 12% of the administered dose was absorbed. The results of these studies must be interpreted with caution, as direct measurement of calcipotriol levels was not performed. Radiolabeled calcipotriol (^{3}H-calcipotriol) was used, and urine, feces, and serum were measured at frequent intervals for 21 days for radioactivity and tritiated water. A sensitive assay of calcipotriol has recently been developed [23] and levels have been measured in patients using large amounts of calcipotriol topically. Using this method, it should be possible to study the absorption and metabolism of calcipotriol accurately in humans.

No direct comparative studies to assess metabolism of 1,25-dihydroxyvitamin D_3 and calcipotriol have been carried out in human subjects. One study compared the effects on systemic calcium homeostasis in psoriatic patients taking oral 1,25-dihydroxyvitamin D_3 and an equivalent amount of topical calcipotriol (assuming 1% absorption) [24]. Patients using calcipotriol showed no alteration in serum total adjusted calcium, ionized calcium, creatinine, alkaline phosphatase, osteocalcin, intact parathyroid hormone (PTH), calcidiol, and 1,25-dihydroxyvitamin D_3 or in daily or fasting urinary excretion of calcium or cAMP. Patients taking oral 1,25-dihydroxyvitamin D_3 showed a rise in serum total adjusted calcium, serum 1,25-dihydroxyvitamin D_3 levels, 24-hr urine calcium excretion, and a fall in serum PTH. The study was poorly designed and makes several assumptions that leave it open to error. Further studies are needed using direct measurement of calcipotriol absorption, which is now available [23], to confirm that the weaker effects in animal studies can be extrapolated to humans.

B. Systemic Effects of Topical Calcipotriol

It is important to consider the evidence for calcipotriol toxicity in licensed and unlicensed usage separately. Calcipotriol is licensed for use in mild to moderately severe chronic plaque psoriasis provided that no more than 100 g of the 50 μg/g ointment or cream is used per week. Calcipotriol is not licensed for use in severe or unstable psoriasis or in other unrelated disorders.

1. Therapeutic doses ($\leq$100 g per Week)

Serum Calcium

Most studies on calcipotriol involved measurement of serum total adjusted calcium. Published safety data are available on approximately 2500 patients with mild to moderate chronic plaque psoriasis requiring less than 100 g of calcipotriol (50 μg/g) ointment per week. In these studies, mostly multicenter, no short-term (6–8 weeks) effect on serum calcium could be demonstrated [25–31]. Long-term toxicity has also been examined. No effect on serum calcium was demonstrated in 15 patients using calcipotriol for 6 months [32] and, in a separate study, in 161 patients using calcipotriol for 1 year [33]. Most of these studies assessed patients using small amounts of calcipotriol (30–40 g of ointment per week). A small number of studies have assessed patients using larger amounts of ointment within the recommended maximum of 100 g per week. Guzzo et al. [34] assessed 39 patients using a mean of 81 g per week and found no alteration in serum calcium. Gumowski-Sunek et al. [35] assessed 10 patients applying approximately 90 g per week. They found no alteration in serum calcium. We examined 12 patients using exactly 90 g of calcipotriol during a double-blind comparison with calcitriol [36]. We demonstrated a small rise in serum ionized calcium within normal limits over an 8-week period. There was no change in serum total adjusted calcium. We also examined 10 patients using 100 g per week and demonstrated no change in serum calcium over a 4-week period [37]. This was confirmed in another study involving 11 patients (Bourke JF, M.D. thesis, Leicester University 1996).

There is one report describing 2 patients using 70–80 g of calcipotriol 50 $\mu g/g$ ointment who developed hypercalcemia [38]. However, in one case, the level was measured 2 weeks after stopping calcipotriol and was only just above the normal limit. In the other, hypercalcaemia developed after prolonged use of calcipotriol (11 weeks). It is possible that these patients represent a small subgroup of patients who are particularly susceptible to calcipotriol toxicity.

There is also one surprising report from a study comparing the efficacy of tar and calcipotriol. A 74-year-old man developed hypercalcemia after using 180 g of ointment over a 6-week period. That study also detected a significant rise in serum calcium and phosphate over the 6-week period, although the maximum amount of calcipotriol used was only 60 g of the ointment per week. These figures are very much at variance with the experience of others with calcipotriol.

Urine Calcium

Hypercalciuria is one of the main concerns when using vitamin D and its analogs. A persistent rise in urine calcium excretion could give rise to the development of renal calculi. We examined 20 patients using on average 30–40 g of calcipotriol per week over a 1-year period. We demonstrated no effect on serum total adjusted calcium or 24-hr urine calcium. [35] Guzzo et al. [34] found no change in 24-hr urine calcium in 39 patients using a mean of 81 g of ointment per week over an 8-week period. Gumowski-Sunek et al. [35] studied 10 patients using a mean of 383 g of calcipotriol ointment per month over a mean 6.5-week period and found no significant alteration in 24-hr urine calcium.

In our study assessing patients using 90 g per week, we also found no effect on 24-hr urine calcium [36]. When we examined 10 patients using 100 g per week over 4 weeks [37], we did demonstrate a small rise in 24-hr urine calcium.

Other Parameters of Systemic Calcium Homeostasis

Other sensitive parameters of calcium homeostasis have been measured in a small number of studies. No short-term effects on serum alkaline phosphatase, osteocalcin, PTH, 25-vitamin D, 1,25-vitamin D, 24-hr urine calcium, urine calcium/creatinine ratio, or tubular reabsorption of phosphate and calcium could be demonstrated in patients using on average 25 and 40 g of the ointment per week [39,40]. Guzzo et al. [34] detected no change in serum PTH levels, bone-specific alkaline phosphatase, urine hydroxyproline, and bone densitometry in patients using an average of 81 g per week over an 8-week period. In our study assessing 90 g of ointment per week for 8 weeks [36], we detected no change in serum phosphate, serum alkaline phosphatase, serum osteocalcin, serum 25-hydroxyvitamin D_3, serum 9 a.m. PTH, and 24-hr urine calcium, phosphate, creatinine, and hydroxyproline. Gumowski-Sunek et al. [35] assessed 10 patients using a mean of 383 g per month over a mean of 6.5 weeks and found no change in serum PTH, alkaline phosphatase, osteocalcin, 25-hydroxyvitamin D_3 and 1,25-dihydroxyvitamin D_3. We also assessed patients using exactly 100 g of calcipotriol ointment per week and found a significant change in serum phosphate but no alteration in serum 9 a.m. PTH, serum osteocalcin, serum C-terminal propeptide of type I collagen, or serum bone-specific alkaline phosphatase over a 4-week period (Bourke JF, M.D. thesis, Leicester University, 1996).

2. High Doses

Serum Calcium

There are four reported cases [25,41] of hypercalcaemia in patients treating extensive chronic plaque psoriasis with excessive amounts of calcipotriol (200–700 g per week).

   Van de Kerkhof et al. [42] assessed 41 patients using a mean of 94 g of calcipotriol ointment plus 14 g of scalp application per week for 4 weeks. This was compared with a control group of 47 patients using dithranol or tar. No change in serum calcium was detected. We have examined 30 patients using up to 360 g per week as inpatients in a dose tailored to the extent of psoriasis. There was a significant rise in mean serum total adjusted calcium which was dose-dependent, and 5 patients developed hypercalcemia. These were the patients who were using doses greater than 5.5 g per kg body weight per week of the calcipotriol 50 μg/g ointment [43].

Urine Calcium

There is one report of a patient who developed hypercalciuria without any change in serum calcium while using 150 g per week [44]. Van de Kerkhof et al. [42]

found no change in urine calcium excretion in patients using a mean of 94 g of ointment plus 14 g of scalp application. We have demonstrated a rise in mean 24-hr urine calcium in 30 patients using doses of up to 360 g of calcipotriol per week, which was dose-dependent [40]. Of these, 12 became hypercalciuric during treatment and 2 more patients developed hypercalciuria after withdrawal of treatment.

Other Parameters of Systemic Calcium Homeostasis

Van de Kerkhof et al [42] found no change in serum parathyroid hormone, serum 25- and 1,25-vitamin D, serum osteocalcin, serum bone specific alkaline phosphatase, and serum C-terminal propeptide of collagen I levels or in urinary excretion of pyridinoline in patients using a mean of 94 g of ointment plus 14 g of scalp application. We examined the effects of up to 360 g of calcipotriol ointment in 30 patients with extensive chronic plaque psoriasis on a comprehensive range of parameters of systemic calcium homeostasis. The results are summarized in Table 1. We found that the effects of calcipotriol were as would be expected in vitamin D toxicity, with the exception that we demonstrated no effect on bone. The duration of the study was only 2 weeks which may explain the lack of any demonstrable effect on bone.

Table 1 Effects of High-Dose Topical Calcipotriol on Various Indices of Systemic Calcium Homeostasis in Patients with Chronic Plaque Psoriasis

Parameter measured	Effect of calcipotriol
Serum total adjusted calcium	Increased
Serum ionized calcium	Increased
Serum phosphate	Increased
Serum total alkaline phosphatase	Reduced
Serum bone–specific alkaline phosphatase	No change
Serum osteocalcin	No change
Serum C-terminal propeptide of collagen I	No change
Serum parathyroid hormone	Reduced
Serum 1,25 dihydroxyvitamin D_3	Reduced
Serum calcipotriol	Increased
24-hr urine calcium	Increased
Morning urine hydroxyproline	No change
Morning urine calcium	No change
Morning urine deoxypyridinoline X-links	No change
Intestinal strontium absorption	Increased

3. Unstable or Pustular Psoriasis

There have been reports of hypercalcaemia in patients with unstable psoriasis, published [45,46], and one unpublished (Personal communication, Leo Laboratories Ltd.). In 2 of these patients, less than 100 g per week were used. It is likely that excessive absorption of calcipotriol through inflamed skin was the cause of toxicity in these patients.

4. Other Uses

Because of enhancement of cell differentiation, there has been considerable interest in the effects of vitamin D and its analogs on cancer cells. Bower et al. [47] studied the effects of topical calcipotriol in patients with metastatic breast cancer. Of nineteen patients who used 1 g of calcipotriol 100 μg/g ointment under occlusion, 2 developed hypercalcaemia after 2 and 8 days of therapy. One patient required rehydration and a biphosphonate as well as withdrawal of calcipotriol. Whether this was a genuine effect of such a small dose of calcipotriol and how much of the hypercalcemia was related to bony metastases are difficult questions to answer. Patients with bony metastases may possibly be hypersensitive to vitamin D and/or its analogs.

There has also been some interest in the treatment of congenital ichthyosis with topical calcipotriol [48]. One patient treated with 80–100 g/day of calcipotriol (50 μg/g) ointment for 1 week developed vomiting and weight loss and a serum calcium 3.55mmol/L [49]. Levels returned to normal 8 days after withdrawal of calcipotriol.

C. Other Toxic Effects

There is one report of precipitation of pustular psoriasis presumably due to irritation from calcipotriol.

In general, the combination of calcipotriol with other antipsoriatic therapies has been beneficial [50,51]. However, there have been reports of adverse interaction with ultraviolet light. This has taken two forms—inhibition of the effect of ultraviolet light if applied before therapy [52] and enhancement of photosensitivity [53].

V. SUMMARY

The principal concern with the use of calcipotriol is the possibility of vitamin D toxicity leading to hypercalcemia and hypercalciuria. Both of these side effects have been reported following the use of topical calcipotriol. However, within recommended guidelines, calcipotriol appears to be very safe. At the upper limit of the recommended dose in adults (100 g/week), a small effect on urine calcium may be demonstrated; this could be of importance in patients at risk for renal calculi. Patients with unstable of pustular psoriasis are also at increased risk of toxicity and should be carefully monitored even when staying under 100 g/week.

In general, calcipotriol is well tolerated as an adjunctive therapy with other antipsoriatic treatments. Patients receiving ultraviolet light should not apply it before phototherapy and dermatologists should be aware of the possibility of photosensitivity.

REFERENCES

1. Binderup L, Bramm E. Effects of a novel vitamin D analogue MC903 on cell proliferation and differentiation in vitro and on calcium metabolism in vivo. Biochem Pharmacol 1988; 37:889–895.
2. Calverley MJ. Synthesis of MC903 a biologically active vitamin D analogue. Tetrahedron 1988; 43:4609–4619.
3. Mezzetti G, Bagnara M, Monti MG, Bonsi L, Brunelli MA, Barbiroli B. 1 alpha,25-dihydroxycholecalciferol and human histiocyte lymphoma cell line (U-937): The presence of receptor and inhibition of proliferation. Life Sci 1984; 34:2185–2191.
4. Kragballe K, Wildfang IL. Calcipotriol (MC903), a novel vitamin D_3 analogue, stimulates terminal differentiation and inhibits proliferation of human keratinocytes. Arch Dermatol Res 1990; 282:164–167.
5. Evans DB, Thavarajah M, Binderup L, Kanis JA. The regulatory actions of MC903, a novel vitamin D_3 analogue, on human osteoblast-like cells in culture. Bone 1990; 11:223.
6. Marie PJ, Connes D, Hott M, Miravet L. Comparative effects of a novel vitamin D analogue MC903 and 1,25-dihydroxyvitamin D_3 on alkaline phosphatase activity, osteocalcin and DNA synthesis by human osteoblastic cells in culture. Bone 1990; 11:171–179.
7. Thavarajah M, Evans DB, Binderup L, Kanis JA. $1,25(OH)_2D_3$ and calcipotriol (MC903) have similar effects on the induction of osteoclast-like cell formation in human bone marrow cultures. Biochem Biophys Res Comm 1990; 171:1056–1063.
8. Norman AW, Nemere I, Zhou LX, Bishop JE, Lowe KE, Maiyar AC, Collins ED, Taoka T, Sergeev I, Farach, Carson MC. $1,25(OH)_2$-vitamin D_3, a steroid hormone that produces biologic effects via both genomic and nongenomic pathways. J Steroid Biochem Mol Biol 1992; 41:231–240.
9. Naveh-Many T, Silver J. The effects of calcitriol, 22-oxacalcitriol and calcipotriol on serum calcium and parathyroid hormone gene expression. Endocrinology 1993; 133:2724–2728.
10. Kitagi T, Oguma Y, Yokota F, Ono M, Shirakawa K, Nagata M, Konishi R. A Mutagenicity study of calcipotriol. J Toxicol Sci 1996; 21(suppl 2):465–474.
11. Binderup L. Comparison of calcipotriol with selected metabolites and analogues of vitamin D_3: Effects on cell growth regulation in vitro and calcium metabolism in vivo. Pharmacol Toxicol 1993; 72:240–244.

12. Mortensen JT, Lichtenberg, Binderup L. Toxicity of 1,25(OH)$_2$D$_3$, tacalcitol and calcipotriol after dermal treatment of rats. J Invest Dermatol Symp Proc 1996; 1: 60–63.

13. Bouillon R, Allewaert K, Xiang DZ, et al. Vitamin D analogues with low affinity for the vitamin D binding protein: Enhanced in vitro and decreased in vivo activity. J Bone Min Res 1991; 6:1051–1057.

14. Kissmeyer A-M, Mathiasen IS. The affinity of vitamin D analogues for the vitamin D binding protein correlated with the serum level and the serum half-life (T$_2$). In: Norman AW, Bouillon R, Thomasset M, eds. Proceedings of the Ninth Workshop on Vitamin D. Berlin: de Gruyter, 1994:178–179.

15. Sorensen H, Binderup L, Calverley MJ, Hoffmeyer L, Andersen NR. In vitro metabolism of calcipotriol (MC 903), a vitamin D analogue. Biochem Pharmacol 1990; 39:391–393.

16. Kissmeyer AM, Binderup L. Calcipotriol (MC903): Pharmacokinetics in rats and biological activities of metabolites. Biochem Pharmacol 1991; 41:1601–1606.

17. Uchiyama H, Suzuki T, Koike Y, Ono M, Shirakawa K, Nagata M. Reproductive and developmental toxicity studies of calcipotriol (MC903): (4)—A perinatal and postnatal study in rats by subcutaneous administration. J Toxicol Sci 1996; 21(suppl 2):439–455.

18. Uchiyama H, Suzuki T, Koike Y, Konishi R. Reproductive and developmental toxicity studies of calcipotriol (MC903): (2)—A teratogenicity study in rats by subcutaneous administration. J Toxicol Sci 1996; 21(suppl 2):403–424.

19. Suzuki T, Uchiyama H, Koike Y, Ono M, Shirakawa K, Nagata M, Konishi R. Reproductive and developmental toxicity studies of calcipotriol (MC903): (1)—A fertility study in rats by subcutaneous administration. J Toxicol Sci 1996; 21(suppl 2):389–401.

20. Uchiyama H, Suzuki T, Koike Y, Ono M, Shirakawa K, Nagata M, Konishi R. Reproductive and developmental toxicity studies of calcipotriol (MC903): (3)—A teratogenicity study in rabbits by subcutaneous administration. J Toxicol Sci 1996; 21(suppl 2):425–438.

21. Leo Laboratories. Dovonex: Investigators Handbook.

22. Delaney C, Liao W, Cohen M, et al. Percutaneous absorption of calcipotriene (calcipotriol) in normal volunteers and psoriatic patients after a single dose of ^{3}H-calcipotriene and in psoriatic patients after a single dose of ^{3}H-calcipotriene following multiple dose treatment with non-radiolabeled calcipotriene 0.005% ointment. J Invest Dermatol Symp Proc 1996; 1:112.

23. LeVan LW, Knutson JC, Valliere CR, Bishop CW. A sensitive and specific assay for calcipotriol (MC903) in serum or plasma. In: Book of Abstracts from the Ninth Workshop on Vitamin D, Florida, May 28–June 2, 1994, p. 204.

24. Gumowski-Sunek-D; Rizzoli-R; Saurat JH. Effects of topical calcipotriol on calcium metabolism in psoriatic patients: Comparison with oral calcitriol. Dermatologica 1991; 183:275–279.

25. Cunliffe WJ, Berth-Jones J, Claudy A, Fairiss G, Goldin D, Gratton D, Henderson CA, Holden CA, Maddin SW, Ortonne J-P, Young M. Comparative study of calcipotriol (MC903) ointment and betamethasone 17-valerate ointment in patients with psoriasis vulgaris. J Am Acad Dermatol 1992; 26:736–743.

26. Berth-Jones J, Chu AC, Dodd WA, Perussel M, Kalis B, Meynadier J, Chevrant-Breton J, Beylot C, Bazex JA, Jurgensen HJ. A Multicentre, parallel group comparison of calcipotriol ointment and short-contact dithranol therapy in chronic plaque psoriasis. Br J Dermatol 1992; 127:266–271.

27. Dubertret L, Wallach D, Souteyrand P, Perussel M, Kalis B, Meynadier J, Chevrant-Breton J, Beylot C, Bazex JA, Jurgensen HJ. Efficacy and safety of calcipotriol (MC903) ointment in psoriasis vulgaris: A randomized, double-blind, right/left comparative, vehicle-controlled study. J Am Acad Dermatol 1992; 27:983–988.

28. Mortensen L, Kragballe K, Wegmann E, et al. Treatment of psoriasis vulgaris with topical calcipotriol has no short-term effect on calcium or bone metabolism: A randomized, double-blind, placebo-controlled study. Acta Derm Venereol 1993; 73: 300–304.

29. Kragballe K, Gjertsen BT, de Hoop D, Karlsmark T, Van de Kerkhof PCM, Larko O, Niebor C, Roed-Petersen J, Strand A, Tikjob G. Double-blind, right/left comparison of calcipotriol and betamethasone valerate in treatment of psoriasis vulgaris. Lancet 1991; 337:193–196.

30. Kragballe K, Beck HI, Soggard H. Improvement of psoriasis by a topical vitamin D analogue (MC903) in a double-blind study. Br J Dermatol 1988; 119:223–230.

31. Kragballe K. Treatment of psoriasis by the topical application of the novel cholecalciferol analogue calcipotriol (MC903). Arch Dermatol 1989; 125:1647–1652.

32. Kragballe K, Fogh K, Sogaard H. Long-term efficacy and tolerability of topical calcipotriol in psoriasis. Acta Derm Venereol (Stockh) 1991; 71:475–478.

33. Ramsay CA, Berth-Jones J, Brundin G, Cunliffe WJ, Dubertret L, Van de Kerkhof PCM, Menne TG, Wegmann E. Long-term use of topical calcipotriol in chronic plaque psoriasis. Dermatology 1994; 189:260–264.

34. Guzzo C, Lazarus G, Goffe BS, Katz HI, Lowe NJ, Pincus SH. Topical calcipotriene has no short-term effect on calcium and bone metabolism of patients with psoriasis. J Am Acad Dermatol 1996; 34:429–433.

35. Gumowski-Sunek D, Rizzoli R, Saurat J-H. Oral calcium tolerance test in extensive psoriasis treated with topical calcipotriol. Dermatology 1995; 190:43–47.

36. Bourke JF, Iqbal SJ, Hutchinson PE. A randomized double-blind comparison of the effects on systemic calcium homeostasis of topical calcitriol (3 micrograms/g) and calcipotriol (50 micrograms/g) in the treatment of chronic plaque psoriasis vulgaris. Acta Derm Venereol 1997; 77:228–230.

37. Berth-Jones J, Bourke JF, Iqbal SJ, Hutchinson PE. Urine calcium excretion during treatment of psoriasis with topical calcipotriol. Br J Dermatol 1993; 129:411–414.

38. Hardman KA, Heath DA, Nelson HM. Hypercalcaemia associated with calcipotriol (Dovonex) treatment. Br Med J 1993; 306:896.

39. Mortensen L, Kragballe K, Wegmann E, et al. Treatment of psoriasis vulgaris with topical calcipotriol has no short-term effect on calcium or bone metabolism: A randomised, double-blind, placebo-controlled study. Acta Derm Venereol (Stockh) 1993; 73:300–304.

40. Gumowski-Sunek D, Rizzoli R, Saurat JH. Effects of topical calcipotriol on calcium metabolism in psoriatic patients: Comparison with oral calcitriol. Dermatologica 1991; 183:275–279.

41. Bourke JF, Berth-Jones J, Hutchinson PE. Hypercalcaemia with topical calcipotriol. Br Med J 1993; 306:1344–1345.
42. Van de Kerkhof PCM, Van der Vleuten C, Hamberg K. High dose calcipotriol (calcipotriene) in psoriasis does not affect bone turn-over or calcium metabolic profile. Poster at American Academy of Dermatology meeting, Orlando, FL, 1998.
43. Bourke JF, Mumford R, Iqbal SJ, Whittaker P, Le Van LW, Trevellyan A, Hutchinson PE. The effects of high dose topical calcipotriol on systemic calcium homeostasis. J Am Acad Dermatol 1997; 37:929–934.
44. McKenna KE, Burrows D. Hypercalciuria and topical calcipotriol therapy. Br J Dermatol 1994; 131:588–589.
45. Dwyer C, Chapman RS. Calcipotriol and hypercalcaemia. Lancet 1991; 338: 764–765.
46. Russell S, Young MJ. Hypercalcaemia during treatment of psoriasis with calcipotriol. Br J Dermatol 1994; 130:795–796.
47. Bower M, Colston KW, Stein RC, et al. Topical calcipotriol in advanced breast cancer. Lancet 1991; 357:701–702.
48. Lucker GPH, Van de Kerkhof PCM, Van Dijk MR, Steijlen PM. Effect of topical calcipotriol on congenital ichthyoses. Br J Dermatol 1994; 131:546–550.
49. Hoeck HC, Laurberg G, Laurberg P. Hypercalcaemic crisis after excessive use of a vitamin D derivative. J Intern Med 1994; 235:281–282.
50. Grossman RM, Thivolet J, Claudy A, Souteyrand P, Guilhou JJ, Thomas P, Amblard P, Belaich S, Belilovsky C, de la Brassine M. A novel therapeutic approach to psoriasis with combination calcipotriol ointment and very low-dose cyclosporine: Results of a multicenter placebo-controlled study. J Am Acad Dermatol 1994; 31:68–74.
51. Vazquez-Lopez F, Perez-Oliva N, Hernandez-Mejia R. Topical calcipotriene ointment and etretinate: Another combination therapy for psoriasis vulgaris. J Am Acad Dermatol 1997; 36:803.
52. Marsico RE, Dijkstra JW. UVB blocking effect of calcipotriene ointment 0.005%. J Am Acad Dermatol 1996; 34:539–540.
53. McKenna KE, Stern RS. Photosensitivity associated with combined UV-B and calcipotriene therapy. Arch Dermatol 1995; 131:1323–1324.

19

Safety and Efficacy of Calcipotriol in Children

Charles R. Darley
Brighton Health Care NHS Trust, Brighton, England

I. INTRODUCTION

Psoriasis is seen in about 1–3% of the population. The incidence in children is much lower than that in adults. The point prevalence at the age of 11 years has been reported to be 0.5% [1].

There are certain patterns of psoriasis that are seen particularly in children. Diaper psoriasis occurs as a Koebner phenomenon in a genetically predisposed child. It can be very resistant to standard therapy for diaper dermatitis but usually responds to a moderately potent topical steroid such as clobetasone butyrate. Guttate psoriasis is seen most commonly after a streptococcal sore throat. There are many small lesions present, which make topical treatment impractical. Phototherapy can be used, but fortunately, in most cases, this pattern of psoriasis is self-limiting after several weeks.

Typical plaque psoriasis of the body and limbs is more difficult to treat in children than in adults. Anthraline is generally too irritant and messy for outpatient use in children. Coal tar–containing preparations are of some value, but they are also messy. Topical steroids have a beneficial effect, but it is often necessary to use a potent steroid. There is always concern about using such preparations long-term in children, and bearing in mind that psoriasis may be a chronic condition, the amount used should be closely monitored.

In many countries, calcipotriol now has a product license for the treatment of plaque psoriasis in children. The evidence for its safety and efficacy is based predominantly on two trials, one undertaken in the United Kingdom [2] and the other an international study [3].

II. EFFICACY

The U.K. study was a multicenter prospective, noncontrolled open-label trial of calcipotriol (50 μg/kg). Children between 2 and 14 years of age with stable mild to moderate plaque psoriasis on the body and limbs involving less than 30% of the total body surface were included. Calcipotriol was applied twice daily. A maximum amount of ointment for each patient was calculated based on body surface area. The psoriasis area severity index (PASI) score was used to assess the severity of the psoriasis and was measured before and after a 2-week washout period and every 2 weeks during the 8 weeks of the trial. Overall efficacy was also assessed by the investigator and either the child or his or her parent.

A total of 66 children were enrolled and 58 completed the study (2 withdrew because of side effects, 2 because of worsening psoriasis, and 4 defaulted). There was a significant reduction in the PASI score compared with baseline at weeks 2,4,6, and 8 (Figure 1). There was a similar significant fall in each component of the PASI score. The mean PASI score fell from 6.1–2.4 after 8 weeks.

Clearance or marked improvement was seen in 65% of cases as judged by the investigator and 62% as judged by the patient and/or parent (Figure 2).

The international study was a prospective double-blind, randomized, placebo-controlled, parallel-group trial comparing calcipotriol ointment with the

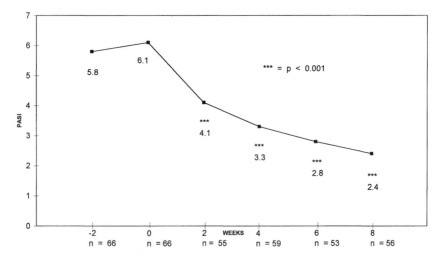

Figure 1   Mean PASI (+/− standard error of the mean) before and during treatment.

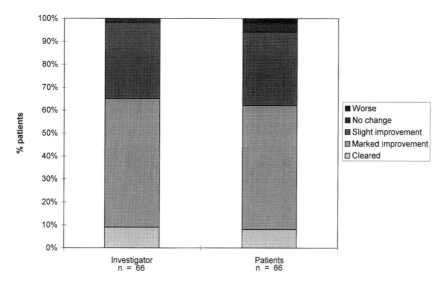

Figure 2   Patients' and investigators' overall efficacy assessment at the end of treatment.

ointment vehicle. Inclusion and exclusion criteria, treatment schedule, and assessment were identical in the U.K. and international studies.

Of the 81 children (mean age 10 years) recruited, 3 cleared during the washout period and 1 had abnormal liver function tests; 43 children were randomized into the calcipotriol group (6 withdrawals) and 34 into the placebo group (3 withdrawals). There was a 52% reduction in the mean PASI score in the calcipotriol group by the end of the study compared with a 37% reduction in the vehicle group, but the difference was not statistically significant (Figure 3). However there was a significant reduction in redness and scaliness but not in thickness when the two groups were compared (Table 1). The investigators judged 60.5% of patients in the treated group as clear or markedly improved, compared with 44.1% in the control group (Figure 4). This difference was statistically significant. Patients' and/or parents' assessment of the two treatments did not differ significantly (Table 2).

In a small double-blind study published as an abstract [4], 29 children were enrolled; 16 received calcipotriol ointment and 13 placebo (vehicle). Among the 25 patients who completed the 6-week study, 73% of those receiving calcipotriol showed marked improvement or better, compared with 40% of the control group.

In an open study [5] of calcipotriol ointment in 12 children, the mean PASI score fell from 3.28 pretreatment to 0.28 at the end of 6 weeks.

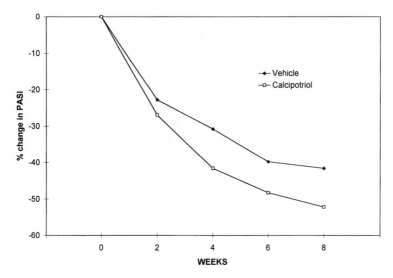

Figure 3   Percentage change (mean) in PASI from baseline in a double-blind calcipotriol study in children with psoriasis. Difference was not statistically significant ($p - 0.14$).

Table 1   Change in Scores (PASI, Redness, Thickness, Scaliness, and Extent) from Baseline (Visit 2) to End of Calcipotriol or Vehicle Treatment in 77 Children with Psoriasis

| | Treatment | | | |
	Calcipotriol ($n = 43$)	Placebo ($n = 34$)	Difference[a]	p Value[b]
Redness	−0.84 (0.13)	−0.46 (0.12)	−0.35 (0.16)	0.037[c]
Thickness	−1.05 (0.14)	−0.72 (0.13)	−0.31 (0.17)	0.075
Scaliness	−1.09 (0.12)	−0.70 (0.15)	−0.41 (0.17)	0.018[c]
PASI	−52.0 (6.9)	−37.1 (6.8)	−14.9 (9.8)	0.14
Extent of disease	−0.40 (0.12)	−0.24 (0.09)	−0.18 (0.13)	0.17

[a] Difference between groups after adjustment for baseline severity score by analysis of covariance (ANCOVA).
[b] Between-group probability (ANCOVA, *F* test).
[c] Differences were statistically significant.

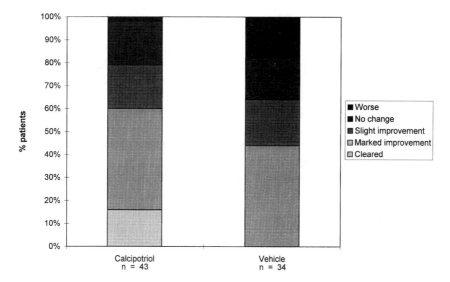

Figure 4   Investigators' overall assessment of treatment response at end of treatment.

Table 2   Overall Assessment by Patient and Investigator of Response to Calcipotriol or Vehicle Treatment in 77 Children with Psoriasis at End of Treatment[a]

	Investigator		Patient	
	Calcipotriol	Vehicle	Calcipotriol	Vehicle
Worse	1	6	2	8
No change	8	6	6	3
Slight improvement	8	7	14	7
Marked improvement	19	15	16	16
Cleared	7	0	5	0
Total	43	34	43	34
Wilcoxon test				
Exact *p* value	0.023[b]			0.19

[a] Data expressed as number of patients.
[b] Difference was statistically significant.

III. ADVERSE EFFECTS

In the U.K. study, 16 patients out of 66 (24%) experienced 18 side effects (Table 3), of which 15 were possibly related to treatment. Lesional and perilesional irritation was the commonest problem, occurring in 7 (11%) of children, 2 of whom withdrew because of it. Unexplained facial irritation was seen in 4 children (6%). Worsening of psoriasis necessitated withdrawal in two other cases. Cosmetic acceptability of the treatment was judged to be excellent or good by 79% of patients and/or parents.

In the international study, the profile of side effects was very similar. There was no significant difference between treatment and placebo groups with regard to adverse effects or between patients' and/or parents' assessment of acceptability of the two treatments. In the calcipotriol group, acceptability was found to be excellent or good by 79.1%.

IV. SAFETY

In the U.K. study, the amount of calcipotriol ointment used each week fell from 16.9 g (range, 0.1–71.5 g) to 12.4 g (range, 0.2–53.8 g) at the end of 8 weeks.

The mean amount of calcipotriol ointment used each week was 15.0 g in the U.K. study and 15.2 g in the international study. When body surface area is taken into account, the amount used equates to less than 20.0 g/week/m^2 (range, 0.15–45.0 g/week/m^2) in the U.K. study and to 12.9 g/week/m^2 (maximum 42.4 g/week/m^2) in the international study.

Probably the main concern, particularly in children, has been whether topical calcipotriol was absorbed and could affect calcium homeostasis. In the U.K. study, ionized calcium and phosphate were measured at the beginning of the study and after either 2 weeks when the amount of ointment used was likely to be great-

Table 3   Adverse Events in 66 Patients

	No.	%
Lesional/perilesional irritation	7	11
Irritation of face/scalp	4	6
Various skin rashes	4	6
Psoriasis worsening	1	2
Noncutaneous	2	3
Total no. of adverse events	18	
Total no. of patients	16	24

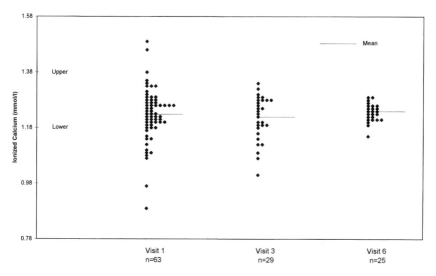

Figure 5   Mean serum ionized calcium from baseline to end of treatment.

est or at 8 weeks (at the end of the study). There was no significant change in the mean serum ionized calcium from baseline to 2 weeks or 8 weeks of treatment (Figure 5). Serum phosphate, liver function tests, serum creatinine, and routine hematology were normal at the beginning of the study and did not change during it.

In the international study, laboratory monitoring was undertaken at the beginning of the study and at 2 and 8 weeks. Routine hematology, liver function, and renal function were measured. Total calcium and phosphate, markers of calcium metabolism (osteocalcin, bone-specific alkaline phosphatase, procollagen type 1, C-terminal propeptide, procollagen, and collagen telopeptide) and 12-hr fasting morning urine for analysis of calcium, phosphate, creatinine, and hydroxyproline were also measured. Although there was considerable variation in measurement of calcium homeostasis, there was no significant difference in the treatment group as compared with the placebo group.

There was no evidence of a positive correlation between serum calcium levels and the amount of calcipotriol ointment used in either the U.K. or the international study.

V.   CONCLUSION

It is clear that calcipotriol is as effective in the treatment of psoriasis in children as it is in adults. In the international study, it is surprising that the vehicle had such a beneficial effect, and this emphasizes the fact that simple emollients are of some value in the treatment of psoriasis. On the basis of these studies, one can expect a better than 50% improvement in mean PASI score when prescribing calcipotriol ointment over a 6- to 8-week period. Most improvement is likely to be in redness and scaliness. Some 50–60% of parents will report marked improvement or clearance.

The side effects seen in children are similar in type and frequency to those seen in adults. They are not usually a problem, although local irritation may occasionally require cessation of treatment.

It is now recommended that children between 6 and 12 years of age should use no more than 50 g/week. Although the two main studies included 10 children between the ages of 2 and 6 years, safe quantities for children in this age group are not yet established. However, the quantities used in the studies referred to did not result in any disturbance of calcium metabolism.

REFERENCES

1. Williams HC, Strachan DP. Psoriasis and eczema are not mutually exclusive diseases. Dermatology 1994; 189:238–240.
2. Darley CR, Cunliffe WJ, Green CM, Hutchinson PE, Klaber MR, Downes N. Safety and efficacy of calcipotriol ointment (Dovonex) in treating children with psoriasis vulgaris. Br J Dermatol 1996; 135:390–391.
3. Oranje AP, Marcoux D, Svensson A, Prendiville J, Krafchik B, Toole J, Rosenthal D, de Waard-van der Spek F, Molin L, Axelsen M. Topical calcipotriol in childhood psoriasis. J Am Acad Dermatol 1997; 36:203–208.
4. Siskin SB, Kosowski M. A pilot study to assess the safety and efficacy of calcipotriene 0.005% ointment in a pediatric population. Br J Dermatol 1996; 135:848.
5. Fabrizi G, Vultaggio P. Calcipotriol and psoriasis in children. J Dermatol Treat 1997; 8:221–223.

20

Clinical Use of Topical and Oral Calcitriol for Treating Psoriasis

Michael F. Holick
*Boston University School of Medicine,
Boston, Massachusetts*

I. INTRODUCTION

In the 1940s, vitamin D was touted as a miracle drug for treating a wide variety of systemic and skin diseases [1]. However, after careful scrutiny, it was found that high doses of vitamin D often caused vitamin D intoxication but had little beneficial effect, including for the treatment of psoriasis. The concept of using vitamin D for the treatment of psoriasis resulted from the initial observation in 1979 that the activated form of vitamin D, 1,25-dihydrovitamin D [1,25(OH)$_2$D], was recognized by specific receptors found in a wide variety of tissues, including the brain, stomach, pancreas, gonads, and skin [2]. In the early 1980s, it was demonstrated that human skin fibroblasts [3] and keratinocytes had a vitamin D receptor [VDR] and that 1,25(OH)$_2$D inhibited the proliferation of cultured human fibroblasts; it also inhibited the proliferation and induced terminal differentiation of cultured human keratinocytes [4]. In 1985, McLaughlin et al. [5] reported that cultured fibroblasts from psoriatic patients had a partial resistance to the antiproliferative activity. This prompted the recommendation that pharmacological does of 1,25(OH)$_2$D$_3$ (calcitriol) or its analogs could be developed for the treatment of psoriasis.

II. TOPICAL TREATMENT OF PSORIASIS WITH CALCITRIOL

Although it was theoretically feasible to treat psoriasis with topical calcitriol [1,25(OH)$_2$D$_3$] because of its potent antiproliferative activity, there was concern that the topical application of calcitriol could cause serious hypercalciuria and hypercalcemia. The kidney produces approximately 2 μg of 1,25(OH)$_2$D a day [6]. Thus, even if only a few percent of several hundred micrograms of calcitriol applied topically were absorbed into the circulation, it could have disastrous consequences. One of the first topical studies with calcitriol was reported by Smith et al. [7]. They formulated calcitriol in a petrolatum-based ointment (3 μg of calcitriol per gram of petrolatum) and had psoriatic patients apply 0.1 g once daily over an area of 50 cm^2. A comparable contralateral lesion received in a blinded fashion the petrolatum-based ointment alone. After 2 months, there was significant thinning of psoriatic plaques as well as reduced scaling and erythema as compared with the placebo-treated lesions. No hypercalciuria or hypercalcemia was noted in the treated patients. At the same time, Morimoto et al. [8] reported that the topical application of 0.1–0.5 μg of calcitriol per gram of base resulted in five of five patients having some improvement of their lesions. The serum calcium remained normal in all the patients. Two years later, however, Van de Kerkhof et al. [9] reported no therapeutic efficacy when calcitriol was applied twice daily in a formulation of 2.0 μg/g, using medium-chain fatty acids as the vehicle. Compared with the placebo treated lesions, there was no significant change in either psoriatic plaque thickness, scaling, or erythema.

With the experience that a topical application of 0.3 μg daily had some partial benefit and had no effect on urinary or serum calcium concentrations, it was decided that in order to gain better clinical efficacy, the concentration of the drug should be increased by fivefold to 15 μg/g ointment. A total of 84 patients (55 men and 25 women, mean age 46 years, range 19–76 years) with either stable plaque or erythrodermic psoriasis involving at least 10% of the body surface were recruited. They had not responded satisfactory to at least one of the standard treatments for psoriasis. The study design was a double-blind randomized intrapatient comparison. In each patient, two similar psoriatic lesions approximately 50 cm^2 in size, were selected for treatment.All 84 patients applied, in a randomized double-blind manner for 2.4 $\pm$ 0.1 month, 0.1 g of petrolatum-based ointment containing calcitriol (15 μg/g of petrolatum) on one lesion as a single application at night. The other lesion received 0.1 g of petrolatum ointment. The treated areas were not occluded and the lesions were evaluated every 2 weeks. A 4-mm punch biopsy was taken from both lesions at the completion of the study. It was then found that 96.5% of the patients had responded to topical calcitriol therapy, compared with 15.5% whose lesions improved with petrolatum ointment alone after 2.4 months. None of the patients experienced any alteration in their 24-hr urine calcium or serum calcium levels [10].

At the end of the 2.4-month study, the lesions treated with topical calcitriol showed a decrease of 60.8 $\pm$ 3% in the mean global severity score, whereas placebo-treated areas showed a decrease of only 4.7 $\pm$ 1.0%. The improvement in the lesions receiving topical calcitriol was significantly greater than that of the lesions receiving petrolatum alone. The major effect observed in the lesions treated with petrolatum alone was decreased scaling (6.7 $\pm$ 1.6% from baseline). Erythema and plaque thickness changed by only 3.5 $\pm$ 1.0% and 3.1 $\pm$ 1.2%, respectively. Lesions receiving topical calcitriol showed a marked decrease in scaling, erythema, and plaque thickness of 66.3 $\pm$ 3.2%, 54.2 $\pm$ 3.3%, and 60.5 $\pm$ 3.3%, respectively (Figure 20.1, see color insert). Histological examination of skin biopsies taken from the petrolatum-treated plaque showed focal parakeratosis and intracorneal neutrophilic infiltrate, psoriaform epidermal hyperplasia, hypogranulosis, dermal papillary edema, telangiectasia, and superficial perivascular lymphocytic infiltrates (Figure 20.1). These changes are typical of psoriasis. In contrast, the skin biopsy of the lesion treated with topical calcitriol showed orthokeratosis, a marked reduction in epidermal thickness, a prominent granular layer without a neutrophilic infiltrate, and minimal perivascular lymphocytic infiltration.

The overall clinical assessment showed that 96.5% of patients responded to topical calcitriol therapy, compared with 15.5% of those whose lesions improved with petrolatum treatment alone. Excellent and moderate improvement was observed in 44.1 and 35.7%, respectively, after 2.4 $\pm$ 1 months of topical calcitriol therapy. Of the 96.5% of patients who responded to topical calcitriol, only 16.7% showed slight improvement. No benefit was observed in 3.5% of the patients on topical calcitriol treatment. Slight improvement in scaling and plaque thickness was observed in 15.5% of patients treated with petrolatum alone. None showed moderate or excellent improvement. A total of 83.3% had no significant change in lesional activity, and 1.2% showed deterioration in the lesions treated with petrolatum alone [10].

III. EFFICACY AND SAFETY OF LARGE-AREA TOPICAL ADMINISTRATION OF CALCITRIOL

Once it was demonstrated that topical calcitriol was efficacious for treating psoriasis [7,8], it was of great interest to determine whether the area of application could be increased without causing any untoward effect on calcium metabolism. Twenty-two patients from the original study agreed to participate for at least 6 months in the study to evaluate the effect of treating an increasing area with topical calcitriol. These 22 patients had at least 25% of their body surface involved with skin lesions. They applied calcitriol ointment (15 μg/mg of petrolatum) in the same amount (0.1 g/50 cm^2) to areas ranging from 2500–5000 cm^2 each night for the duration of the study. An area of 50 cm^2, which received 0.1 g of petrolatum, served as a control site. The patients' lesions were evaluated at monthly intervals. In addition, their calcium metabolism was carefully evaluated. At the end of 12 months, the global severity score was reduced by 84.2 $\pm$ 3.7% from baseline, whereas the area treated with petrolatum alone showed only a 4.3 $\pm$ 2.0% change. At 12 months of treatment, scaling, plaque thickness, and erythema decreased by 75.0 $\pm$ 4.1, 86.2 $\pm$ 5.5, and 94.4 $\pm$ 4.9%, respectively, in those lesions treated with topical calcitriol ($p <$

0.0001) (Figure 2). By comparison, the lesion treated with petrolatum showed a minimal decrease in erythema and plaque thickness of 1.6 ± 1.0% and 3.9 ± 2.7%, respectively, and a 7.1 ± 3.3% decrease in scaling. The mean pretreatment psoriasis area severity index (PASI) score was 10.8 ± 2.2. After 3 months of treatment, the mean PASI score was significantly decreased to 4.9 ± 1.4. A follow-up indicated that the patients were able to maintain a mean PASI score of 3.0 ± 1.5 during 12 months of topical treatment (Figure 3). Ninety-one percent of the patients showed either excellent or moderate improvement in their lesions. The remaining 9.1% demonstrated slight improvement. None of the patients experienced any local cutaneous side effect, including six who applied the calcitriol ointment to their faces.

The 24-hr urinary calcium/creatinine ratio and serum calcium did not increase above the normal range. There was no alteration in renal function, parathyroid hormone levels, alkaline phosphatase, or circulating concentrations of $1,25(OH)_2D_3$ (Figure 4).

A similar study whereby patients received an application of 15 $\mu g/g$ of $1,25(OH)_2D_3$ ointment twice daily showed significant improvement in 15 of 32 patients, with complete clearance of their psoriatic lesions [11].

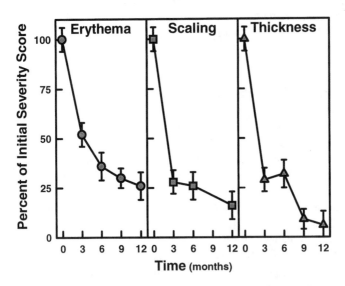

Figure 2   Changes in severity scores during calcitriol ointment. Vertical range bars indicate ± standard error of mean (SEM). The severity scores during treatment with calcitriol showed a statistically significant improvement ($p < 0.001$) in comparison with baseline values. The number of subjects studied at 0, 3, 6, 9, and 12 months were 22, 18, 13, 7, and 6, respectively. (From Ref. 10.)

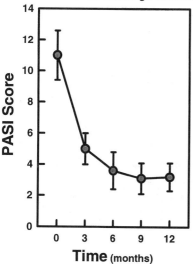

Figure 3 Mean psoriasis area and severity index (PASI) scores before and during treatment with calcitriol ointment. Vertical range bars indicate ± standard error of mean (SEM). The changes in PASI scores during treatment with calcitriol were statistically significant ($p < 0.001$) in comparison with baseline values. The number of subjects studied at 0, 3, 6, 9, and 12 months were 22, 18, 13, 7, and 6, respectively. (From Ref. 10.)

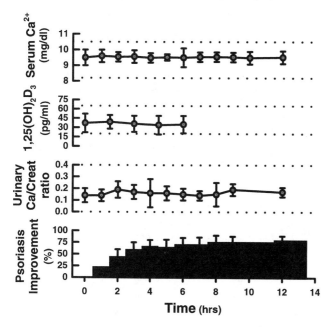

Figure 4 Sequence of clinical events over time. Changes in blood and urine calcium and serum calcitriol concentrations are shown a long with the improvement in psoriasis. (From Ref. 10.)

IV. EFFICACY OF ORALLY ADMINISTERED CALCITRIOL

In 1985, Morimoto et al. [12] reported a fortuitous clinical observation of a patient receiving oral 1α-hydroxyvitamin D_3 (a calcitriol analog) for the treatment of osteoporosis. They observed that this woman's psoriasis also improved after 10 weeks of treatment.

Although oral calcitriol was available for the treatment of renal osteodystrophy, hypoparathyroidism, and osteoporosis [6], most physicians and dermatologists were reluctant to use oral calcitriol for the treatment of psoriasis. The major concern was that oral calcitriol had a low therapeutic window and could cause severe hypercalciuria, hypercalcemia, and increased risk of kidney stones. Furthermore, since calcitriol increased mobilization of bone calcium, there was further concern that it might also exacerbate osteoporosis.

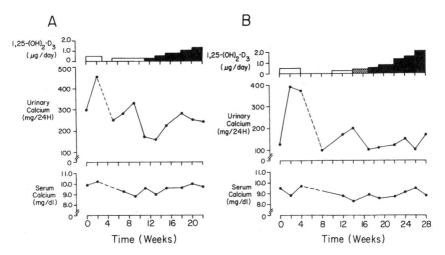

Figure 5   Effect of daytime versus bedtime oral dosing with $1,25(OH)_2D_3$ on urinary and serum calcium concentrations of a patient with psoriasis. A. Initially patient 1 had a high normal excretion of calcium in the urine, which was increased when he began receiving 0.5 μg of $1,25(OH)_2D_3$ in divided doses during the daytime (solid line). The medication was discontinued (dotted line) and was later restarted at 0.25 μg once a day. Once again hypercalciuria was observed and the patient was switched to a single dose of $1,25(OH)_2D_3$ at bedtime (solid block). B. Initially this second patient was taking oral $1,25(OH)_2D_3$ during the daytime in divided doses. Medication was discontinued (dotted line) with the onset of hypercalciuria, and daytime dosing every other day was resumed when the patient became normocalciuric (dashed block). The patient was then switched to a single dose of $1,25(OH)_2D_3$ at bedtime (solid block). Points represent times at which 24-hr urinary calcium concentrations were measured. (From Ref. 7.)

Initially, we began an open trial whereby patients were given 0.25 μg of calcitriol once a day. The dose was increased once every 2 weeks as long as the serum and urine calcium remained within the normal range. However, we quickly observed that patients developed hypercalciuria on as little as 0.5 μg a day (Figure 5) [7]. We reasoned that it was likely that the calcitriol was stimulating intestinal calcium absorption throughout the day. As a result, the drug was given at night, before bedtime. During the night, there was no ingestion of calcium; therefore, there would be a limit on intestinal calcium transport for the 8–12 hr after the dose. By using this simple method, we were able to increase the dose in 0.5-μg increments. In our initial pilot study, it appeared that oral calcitriol was effective in treating psoriasis [7]. To determine the therapeutic efficacy of oral calcitriol, 84 patients with psoriasis vulgaris or erythrodermal psoriasis were treated with 0.5 μg of calcitriol at night. The dose was increased every 2 weeks as long as the urine calcium/creatinine ratio was less than 0.35 and the serum calcium remained in the normal range. The usual dose was 1–3 μg each night, but some patients could tolerate as much as 5 μg each night without evidence of hypercalciuria or hypercalcemia [13]. The mean global severity score decreased by 58.7 ± 12.8%. The mean PASI score at the start of therapy was 18.4 ± 1.0; at 6 and 36 months of treatment, the PASI score had decreased to 9.7 ± 0.8 and 7.0 ± 1.3, respectively (Figure 6). Overall, clinical assessment

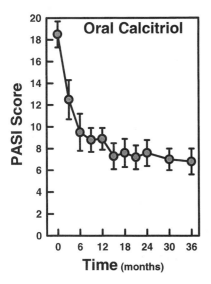

Figure 6 Mean values of the psoriasis area and severity index (PASI) scores using oral calcitriol before and during treatment are shown. Vertical range bars indicate mean ± SEM. PASI scores during treatment with calcitriol were statistically significant ($p < 0.001$) in comparison with baseline values. (From Ref. 13.)

showed that 88% of patients taking calcitriol showed some improvement in their disease. Of these, 26.5% had complete clearing, 36.2% had moderate improvement, 25.5% had slight improvement, and 12% had no change in their disease status. A majority of the patients reporting even only moderate to slight improvement noted a significant increase in the elasticity of their skin, with decreased itching and scaling; overall, they felt that their skin was more comfortable to live with. Most patients did not show any increase in serum calcium levels above the normal range. The 24-hr urinary calcium/creatinine ratio increased but was usually within the normal range (Figure 7). Measurements of bone mineral density and ultrasound scans for renal stones at 6-month intervals for up to 4 years were unchanged from baseline. Two

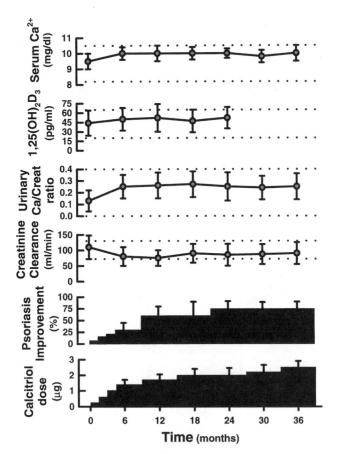

Figure 7 Sequence of clinical events over time. Changes in blood and urine calcium as well as serum calcitriol concentrations are shown at the same time as the clinical improvement occurred. (From Ref. 13.)

patients who had evidence of renal calculi did not show any change in the size or number after oral calcitriol therapy.

V. ORAL TREATMENT FOR PSORIATIC ARTHRITIS

Approximately 10% of patients with psoriasis developed psoriatic arthritis. Although there are several treatment strategies for psoriatic arthritis, most are potentially toxic and none are completely safe and effective. Since calcitriol has marked effects on the immune system, it was reasoned that oral calcitriol may be of some therapeutic value for treating psoriatic arthritis. A 6-month trial was conducted in which 18 patients with psoriatic arthritis received, in a stepwise fashion, 0.5 μg of calcitriol orally each night. A statistically significant improvement in tender joint count and physician global assessment was observed. Of the 10 patients, 4 displayed substantial (greater than 50%) improvement and 3 had moderate (greater than 25%) improvement in tender joint count (Figure 8).

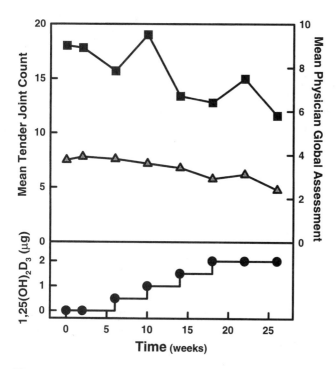

Figure 8 Changes in the mean tender joint count ($\triangle$) and the mean physician global assessment ($\bullet$) in six psoriatic arthritis patients who completed the 6-month oral trial of 1,25-dihydroxycholecalciferol (Rocaltrol; Hoffmann-La Roche, Nutley, NJ) ($\bullet$), according to the mean daily dosage. (From Ref. 14.)

VI. CONCLUSION

There are many therapies for psoriasis, but most are associated with significant side effects. The topical use of activated vitamin D analogs for the treatment of psoriasis is a major step forward in treating this difficult disease. However, since many patients have more than 30% of their bodies affected with the disease, it is reasonable to consider oral calcitriol therapy, which is more user-friendly than topically application of an activated vitamin D. Clearly, we and others have demonstrated that oral treatment with calcitriol or its 25-deoxy derivative, 1α-hydroxyvitamin D_3, is effective for treating psoriasis [7,8,13]. Patients with erythrodermic psoriasis appear to have the most dramatic response (Figure 20.9, see color insert). However, it is not surprising that the response was not as impressive as that from topical therapy. This is because a relatively small amount of calcitriol ultimately gets to the skin when the drug is taken orally compared to the topical route. However, despite this limitation, some patients clearly benefit from oral calcitriol therapy, and this should be considered as part of the armamentarium for treating the disease, especially in patients who have more than 30% involvement. Oral calcitriol for treating psoriatic arthritis is also a relatively safe and effective new approach for treating this difficult disorder.

ACKNOWLEDGMENT

This work was supported in part by grants from NIH M01 00533 and AR 36963.

REFERENCES

1. Holick MF. Clinical efficacy of 1,25-dihydroxyvitamin D_3 and its analogs in the treatment of psoriasis. Retinoids 14:12–17, 1998.
2. Stumpf WE, Sar M, Reid FA, et al. Target cells for 1,25-dihydroxyvitamin D_3 in intestinal tract, stomach, kidney, skin, pituitary, and parathyroid. Science 206:1188–1190, 1979.
3. Feldman D, Chen T, Cone C, Hirst M, Shani S, Benderli A, Hochberg Z. Vitamin-D resistant rickets with alopecia: cultured skin fibroblasts exhibit defective cytoplasmic receptors and unresponsiveness to $1,25(OH)_2D_3$. J Clin Endocrinol Metab 55: 1020–1022, 1982.
4. Smith EL, Walworth ND, Holick MF. Effect of 1,25-dihydroxyvitamin D_3 on the morphologic and biochemical differentiation of cultured human epidermal keratinocytes grown in serum-free conditions. J Invest Dermatol 86:709–714, 1986.
5. MacLaughlin JA, Gange W, Taylor D, Smith E, Holick MF. Cultured psoriatic fibroblasts from involved and uninvolved sites have a partial but not absolute resistance to the proliferation-inhibition activity of 1,25-dihydroxyvitamin D_3. Proc Natl Acad Sci USA 82:5409–5412, 1985.

6. Holick MF. Vitamin D: Photobiology, metabolism, and clinical applications. In: De-Groot L et al. eds. Endocrinology, 3d ed. Philadelphia: Saunders, 1995, pp. 990–1013.
7. Smith EL, Pincus SH, Donovan L, Holick MF. A novel approach for the evaluation and treatment of psoriasis. J Am Acad Dermatol 19:516–528, 1988.
8. Morimoto S, Onishi T, Imanaka S, Yukawa H, Kozuka T, Kitano Y, Yoshikawa K, Kumahara Y. Topical administration of 1,25-dihydroxyvitamin D_3 for psoriasis: report of five cases. Calcif Tissue Int 38:119–122, 1986.
9. Van de Kerkhof PCM, Van Bikhoven M, Zultak M, Czarnetzki BM. A double-blind study of topical 1,25-dihydroxyvitamin D_3 in psoriasis. Br J Dermatol 120:661–664, 1989.
10. Perez A, Chen TC, Turner A, Raab R, Bhawan J, Poche P, Holick MF. Efficacy and safety of topical calcitriol (1,25-dihydroxyvitamin D_3) for the treatment of psoriasis. Br J Dermatol 134:238–246, 1996.
11. Langner A, Verjans H, Stapór V, Mol M, Fraczykowska M. Topical calcitriol in the treatment of chronic plaque psoriasis: a double-blind study. Br J Dermatol 128:566–571, 1993.
12. Morimoto S, Kumahara Y. A patient with psoriasis cured by 1α-hydroxyvitamin D_3. Med J Osaka U 35:51, 1985.
13. Perez A, Raab R, Chen TC, Turner A, Holick MF. Safety and efficacy of oral calcitriol (1,25-Dihydroxyvitamin D_3) for the treatment of psoriasis. Br J Dermatol 134:1070–1078, 1996.
14. Holick MF. McCollum Award Lecture, 1994: Vitamin D: new horizons for the 21st century. Am J Clin Nutr 60:619–630, 1994.

21
Long-Term Therapy and Safety of Calcitriol

Andrzej W. Langner and Wadim Stapór
Medical University of Warsaw, Warsaw, Poland

I. INTRODUCTION

Dermatological interest in vitamine D_3 and its active metabolites in the treatment of psoriasis dates to 1985, when Morimoto et al. described a patient with senile osteoporosis and psoriasis who benefited from oral administration of 1α-hydroxy-vitamin D_3 [$1\alpha\,(OH)\,D_3$] at a dosage of 0.75 g/day [1]. After 2 months of therapy, the investigators observed pronounced improvement of psoriatic lesions. In 1986 the same authors published the results of oral treatment with 1 μg/day of alphacalcidiol in 17 patients suffering from chronic plaque psoriasis [2]. In 13 of them, psoriasis improved significantly, with no influence on calcium-phosphorus metabolism. Holland et al. described clinical and immunohistochemical results following oral administration of 1 μg of alphacalcidiol in 15 patients with chronic plaque psoriasis during 4–6 months. In 2, complete resolution of psoriasis occurred within 6 weeks and in 5 after 4–6 months; 3 showed moderate improvement, whereas the rest were judged to be "nonresponders" [3].

The results of open clinical trials with oral calcitriol in chronic plaque psoriasis were published by Morimoto et al. [4]. $1,25(OH)_2D_3$ given orally in dosage of 0.5 μg/day for 6 months was accompanied by moderate improvement in only 25% of patients. In order to diminish the calciuretic influence of calcitriol, Smith et al. administered 0,25–0,75 μg of the drug in divided doses (lower doses) or in a single dose at bedtime accompanied by a low-calcium diet (<800 mg/day). This approach aimed at minimizing the absorption of calcium from the gastrointestinal tract. Hypercalciuria was usually observed when the divided daytime dosage exceeded 0.75 μg/day. Despite almost double the normal concentration of calcitriol in serum 6 hr after ingestion in a patient receiving 2 μg of calcitriol per day, no signs of hypercalciuria or hypercalcemia were found [5].

Since the treatment of an area of more than 10% of the body area with ointments could be inconvenient to a patient, Holick et al. treated 84 patients with oral calcitriol starting with a dose of 0,5 μg/day given at night with a gradual increase in dose [6]. The study group also included patients with erythrodermic psoriasis. After 36 months of therapy, the mean psoriasis area severity index (PASI) score decreased from 18.4 to 9.7 and 7.0 after 6 and 36 months respectively; 25.3% of the patients experienced complete clearing and 36.2% improved moderately; while 12% did not respond to the therapy. Serum calcium concentration was usually normal; however, 24-hr urine calcium excretion increased but remained within the normal range.

II. TOPICAL TREATMENT

In 1986 Morimoto et al. described good clinical results in chronic plaque psoriasis after topical application of 0.1–0.5 μg/g of 1,25-dihydroxyvitamin D_3 in ointment form [7]. In a double-blind contralateral study, 16 of 19 patients applying 0.5 μg/g of 1,25(OH)$_2$D$_3$ or placebo experienced very good or good improvement on the side treated with active compound, whereas the placebo side remained unchanged. During this study, no patient showed any abnormalities in calcium-phosphorus homeostasis and the concentrations of endogenous vitamin D_3 metabolites, calcitonin, and parathyroid hormone (PTH) remained within normal ranges.

Smith et al. applied 3 μg/g of calcitriol in a petroleum jelly (Vaseline) base or placebo ointment to the extensor surfaces of the limbs of 3 patients, under occlusion with plastic wrap [5]. After 6 weeks of therapy, the clinical results were encouraging, but the limited number of patients and small areas of application (5–10 cm^2) made it impossible to draw any significant conclusions.

Holick et al. described their 3-year experience with higher concentrations of calcitriol ointment in a Vaseline base (15 μg/g) in 57 patients in a double-blind, contralateral controlled trial [8]. In this study, the ointment was applied once daily under occlusion, starting from small amounts of the ointment to a limited psoriatic lesion area (0.1 g on <100 cm^2), amounting to 1.5 μg of 1,25(OH)$_2$D$_3$ daily. Complete clearance of psoriasis was observed in 60% of cases without any signs of hypercalciuria or hypercalcemia despite the fact that in two cases the total area under the treatment reached 1000 cm.^{2} It was estimated that in these two patients the total daily dose of calcitriol applied on the skin reached 30–45 μg and was over 20 times higher than a maximal oral dose of 2.0 μg/day, as reflected in the physiological biosynthesis of this hormone in the kidneys.

The use a correct base plays a crucial role in efficacy of calcitriol preparations because it must promote the penetration of the drug into viable compartments of epidermis and upper dermis. In 1989, van de Kerkhof et al. and Henderson et al. published negative results in a total of 57 patients who used either 2 μg/mL of calcitriol solution in medium-chain triglyceride (MCT) vehicle or placebo for a maximum of 28 days [9,10]. The active solution was prepared extemporaneously by dissolving 0.5 μg of calcitriol in 0.25 mL of MCT. The results of these trials showed no statistically significant differences between the treatments. In some patients, however, the vehicle alone resulted in some degree of improvement, but only in the degree of scaling. In addition, the MCT base was too fluid and many patients found it difficult to apply the full quantity of medicine to the psoriatic plaques; thus they received less than 1 μg of calcitriol on the plaque each day. These results prompted the forming of a negative opinion on the efficacy of topical calcitriol in psoriasis [11].

In the next years only vehicles based on petrolatum or synthetic compounds were preferred as being the most efficacious delivery systems.

In 1991 we initiated clinical trials with ointments containing 3 μg/g calcitriol in petrolatum. Initially only limited symmetrical areas ($<$300 cm^2) localized on the contralateral sides of the body were treated for up to 6 weeks, twice daily in 29 patients [12]. Clearance or significant improvement was observed in 48 and 24% respectively on the sides treated with calcitriol ointment and in 7 and 24% respectively on the sides treated with the placebo ointment. The difference in clinical efficacy between 3 μg/g 1,25(OH)$_2$D$_3$ ointment and placebo ointment was already highly statistically significant as early as 1 week after the start of treatment ($p < 0.001$) and was maintained over the entire study period.

Mean serum levels of 1,25-dihydroxyvitamin D$_3$, 25-hydroxyvitamin D$_3$, albumin-adjusted total calcium, phosphorus, creatinine, mean 24-hr urinary calcium excretion, and mean urinary calcium/creatinine ratio remained unchanged during the treatment.

Only one patient complained of mild redness at the application sites on both treated sides of the body during the last 2 weeks of treatment.

In order to evaluate whether the application of higher topical calcitriol concentrations would increase the clearance ratio of psoriatic lesions, the clinical study with 15 μg/g calcitriol ointment bid was performed in 32 patients with symmetrical skin lesions covering up to 1200 cm^2 of the body [13]. Clinical results revealed clearance or significant improvement of psoriasis in 47 and 28% of patients treated with calcitriol ointment compared with 13 and 31% on the sites treated with the placebo ointment. A statistically significant difference between 15 μg/g calcitriol ointment and placebo ointment could be observed as soon as 1 week in global severity, erythema, and induration ($p < 0.005$) and after 4 weeks of treatment in scaling and pruritus ($p < 0.02$). Mean serum levels of 1,25(OH)$_2$D$_3$, 25(OH)D$_3$, albumin adjusted serum calcium, phosphorus, creatinine, and mean 24-hr urinary calcium excretion did not change during the treatment. Two patients had transient hypercalcemia without symptoms at week 1 (lesions of 450 and 600 cm^2) and one patient also without symptoms at week 6 (1000 cm^2); this normalized 3 days after discontinuation of treatment. In the group of patients applying the ointments over the largest areas of the body (600–1200 cm^2), an increase in mean 24-hr urinary calcium excretion was observed, but this was also within the normal range. One patient had a transient skin irritation at the calcitriol-treated site and another experienced erythema multiforme–like lesions and subjective skin symptoms on distant, untreated, and uninvolved skin areas (Figure 21.1, see color insert).

Comparison of these two concentrations of calcitriol ointment to placebo ointment applied twice daily on contralateral, symmetrical psoriatic plaques revealed no significant advantage to the higher concentration of 1,25(OH)$_2$D$_3$ in respect of clinical activity. In view of the fact that 15 μg/g calcitriol ointment applied twice daily can provoke hypercalciuria and asymptomatic hypercalcemia, especially in the treatment of larger skin areas, this concentration was judged unsuitable for further investigation; however, Wishart in 1994 described no significant alteration in calcium homeostasis during once-daily application of 15 μg/g calcitriol ointment [14]. Nevertheless, the clearance rate in this study was lower than that after twice-daily application.

The next studies with 3 μg/g calcitriol ointment confirmed its beneficial action in chronic plaque psoriasis and safety in respect to calcium-phosphorus homeostasis even when used on larger areas. A study comparing 3 μg/g calcitriol, betamethasone valerate 0.1%, and placebo ointments revealed slightly superior results of treatment with 3 μg/g calcitriol ointment to betamethasone valerate ointment and significantly better results in comparison to placebo ointment (unpublished data) (Figure 21.2A and B, see color insert). This was in agreement with the results obtained by Kragballe et al. and Cunliffe et al. for calcipotriol ointment [15,16]. Posttreatment observation of 8 patients who cleared or improved significantly after the 6-week period of the therapy, showed that relapse of psoriasis occurred after 42 days on average (5 patients). In only one was the relapse of moderate intensity, the remainder experienced only mild worsening of their skin condition.

Calcitriol ointments in a concentration of 3 μg/g possess less irritation potential than the vitamin D$_3$ analog calcipotriol [1,24(OH)$_2$D$_3$]. Irritation was observed in approximately 20% of patients during a long-term efficacy and tolerability study with topical calcipotriol and was attributed to the lower concentration of calcitriol than calcipotriol in the ointments (3 μg/g versus 50 μg/g) [17,18].

For this reason, calcipotriol ointment is contraindicated for scalp application. Results in 10 patients participating in an open study showed that calcitriol can be effectively used in hairline, retroauricular, and facial psoriasis (Figure 21.3A and B, see color insert) [19]. Clearance or significant improvement was obtained in 40 and 50% of patients respectively, but two patients developed transient and mild skin irritation during the treatment. Laboratory results reflecting calcium-phosphorus homeostasis and concentration of 1,25(OH)$_2$D$_3$ and 25(OH)D$_3$ in serum remained unchanged. Patients considered this mode of therapy as convenient or very convenient; but from a cosmetic and practical point of view, a less greasy vehicle would be better for scalp application. Comparative studies with calcipotriol and steroid preparations showed comparable efficacy, but vitamin D_3 metabolites or analogs show a lower risk of skin atrophy even after prolonged treatment. Nevertheless skin irritation was observed in 26% of patients [20].

III. LONG-TERM STUDY

It was still unknown whether prolonged treatment with topical calcitriol preparations could influence endogenous levels of this metabolite in patients. The aim of the long-term calcitriol study was to assess the safety, tolerability, and efficacy of 3 $\mu g/g$ calcitriol ointment when applied twice daily on an unlimited skin area in patients with chronic plaque psoriasis [21].

A total of 257 outpatients with chronic plaque psoriasis were included in an open, long-term, multicenter study conducted to assess safety and efficacy of 3 $\mu g/g$ calcitriol ointment applied twice daily. Patients were selected at the screening visit and were excluded from the study if they were suffering from other types of psoriasis, had received any systemic or intralesional photo (chemo) therapy for psoriasis during the previous 2 months, had used topical antipsoriatic therapy (with the exception of emollients and tar shampoos during the week before the start of therapy), were receiving any concomitant medication, or were suffering from any other disease that might interfere with the assessment of the study drugs. Pregnant women or patients with known hypersensitivity to vitamin D_3 or its analogs were also excluded.

At the screening visit, the general health of the patients was assessed; 1 week later, at the baseline, visit patients were provided with ointments containing 3 $\mu g/g$ of calcitriol for twice-daily application to all psoriatic lesions on the body except those on the scalp. No occlusion was used, and the patients could wash the ointment off 8–12 hr after application. A cutoff date was defined 18 months after enrollment of the first patient, which meant that not all participating patients received treatment for a full 18 months.

Laboratory assessments of the parameters reflecting calcium and phosphorus homeostasis were performed at each visit. Creatinine clearance and urinary calcium/creatinine ratio were calculated. In addition in one center, the serum levels of PTH and 25-hydroxyvitamin D_3 and urinary hydroxyproline excretion were also measured at the endpoint. A full general health assessment was carried out at the final visit.

The primary efficacy variable was the overall global improvement rating. Changes in psoriatic lesions were scored on a 6 point rating scale at weeks 2, 4, 8, 13, and on, up to a maximum of 78 weeks of treatment, always including comparison with baseline. In addition, the PASI was modified (head not included) and scores were recorded at baseline as well as at each assessment visit. Pruritus and overall global severity of the treated lesions were also scored. At one center, skin biopsies were taken to investigate how and to what extent the inflammatory, proliferative, and differential components of psoriasis were affected by calcitriol treatment.

Another objective of this study was to assess the relapse rate in patients whose chronic psoriasis had cleared or considerably improved with treatment. Patients reporting a relapse were asked to come to the clinic for assessment of the PASI score, pruritus, and overall global severity. According to the protocol of the trial, only patients showing a relapse within 3 months could reenter the study.

The nonparametric, two-sided Wilcoxon signed-rank test was used to compare baseline safety (laboratory and vital signs) data with the endpoint data.

Of the 257 patients who entered the study, 4 had neither safety nor efficacy data after receiving study medication and were excluded from all analyses. A total of 219 patients were treated continuously for at least 3 months, 149 for at least 6 months, 75 for at least 12 months, and 16 for at least 18 months.

A total of 46 patients (18%) withdrew from the study prematurely because their psoriasis improved or cleared, 7 (2.8%) withdrew due to local intolerance, and one (0.4%) withdrew due to hypercalcemia. A total of 108 patients (42.7%) were excluded due to lack of efficacy; however, among this relatively large group were patients who showed improvement during the first weeks or months of treatment but then showed no further improvement or some deterioration upon continued treatment.

The actual amount of ointment applied was dependent on the size of the lesions and the thickness of the applied layer of ointment. Patients were asked to return all tubes at the end of the study. Of the 80 patients who returned all tubes dispensed, the mean quantity of ointment used was 6 g/day (range, 1–24 g/day); 24 patients (30% of those who returned tubes) used more than 1000 g calcitriol ointment; and 8 (10%) used more than 2000 g during the entire study period. Five patients (6%) used on average more than 15 g of ointment daily, and 13 patients (16%) used more than 10 g daily.

No serious adverse events occurred during the course of the study. Transient skin irritation was experienced by 15% of patients, but these reactions were generally mild. Eight patients withdrew from the study due to adverse events, which, although not serious, were thought to be related to the study medication. Seven of them were considered to be skin irritation reactions and one patient developed a transient, asymptomatic, slight hypercalcemia. Blood biochemistry analyses for calcium, phosphorus, creatinine, calcitriol, 25(OH)D$_3$ and PTH are summarized in Table 1. The mean values of 24-hr urinary calcium, phosphorus, creatinine, and hydroxyproline excretion, calcium/creatinine ratio, and creatinine clearance did not show clinically relevant changes in the baseline/endpoint analyses.

Table 1 Blood Biochemistry During Long-Term Study with 3 μg/g Calcitriol Ointment: Baseline/Endpoint Analyses

Parameter	n	Baseline mean ± SD	n	Endpoint mean ± SD	P Value
Calcium—total (mmol/L)	247	2.353 ± 0.108	224	2.343 ± 0.112	0.5016
Calcium—total adjusted (mmol/L)	244	2.222 ± 0.112	223	2.216 ± 0.119	0.3795
Phosphorus (mmol/L)	238	1.137 ± 0.193	222	1.114 ± 0.203	0.4064
Calcitriol (pg/mL)	228	40.29 ± 15.62	250	42.12 ± 17.14	0.1042
25-hydroxyvitamin D_3 (μg/L)	26	134.69 ± 50.32	30	122.97 ± 56.31	0.1619
Parathomone (pmol/L)	31	0.332 ± 0.115	31	0.325 ± 0.120	0.5500

Ninety-six patients (40.1%) showed definite or considerable improvement at endpoint compared with baseline, and clearance of psoriasis was reported in 39 (16.3%) patients (Figure 21.4A and B, see color insert). Forty-six patients who showed clearing or considerable improvement of psoriasis were withdrawn because of this outcome. Eleven (23%) of these patients relapsed within 3 months and subsequently reentered the study. From the remaining group of 36 patients, a relapse after 3 months was reported in 6 patients, and they were also reentered into the study.

The number of patients with severe or very severe psoriasis fell from 120 (47.4%) at baseline to 54 (21.4%) at endpoint, while the number with no or slight psoriasis increased from 19 (7.5%) to 98 (38.8%). Pruritus also showed a significant improvement over the course of the study. The PASI score showed a marked improvement after 3 months treatment (53.2% reduction in score), which was maintained over the whole course of the study (Table 2).

Table 2 Psoriasis Area Severity Index (PASI) Score

Assessment time	n	Absolute PASI	Percentage reduction
Baseline	253	9.71	—
3 months	253	4.24	53.24
12 months	180	4.23	54.28
18 months	26	4.08	59.59
Endpoint	253	4.32	51.24

These results confirm and extend the findings of previous short-term studies, and they appear to refute suggestions that topical calcitriol treatment may be unsafe due to adverse effects on systemic calcium homeostasis. Even those patients who used large quantities of the ointment for many months showed no relevant changes in levels of serum total calcium, urinary calcium excretion, or vitamin D_3 active metabolites.

The treatment was generally well tolerated and there were no reports of serious adverse events. It is therefore obvious that antipsoriatic therapy with either vitamin D_3 metabolite or analogs permits safe, long-term management of psoriasis. The relapse rate evaluated in 47 patients was considerably lower than that observed after topical corticosteroid therapy.

IV. COMBINED TREATMENT

Combined treatment of chronic plaque psoriasis is widely used in order to diminish the cumulative dose of potentially hazardous methods, increase clearance rate and shorten the duration of therapy. Psoralen plus ultraviolet A (PUVA), re-PUVA, and the Goeckerman or Ingram methods are the most universally accepted methods.

A combined treatment of oral etretinate with topically applied calcitriol was described for the first time in 1989 [22].

Ten patients, representing both sexes, with chronic plaque psoriasis were treated with etretinate at a dose of 1 mg/kg body weight for 3 weeks. Thereafter, a solution of 6 μg/mL 1,25(OH)$_2$D$_3$ in propylene glycol/ethanol (1:1) or the vehicle alone was applied topically once daily. This combined therapy was continued for 5 weeks. In 7 patients with pronounced acanthosis, there was no beneficial effect during initial etretinate therapy; but the addition of topical calcitriol resulted in evident flattening of the psoriatic plaques within a few days. In five patients, the psoriatic lesions on calcitriol-treated sites disappeared completely at the end of a trial; whereas on the vehicle-treated sites, psoriasis was still active despite etretinate therapy. Two patients with less infiltrated lesions improved during initial 3 weeks of etretinate therapy; in one patient, the lesions almost disappeared in the first week of the study.

A similar method and results were described in 1995 after application of a topical calcitriol ointment at a concentration of 3 μg/g with oral etretinate in a moderate dose of 0.5–0.8 mg/kg body weight [23]. Of the 9 patients, 7 cleared completely within 4 weeks of combined therapy; in 1 patient only a slight decrease of induration and erythema was observed, and another single female patient was withdrawn due to local side effects resembling retinoid dermatitis during combined therapy. In our opinion this mode of combined therapy can be especially useful in these patients, who, due to severe, long-lasting psoriasis and previous treatments, should not undergo photochemotherapy, methotrexate, or cyclosporine therapy.

V. MECHANISM OF ACTION

Psoriasis vulgaris affects approximately 2% of the white population and usually improves during the summer period. Therefore, this skin condition was for many years treated with sunbaths or photo (chemo) therapy. Clinical observations prompted investigation into the mechanism of their beneficial action in psoriasis. In 1980, Sommer-Tsilenis et al. described decreased level of 25 (OH) D_3 in 20 patients with psoriasis vulgaris [24]. Treatment with either UVB or UVA irradiation produced a significant increase of the concentration of this metabolite in serum. The same results were obtained by Shuster et al. on the day following initiation of photochemotherapy in all psoriatic patients but not in healthy volunteers [25], whereas Lorenc et al. revealed lowered concentration of $25(OH)D_3$ in 13 psoriatics and low calcitriol level in 12 among 20 patients [26]. The majority (19/20) also showed low circulating calcium levels. Staberg et al. evaluated two different groups of patients: one with eruptive and another with plaque type of psoriasis [27]. Only in those patients with eruptive psoriasis covering more than 20% of the body was the level of $1,25(OH)_2D_3$ decreased significantly ($p < 0.001$). The same authors confirmed normalization of vitamin D_3 metabolite levels after phototherapy, but the main metabolite undergoing changes was $25(OH)D_3$ and not $1,25(OH)_2D_3$, as previously described [28]. Despite an 40% increase in comparison to the baseline, these differences were not statistically significant. Divergent results were also described by other investigators [29,30]. Additionally, it should be noted that in cases of pustular psoriasis and after excision of the parathyroid glands, a significant decrease of circulating calcium was noted in former cases and eruption of psoriatic lesions in the latter.

The mechanism of action of vitamin D_3 metabolites and analogs has been thoroughly investigated. The classical vitamin D action was only one of the proposed mechanisms. Clinical and laboratory observations confirmed that calcium ions play an important role in the development this disease, because decreased serum levels of calcium may provoke pustular eruptions and also stimulate keratinocytes to faster turnover time and abnormal differentiation, whereas normalization of calcium levels abolishes all these events. In vivo, there are two active vitamin D_3 metabolites: $25(OH)D_3$ and $1,25(OH)_2D_3$ (calcitriol). The first may undergo significant fluctuations due to seasonal or dietary changes, whereas the concentration of the second is relatively stable. Its level depends on the calcium and phosphorus requirements of the organism due to short-term needs but also in a long-term fashion during infancy, puberty, and pregnancy.

Vitamin D_3 may have genomic or nongenomic effects. The former is mediated via binding with specific vitamin D_3 receptors (VDR), while the latter is related to its direct effect on calcium. Bittiner et al. described a rapid and significant, dose-dependent increase in free cytosolic calcium levels in keratinocytes and other cell lines [31]. This was due either to increased entry of ions into the cell, decreased transport out of a cell, or mobilization of calcium from intracellular pools. Genomic action of calcitriol mediated via VDR is responsible for activation or deactivation of certain genes responsible for synthesis of a plethora of factors within keratinocytes, Langerhans cells, monocytes, lymphocytes, and other cells. Vitamin D receptors represent the family of nuclear receptors for steroids, thyroid hormones, and retinoic acid.

Keratinocytes are involved in the synthesis of vitamin D_3 under UVB irradiation, its conversion to calcitriol, and utilization to inactive metabolites [32]. 1-Alpha hydroxylase and 24-hydroxylase may play an important role in autocrine regulation the production of active vitamin D_3 metabolites and the differentiation of keratinocytes [33,34].

Calcitriol modifies both the differentiation and inflammation processes within psoriatic papules. Holland et al. described significant changes in keratin expression during oral 1-alpha-hydroxyvitamin D_3 treatment [3]. Keratin 2 increased to levels above those in normal epidermis, while keratins 16 and 18 decreased to normal levels. De Mare et al. partially confirmed these observations during calcipotriol treatment [35].

Cell growth and differentiation could be affected by influence on certain target genes, such as the protooncogenes c-*myc,* c-*myb* and c-*fos.* It was shown that inhibition of the growth of normal human keratinocytes was preceeded by inhibition of c-*myc* mRNA and marked augmentation of c-*fos* mRNA [36]. Keratinocyte kinetics are strongly influenced by calcium and calcitriol concentration in a dose-dependent manner, arresting the cell cycle in a Go/G1 phase.

Results of histological examination of lesional skin biopsies taken before and after the therapy from the sites treated with calcitriol revealed significant normalization of epidermal thickness, disappearance of neutrophils from epidermis, no signs of skin atrophy, but also pronounced infiltrates of polymorphonuclear lymphocytes (PMNs) around superficial skin vessels even after complete clinical clearance of psoriatic lesions. Under high microscopic magnification, pronounced penetration of PMNs through the epidermis is noticeable before therapy, whereas after clearance of psoriatic changes, PMNs were still arrested within dermal papillae (Figures 21.5A and B and 6A and B, see color insert).

It was also demonstrated that calcitriol inhibits early T-cell activation, probably mediated through suppression of the effects of interleukin-2 (IL-2) and interferon gamma production on mRNA level. Further evidence suggest that calcitriol may also affect other cytokines (IL-1α, IL-1R, IL-6, IL-8, TNF-α) and B lymphocytes.

Immunohistochemical observations seem to confirm laboratory results. Gerritsen et al. investigated various aspects of inflammation, epidermal proliferation, and keratinization in vivo [37]. The number of Ki-67–positive cells decreased significantly from 1 week of treatment onward, whereas fillagrin staining in stratum corneum increased from 2 weeks; after an additional 2 weeks it was almost comparable with normal skin. In the granular layer of epidermis, fillagrin returned to practically normal values after 4 weeks of treatment. An opposite trend was observed with involucrin expression. Polymorphonuclear expression in the dermis decreased significantly after 1 week, whereas in the epidermis only slight reduction was seen after week 4. T lymphocytes decreased significantly in the dermis from 2 weeks onward, but in the epidermis the significant decrease took place only after 4 weeks. Similar results were obtained by the same investigators after therapy with tacalcitol ointment [38].

The observed changes reflected normalization of keratinization, return to normal cell kinetics, and diminishing of the inflammatory process.

In our immunofluorescence studies, topical calcitriol treatment in patients who cleared within 6 weeks resulted in diminished numbers of polymorphonuclear neutrophils from the epidermis, a reduction of Ki-67 monoclonal antibody staining, an increased number of Langerhans cells in epidermis, and disappearance of intercellular thrombospondin staining (Figure 21.7A and B, see color insert). However sequential biopses were not performed [39].

In all of the studies of calcitriol and its analogs performed by the authors or other investigators, three distinctive groups of patients were observed: (1) Fast responders, (2) Moderate responders, and (3) Nonresponders. Holick et al. investigated the reason for this phenomenon by analyzing VDR mRNA in psoriatic skin treated with 15 μg/g calcitriol ointment or petroleum jelly (Vaseline) as a placebo [6]. The skin biopsies obtained after 2 months of treatment revealed that those patients who responded to the treatment with calcitriol ointment showed a significant increase of VDR mRNA level ($232 \pm 37\%$) in comparison with the Vaseline-treated site, whereas in nonresponders no differences were disclosed. The authors suggested that those patients resistant to $1,25(OH)_2D_3$ therapy may fail to upregulate or stabilize mRNA for VDR in the skin. Fast responders were also characterized by higher bone mineral density and a lower propensity to develop osteoporosis.

VI. CONCLUSIONS

An accidental clinical observation in 1985 led to the introduction of vitamin D_3 metabolites in the treatment of psoriasis. At present, calcitriol and its analogs are well known by most dermatologists and some are widely used in clinical practice.

This group of preparations possesses pronounced antipsoriatic activity and could be prescribed to almost every patient with chronic plaque psoriasis. The main disadvantage is limited application area or quantity of ointment that can be safely used by a patient, relatively high cost, and skin irritation, which is observed in some patients.

From a cosmetic point of view, calcitriol and its analogs are more acceptable than anthralin or tar preparations. The efficacy of vitamin D_3 derivatives is comparable with that of potent topical steroids, but side effects are not so severe in respect to skin atrophy and influence on the hypothalamus-pituitary-adrenal axis. In the present article we showed, that systemic action of topically applied calcitriol in a concentration of 3 $\mu g/g$ is almost negligible.

Nevertheless, the use of present vitamin D_3 metabolites or analogs does not resolve the problem of psoriasis treatment. However, combination with other treatments such as PUVA and/or retinoids may become the treatment of choice for patients who respond poorly to other treatments.

REFERENCES

1. Morimoto S, Kumahara Y. A patient with psoriasis cured by 1α-hydroxyvitamin D_3. Med J Osaka Univ 1985; 35:51–54.
2. Morimoto S, Yoshikawa K, Kozuka T. An open study of vitamin D_3 treatment of psoriasis vulgaris. Br J Dermatol 1986; 176:1020–1026.
3. Holland DB, Wood EJ, Roberts SG, West MR, Cunliffe WJ. Epidermal keratin levels during oral 1-alpha-hydroxyvitamin D_3 treatment for psoriasis. Skin Pharmacol 1989; 2:68–76.
4. Morimoto T, Yoshikawa K. Psoriasis and vitamin D_3: A review of our experience. Arch Dermatol 1989; 125:231–234.
5. Smith EL, Pincus SH, Donovan L, Holick MF. A novel approach for the evaluation and treatment of psoriasis. J Am Acad Dermatol 1988; 19:516–528.
6. Holick MF, Chen ML, Kong XF, Sanan DK. Clinical uses for calciotropic hormones 1,25-dihydroxyvitamin D_3 and parathyroid hormone-related peptide in dermatology: A new perspective. J Invest Dermatol Symp Proc 1996; 1:1–9.
7. Morimoto T, Yoshikawa K. Psoriasis and vitamin D_3: A review of our experience. Arch Dermatol 1989; 125:231–234.
8. Holick MF, Pochi P, Bhawan J. Topically applied and orally administered 1,25-dihydroxyvitamin D_3 is a novel, safe, effective therapy for the treatment of psoriasis: A three year experience and histologic analysis (abstr). J Invest Dermatol 1989; 92:446.
9. Van de Kerkhof PCM, Van Bokhoven M, Zultak M, Czarnetzki BM. A double-blind study of topical 1,25-dihydroxyvitamin D_3 in psoriasis. Br J Dermatol 1989; 120:661–664.
10. Henderson CA, Papworth-Smith J, Cunliffe WJ, Highet AS, Shamy HK, Czarnetzki BM. A double-blind, placebo-controlled trial of topical 1,25-dihydroxycholecalciferol in psoriasis. Br J Dermatol 1989; 121:493–496.
11. Czarnetzki B. Vitamin D_3 in dermatology: A critical apprisal. Dermatologica 1989; 178:184–188.

12. Langner A, Verjans H, Stapór V, Mol M, Fraczykowska M. 1α, 25-dihydroxyvitamin D$_3$ (calcitriol) ointment in psoriasis. J Dermatol Treat 1992; 3:177–180.

13. Langner A, Verjans H, Stapór V, Mol M, Fraczykowska M. Topical calcitriol in the treatment of chronic plaque psoriasis: A double-blind study. Br J Dermatol 1993; 128:566–571.

14. Wishart JM. Calcitriol (1α,25-dihydroxyvitamin D$_3$) ointment in psoriasis: A safety tolerance and efficacy multicentre study. Dermatology 1994; 188:135–139.

15. Kragballe K, Gjertsen BT, De Hoop D, Karlsmark T, Van de Kerkhof PCM, Larkö O, Nieboer C, Roed-Petersen J, Strand A, Tikjøb G. Double-blind, right/left comparison of calcipotriol and betamethasone valerate in treatment of psoriasis vulgaris. Lancet 1991; 337:193–196.

16. Cunliffe WJ, Berth-Jones J, Claudy A, Fairiss G, Goldin D, Gratton D, Henderson CA, Holden CA, Maddin SW, Ortonne J-P, Young M. Comparative study of calcipotriol (MC903) and betamethasone 17-valerate ointment in patients with psoriasis vulgaris. J Am Acad Dermatol 1991; 26:736–743.

17. Kragballe K, Fogh K, Søgaard H. Long-term efficacy and tolerability of topical calcipotriol in psoriasis: Results of an open study. Acta Derm Venereol 1991; 71: 475–478.

18. Ramsay CA, Berth-Jones J, Brundin G. Long-term use of topical calcipotriol in chronic plaque psoriasis. Dermatology 1994; 189:260–264.

19. Langner A, Verjans H, Stapór W. 3 μg/g Calcitriol ointment in the treatment of facial, hairline and retroauricular chronic plaque psoriasis. Book of Abstracts. Third Congress of the EADV, Copenhagen, Sept 26–30, 1993.

20. Klaber MR, Hutchinson PE, Pedvis-Leftick A, Kragballe K, Reunala TL, Van de Kerkhof PCM, Johnsson MK, Molin L, Corbett MS, Downes N. Comparative effects of calcipotriol solution (50 μg/ml) and betamethasone 17-valerate solution (1 mg/ml) in the treatment of scalp psoriasis. Br J Dermatol 1994; 131:678–683.

21. Langner A, Ashton P, Van de Kerkhof PCM, Verjans H, on behalf of a Multicentre Study Group. A long-term multicentre assessment of safety and tolerability of calcitriol ointment in the treatment of chronic plaque psoriasis. Br J Dermatol 1996; 135:385–389.

22. Langner A, Darmon M, Wolska H, Verschoore M. Combined treatment of psoriasis with oral Tigason and topical 1,25(OH)$_2$D$_3$: Preliminary results. In: Reichert U, Shroot B, eds. Pharmacology of Retinoids in the Skin. Vol. 3: Pharmacology of the Skin. Basel: Karger, 1989:257–258.

23. Langner A, Stapór W, Wolska H. Combined treatment of chronic plaque psoriasis with etretinate and topical 1,25-dihydroxyvitamin D$_3$. J Dermatol Treat 1995; 3:53.

24. Sommer-Tsilenis E, Beykirch W, Kuhlwein A, BTh Rhode. 25-Hydroxycholecalciferol und UV-Bestrahlung der Psoriasis. Z Hautkr 1980; 55:672–677.

25. Shuster S, Chadwick L, Moss C. Serum 25-OH vitamin D after photochemotherapy. Br J Dermatol 1981; 105:421–424.

26. Lorenc R, Szmurło A, Prószyńska K, Gradzka J, Langner A. Evaluation of 25 (OH) D$_3$ and 1,25 (OH)$_2$D$_3$ levels in serum of psoriasis vulgaris patients. Proceedings of the 3rd Psoriasis Symposium, Moscow, 1987:132.

27. Staberg B, Oxholm A, Klemp P, Christiansen C. Abnormal vitamin D metabolism in patients with psoriasis. Acta Derm Venereol 1987; 67:65–68.

28. Staberg B, Oxholm A, Klemp P, Hartwell D. Is the effect of phototherapy in psoriasis partly due to an impact on vitamin D metabolism? Acta Derm Venereol 1988; 68:436–439.
29. Guilhou JJ, Colette C, Manpoint S, Lancrenon E, Guillot B. Vitamin D metabolism in psoriasis before and after phototherapy. Acta Derm Venereol 1990; 70:351–354.
30. Morimoto S, Yoshikawa K, Fukuo K. Inverse relationship between severity of psoriasis and serum 1,25-dihydroxyvitamin D level. J Dermatol Sci 1990; 1:277–282.
31. Bittiner B, Bleehen SS, MacNeil S. $1\alpha,25(OH)_2$ vitamin D_3 increases intercellular calcium in human keratinocytes. Br J Dermatol 1991; 124:230–235.
32. Holick MF. The cutaneous photosynthesis of previtamin D_3: A unique photoendocrine system. J Invest Dermatol 1981; 77:51–58.
33. Pillai S, Bikle DD, Elias PM. 1,25-dihydroxyvitamin D production and receptor binding in human keratinocytes varies with differentiation. J Biol Chem 1988; 11:5390–5395.
34. Smith EL, Walworth NC, Holick MF. Effect of 1a,25-dihydroxyvitamin D_3 on the morphologic and biochemical differentiation of cultured human epidermal keratinocytes grown in serum-free conditions. J Invest Dermatol 1986; 86:709–714.
35. De Mare S, De Jong EGJM, Van de Kerkhof PCM. DNA content and $K_s8.12$ binding of the psoriatic lesion during treatment with the vitamin D_3 analogue MC903 and betamethasone. Br J Dermatol 1990; 123:291–295.
36. Matsumoto K, Hashimoto K, Kiyoki M. Effect of 1,24R-dihydroxyvitamin D_3 on the growth of human keratinocytes. J Dermatol 1990; 17:97–103.
37. Gerritsen M, Rulo H, Van Vlijmen-Willems I, Van Erp PEJ, Van de Kerkhof PCM. Topical treatment of psoriatic plaques with 1,25-dihydroxyvitamin D_3: a cell biological study. Br J Dermatol 1993; 128:666–673.
38. Gerritsen MJP, Boezeman JBM, Van Vlijmen-Willems IMJJ, Van de Kerkhof PCM. The effect of tacalcitol [$1,24(OH)_2D_3$] on cutaneous inflammation, epidermal proliferation and keratinization in psoriasis: A placebo-controlled, double-blind study. Br J Dermatol 1994; 131:57–63.
39. Stapór W, Langner A, Verjans H, Mol M, Chorzelski TP, Elzerman JR. Does topical application of 1,25-dihydroxyvitamin D_3 normalise epidermal differentiation in psoriasis? 18th World Congress of Dermatology, New York, June 1992.

22
Chemistry and Pharmacology of Tacalcitol

Tomohiro Ohta, Masami Fukuoka, Hiroaki Sato, and Keiji Komoriya
Teijin Institute for Bio-Medical Research, Tokyo, Japan

I. INTRODUCTION

Psoriasis is a chronic skin disorder characterized by epidermal hyperproliferation, abnormal keratinization, and cutaneous inflammation [1]. Because it is difficult to cure psoriasis completely, the aim of treatment is to control it by suppressing and alleviating symptoms [2].

The physiologically active metabolite of cholecalciferol (vitamin D_3), calcitriol [$1\alpha,25$-$(OH)_2D_3$], is involved in the regulation of plasma calcium and phosphorus levels and bone homeostasis [3,4]. In addition, $1\alpha,25$-$(OH)_2D_3$ is biologically active in the skin and modulates epidermal proliferation, keratinization, and inflammation [1,5,6].

However, its usefulness as a drug in treating psoriasis is limited by adverse effects on calcium metabolism, which can result in hypercalciuria, hypercalcemia, nephrocalcinosis, nephrolithiasis, and soft tissue calcification [5]. Synthetic vitamin D_3 analogs, tacalcitol [$1\alpha,24R$-$(OH)_2D_3$], and calcipotriol (calcipotriene), have been developed with the aim of maintaining the potent cell-regulating properties of $1\alpha,25$-$(OH)_2D_3$ without the calcium-related adverse effects [5]. Tacalcitol was synthesized by Teijin Ltd. and differs structurally from $1\alpha,25$-$(OH)_2D_3$ due to hydroxylation at the 24 position instead of the 25 position [7]. Tacalcitol is available in Japan as 2 μg/g in an ointment and a cream for twice-daily application; in Western markets it is available as 4 μg/g in an ointment for once-daily application.

II. CHEMISTRY OF TACALCITOL

The vitamin D_3 analog tacalcitol [-1α,3β, 24-(R)-dihydroxy cholecalciferol, (+)-(5Z,7E,24R)-9,10-secocholesta 5,7,10(19)-triene-1α,3β,24 triol monohydrate] has seven asymmetrical carbon atoms and is an optically active substance. The structure of tacalcitol is shown in Figure 1. Tacalcitol is a white crystalline powder. It is very soluble in methanol and ethanol as well as being soluble in chloroform and ether and very slightly soluble in hexane and water. The melting point is 100.3°C. Tacalcitol ointment and cream stored in aluminum tubes were stable for 3 years at room temperature.

III. PHARMACOLOGICAL PROFILES

Table 1 summarizes the pharmacological profiles of tacalcitol.

A. Mechanisms of Action

Calcitriol [1α,25-(OH)$_2$D$_3$] exerts its effects after binding to a specific nuclear receptor, the vitamin D_3 receptor (VDR), which is present in many kinds of cells [6,8]. The binding affinity of tacalcitol for mouse epidermal VDRs was similar to that of 1α,25-(OH)$_2$D$_3$ [9]. In cultured human epidermal keratinocytes, tacalcitol showed higher binding affinity for VDRs than 1α,25-(OH)$_2$D$_3$ did [the concentration required to displace control binding to VDRs by 50% was 3×10^{-11} mol/L for tacalcitol versus 6×10^{-11} mol/L for 1α,25-(OH)$_2$D$_3$] [10].

Both tacalcitol and 1α,25-(OH)$_2$D$_3$ inhibited the mRNA expression of c-*fos* and c-*myc* genes in cultured epidermal sheets. These genes produce nuclear DNA-binding proteins, which may play an important role in cell proliferation [11].

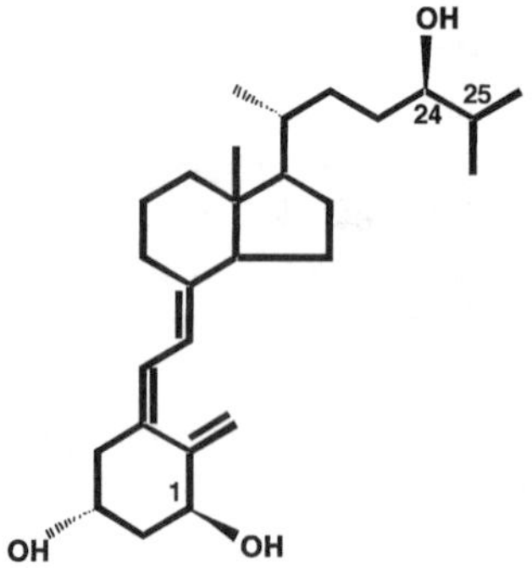

JAPAN;
Bonalfa® Ointment / Cream
(2μg/g base, twice daily)
EUROPE;
Curatoderm® Ointment
(4μg/g base, once daily)

Figure 1   The structure of tacalcitol.

Table 1 Profiles of Tacalcitol

1. Inhibition of cell proliferation	
DNA synthesis, cell number	In vitro
ODC activity, ^{3}H-thymidine uptake	In vivo
2. Induction of cell differentiation	
TGase activity, cornified envelope formation, involucrin synthesis	In vitro
TGase activity	In vivo
3. Inhibition of inflammation in skin	
Inflammatory cell infiltration	In vivo
Chemokine production	In vitro
4. Normalization of skin barrier function	
Transepidermal water loss (TEWL)	In vivo

Nongenomic actions that are involved in a rapid influx of calcium into the cell have also been suggested to account for the activities of vitamin D_3 and its analog [1,5]. Addition of 2.4×10^{-12} mol/L tacalcitol or $1\alpha,25$-$(OH)_2D_3$ to primary mouse epidermal keratinocytes resulted in a significant increase in intracellular calcium levels, from the control level of 1.56×10^{-7} mol/L to 2.19 and 2.07 $\times 10^{-7}$ mol/L, respectively [9].

B. Effects on Cell Proliferation and Differentiation

Tacalcitol has been shown to reduce cell proliferation and to enhance differentiation in vitro, in vivo, and in clinical studies.

To investigate the effects of tacalcitol on psoriasis, various markers of cell proliferation and differentiation have been used.

Tacalcitol inhibited the DNA synthesis in mouse cultured keratinocytes in normal medium, in low-calcium medium, and in epidermal growth factor (EGF)-containing medium in a dose-dependent manner [9,14]. Tacalcitol also inhibited the growth of cultured human keratinocytes from normal and psoriatic lesions at concentrations $\geq 10^{-8}$ mol/L [10,16]. These effects of tacalcitol were comparable to those of $1\alpha,25$-$(OH)_2D_3$.

Hairless mice have been treated with 12-*o*-tetradecanoylphorbol 13-acetate (TPA); this is known as an animal model of psoriasis. In this model, hyperproliferation of keratinocytes results in increased ornithine decarboxylase (ODC) activity and DNA synthesis. Topical application of tacalcitol 1.0 μg per mouse inhibited the TPA-induced ODC activity by 73.1%, whereas the inhibition by $1\alpha,25$-$(OH)_2D_3$ 1.0 μg per mouse was 45.7% and that by betamethasone valerate 0.1 mg per mouse was 18.8% [13]. Topical application of tacalcitol 10 μg per mouse inhibited TPA-stimulated DNA synthesis completely, and $1\alpha,25$-$(OH)_2D_3$ at 10 μg per mouse and betamethasone valerate 0.1 mg per mouse showed the same effect in the same model. Tacalcitol also suppressed the epidermal acanthosis triggered by petroleum jelly (Vaseline) in guinea pigs [15].

Involucrin and filaggrin, together with other proteins, are cross-linked with each other when catalyzed by transglutaminase (TGase) to form the cornified envelope. Formation of the cornified envelope is an important step in the epidermal keratinization process.

Tacalcitol stimulated type I TGase activity at a concentration > 0.12 × 10^{-9} mol/L in cultured mouse keratinocytes as effectively as the same dose of $1\alpha,25$-$(OH)_2D_3$ [9]. Furthermore, tacalcitol dose-dependently increased the number of involucrin-positive cells in cultured human keratinocytes as effectively as $1\alpha,25$-$(OH)_2D_3$ [16].

Tacalcitol ointment (2 μg/g, 30 mg ointment per mouse) significantly increased the epidermal type I TGase activity in hairless mice at 24 hr after application [13].

In a double-blind test (DBT) involving 20 patients with plaque-type psoriasis, tacalcitol ointment (4 μg/g, once daily for 8 weeks) significantly decreased the percentage of basal keratinocytes from 20 to 13.2% [18]. Tacalcitol ointment (4 μg/g once daily for 8 weeks) significantly decreased the number of cycling nuclei; it increased the expression of keratin 16, involucrin, and filaggrin in DBT involving patients with psoriasis [12]. Tacalcitol ointment (2 μg/g, twice daily for 2 weeks) plus psoralen and ultraviolet A (PUVA) therapy decreased both epidermal thickness and the number of cycling (Ki-67 positive) cells much more effectively than betamethasone valerate ointment 0.06% plus PUVA or placebo plus PUVA in patients with psoriasis [17].

C. Effects on Inflammation and Immunological Response

Tacalcitol exerts a suppressive effect on cutaneous inflammation in vitro, in vivo, in clinical studies, and on immunological responses in vitro.

Tacalcitol dose-dependently suppressed RANTES (regulated on activation, normal T expressed and secreted) and interleukin-8 (IL-8) production induced by tumor necrosis factor-α (TNF-α) plus interferon-γ (IFN-γ) in cultured human epidermal keratinocytes at concentrations between 10^{-12} and 10^{-7} mol/L (Figure 2) [21]. Tacalcitol dose-dependently suppressed RANTES and IL-8 production induced by TNF-α in cultured human dermal fibroblasts at concentrations between 10^{-12} and 10^{-7} mol/L [22]. Tacalcitol also significantly inhibited IL-1–induced IL-8 production in cultured peripheral blood mononuclear cells by approximately 50%, as compared with control, at concentrations of 10^{-12} to 10^{-10}

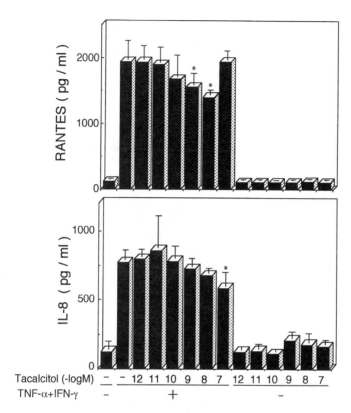

Figure 2 Effects of tacalcitol on RANTES and IL-8 production in cultured human keratinocytes. (From Ref. 21.) Normal human keratinocytes were cultured for 24 hr in the presence of tacalcitol ($10^{-12} - 10^{-7}$ mol/L) with or without stimulation by 5 ng/mL TNF-α and 1 ng/mL IFN-γ. RANTES and IL-8 concentrations were determined by enzyme-linked immunosorbent assay (ELISA). Results are expressed as the mean $\pm$ SD (n = 6). *: $p < 0.05$ vs. the control group (Dunnett test).

mol/L [23]. Furthermore, tacalcitol dose-dependently inhibited IL-1–induced granulocyte-macrophage colony-stimulating factor (GM-CSF) expression in cultured human dermal microvascular endothelial cells from 10^{-11} to 10^{-6} mol/L [24].

Histopathologically, topical application of tacalcitol 0.1 μg per mouse clearly reduced inflammatory cell infiltration to the epidermis in the TPA-treated hairless mouse (Table 2) [13]. Furthermore, tacalcitol decreased the severity of

Table 2 Effect of Tacalcitol on TPA-Induced Cutaneous Inflammation in Hairless Mice (Summary of Histopathological Findings)[a,b]

Item	Vehicle (acetone)					TPA(+)[c]					TPA(+)/tacalcitol(+)[d]				
	−	±	+	++	+++	−	±	+	++	+++	−	±	+	++	+++
Ulcer	3					2		1			3				
Erosion	3					1		2			3				
Epidermal thinness	3							3			2	1			
Epidermal cell atrophy	3							3			2	1			
Epidermal cell degeneration	3							1	2				3		
Epidermal cell necrosis	3						1	2			3				
Inflammatory cell infiltration (~ epidermis)	1	2							3			3			
Inflammatory cell infiltration (~ dermis/hypodermis)		2							3				3		
Edema	3					2	1				3				

[a] Dorsal skin of female SKH1 (hr/hr) hairless mouse was excised at 24 hr following a single topical application of TPA (10 nmol per mouse), TPA plus tacalcitol (0.1 μg per mouse: a dose that significantly inhibited TPA-induced ODC activity), or vehicle acetone. The skin samples were fixed in neutral buffered formalin, embedded in paraffin, sectioned, and stained with hematoxylin and eosin.

[b] Values in table refer to number of animals.

[c] TPA(+); 10 nmol per mouse

[d] Tacalcitol(+); 100 ng per mouse. Histopathological scoring: (−) normal, (±) slight, (+) mild, (++) marked, and (+++) severe.

Source: From Ref. 13.

TPA-induced inflammatory changes, including ulceration, erosion, epidermal thinning, epidermal cell atrophy, degeneration and necrosis, and edema in the same model. Tacalcitol also inhibited TPA-stimulated mast cell degranulation in this model [19]. Tacalcitol (1 ng per mouse applied once daily for 4 days) significantly inhibited hapten-specific and mast cell–dependent biphasic cutaneous reactions induced by intravenous administration of anti-DNP IgE antibodies in a mouse model [20].

Tacalcitol ointment (4 μg/g once daily for 8 weeks) significantly decreased the number of polymorphonuclear leukocytes, T lymphocytes, monocytes, and macrophages in lesions from 10 patients with psoriasis [12]. Tacalcitol ointment (2 μg/g twice daily for 2 weeks) plus PUVA therapy decreased both epidermal leukocyte infiltration and adhesion molecule expression much more effectively than betamethasone valerate ointment 0.06% plus PUVA or placebo plus PUVA in 10 patients with psoriasis [17].

Tacalcitol significantly suppressed the antibody response of mouse splenocytes to sheep red blood cells (SBRC, T cell–dependent antigen) at concentrations between 10^{-10} and 10^{-7} mol/L, in a dose-dependent manner, as effectively as $1\alpha,25\text{-}(OH)_2D_3$ [25]. On the other hand, tacalcitol had no significant effect on the antibody response to T cell–independent (B lymphocyte–dependent) antigen, as is the case with $1\alpha,25\text{-}(OH)_2D_3$ [25].

D. Effect on Transepidermal Water Loss (TEWL)

Transepidermal water loss (TEWL), one of indicators of skin barrier function, was increased after TPA application to the dorsal skin of hairless mice. Tacalcitol dose-dependently inhibited TPA-stimulated TEWL from the dose of 1 ng per mouse to 100 ng per mouse (Figure 3) [26].

IV. PHARMACOKINETIC PROFILES

Pharmacokinetic studies with tritium-labeled tacalcitol were performed following subcutaneous injection into rats [27]. Within 10 days after the injection, 18% of the radioactivity was excreted into the urine and 76% into the feces. Approximately 75% of the total radioactivity was eliminated through the bile, principally excreted in the form of calcitric acid, an inactive metabolite, and only to a very small extent in the unchanged form of tacalcitol. Besides tacalcitol, the only active metabolite, $1\alpha,24,25\text{-}(OH)_3D_3$ ($1\alpha\text{-}24,25$-trihydroxyvitamin D_3) was detected in the plasma. The concentration of unchanged tacalcitol in the plasma peaked 2 hr after the subcutaneous injection and then showed two phases. The half-life of unchanged tacalcitol was 11.1 hr in the later phase.

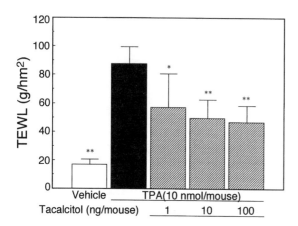

Figure 3   Effects of tacalcitol on TPA-induced TEWL increase in mice. (From Ref. 26.) TEWL was measured on dorsal skin of female SKH1 (hr/hr) hairless mice 72 hr after a single topical application of TPA (10 nmol per mouse), TPA plus tacalcitol, or vehicle acetone. Results are expressed as the mean $\pm$ SD (n = 6). *: $p < 0.05$, **: $p < 0.01$ vs. TPA group (Dunnett test).

The pharmacokinetic studies with subcutaneous injection of tacalcitol in dogs yielded results similar to those in rats [28]. The drug underwent biphasic elimination. The half-lives of unchanged tacalcitol were 8.8 hr for the α phase and 35 hr for the β phase. The only metabolite detected in the plasma was $1\alpha,24,25$-$(OH)_3D_3$.

The pharmacokinetics of tacalcitol following intravenous injection into rats and dogs were investigated [29]. In this case, unchanged tacalcitol and the metabolite $1\alpha,24,25$-$(OH)_3D_3$ proved to be eliminated in the plasma of rats faster than in that of dogs. The study following intravenous injection yielded results very similar to those obtained with subcutaneous injection.

The pharmacokinetic studies following 7 or 21 days of repeated subcutaneous injections of tacalcitol in rats showed results similar to those of a single subcutaneous injection in rats [30]. However, the concentration of unchanged tacalcitol in the plasma following 7 or 21 days of repeated subcutaneous injections of tacalcitol in rats was less than that following a single subcutaneous injection, and its elimination in plasma was accelerated. Furthermore, unchanged tacalcitol did not accumulate in the tissues, including the injected sites, even when subcutaneously injected for 7 or 21 days.

Pharmacokinetic studies following cutaneous application of tacalcitol were performed on rats [31]. The excretion of radioactivity into the urine and feces amounted to 3.6 and 26.4%, respectively, of the dose within 11 days, giving a total absorption rate of approximately 30%. The radioactivities in the treated skin during the topical application or after removal of tacalcitol were detected in unchanged form.

The transfer of tacalcitol to the mother's milk was measured in rats [32]. The unchanged form of tacalcitol was detected in the fetuses and breast milk of pregnant and lactating rats. The concentration of radioactivity in the fetuses was considerably lower than that in the mother animal and the concentration in the milk amounted to 7–19% of that in the mother's plasma.

From a microautoradiographical study following percutaneous application of tacalcitol ointment to rats, it was established that high radioactivity was present in the hair root zone, the cornified layer, and the epidermal cell layer of the skin [33]. The spread of radioactivity into the subcutaneous fatty tissue was very sparse. The results of these observations indicated two routes of skin absorption after percutaneous application of tacalcitol. The first is penetration into the blood through the hair roots, and the second is passage through the cornified and epidermal cell layers and transfer into the blood capillaries.

In cultured human keratinocytes, we investigated whether tacalcitol is metabolized into other compounds [33]. Tacalcitol added to the culture medium was rapidly taken up into cells and then gradually decreased. Other metabolites, such as $1\alpha,24,25\text{-}(OH)_3D_3$, were detected in neither the medium nor the cell fraction.

The plasma protein binding of tacalcitol was calculated to be 100% in human and rat plasma in vitro and 90–98.6% in rat plasma in vivo [34].

Tacalcitol transferred into blood likely binds to vitamin D–binding proteins (DBPs), like $1\alpha,25(OH)_2D_3$. However, the binding affinity of tacalcitol to DBPs was five times weaker than that of $1\alpha,25(OH)_2D_3$ [35]. The weaker induction of hypercalcemia by tacalcitol as compared with $1\alpha,25(OH)_2D_3$ may be explained by its faster turnover, because serum levels of tacalcitol have been found to be lower and to decrease more faster than those of $1\alpha,25\text{-}(OH)_2D_3$ [27,36].

Tacalcitol ointment was applied via an epicutaneous route to study the absorption rate in psoriatic patients [37]. The ointment was topically applied for 8 consecutive days at a dose of 6 μg tacalcitol per subject per day. On days 1 and 8, tritium-labeled tacalcitol ointment was used. Blood and plasma samples were taken immediately before the first and last applications and at different times after the first and last doses (1–96 hr). Furthermore, urine and feces were collected immediately before the first application and for 5 days after the first and the last applications. There were no detectable levels of radioactivity in blood, plasma, or feces of any subject, while traces of radioactivity were found in urine. The absorption rate in psoriatic patients after topical application of tacalcitol was estimated to be less than 0.1% of the dose.

Absorption of tritium-labeled tacalcitol applied to human epidermis mounted on a diffusion cell was approximately one-fiftieth of that through hairless rat epidermis [38]. These results showed the absorption of radioactively labeled tacalcitol through the skin into the circulation to be less than the detection limit.

V. SUMMARY

Tacalcitol inhibits proliferation and induces differentiation of keratinocytes. In addition, tacalcitol inhibits inflammation and immunological mediators in the skin. Furthermore, tacalcitol improves the skin barrier function. These effects of tacalcitol are explained to be mediated through VDRs distributed on cells in the skin.

Tacalcitol was not metabolized into other active metabolites in the skin to which it was applied and was effectively distributed into cells in the skin. The concentration of tacalcitol transferred into plasma is lower and decreased faster than that of $1\alpha,25\text{-}(OH)_2D_3$, because the binding affinity of tacalcitol to DBPs was weaker than that of $1\alpha,25\text{-}(OH)_2D_3$. Furthermore, the absorption rate in psoriatic patients was less than 0.1% of dose. These results account for the reason why tacalcitol rarely causes hypercalcemia in psoriasis patients.

Tacalcitol is useful for the treatment of psoriasis and other keratinizing disorders without causing hypercalcemia.

REFERENCES

1. Van de Kerkhof PCM. Biological activity of vitamin D analogues in the skin, with special reference to antipsoriatic mechanisms. Br J Dermatol 1995; 132:675–682.
2. Williams REA. Guidelines for management of patients with psoriasis. BMJ 1991; 303:829–835.
3. Reichel H, Koeffler, HP, Norman AW. The role of the vitamin D endocrine system in health and disease. N Engl J Med 1989; 320:980–981.
4. Houssler MR, Jurutka PW, Hsieh JC, Thompson PD, Haussler CA, Selznick SH, Remus LS, Hitfield GK. Nuclear vitamin D receptor: Structure-function, phosphorylation, and control of gene transcription. In: Feldman D. Glorieux FH, Pike JW, eds. Vitamin D. New York: Academic Press, 1997:149–177.
5. Bouillon R, Garmyn M, Verstuyf A, Segaert S, Casteels K, Mathieu C. Paracrine role for calcitriol in the immune system and skin creates new therapeutic possibilities for vitamin D analogs. Eur J Endocrinol 1995; 133:7–16.
6. Suda T, Miyaura C, Abe E, Kuroki T. Modulation of cell differentiation, immune responses and tumor promotion by vitamin D compounds. In: Peck WA, ed. Bone and Mineral Research. Vol. 4. Amsterdam: Elsevier, 1986:1–48.
7. Koizumi N, Morisaki M, Ikekawa N, Suzuki A, Takeshita T. Absolute configurations of 24-hydroxycholesterol and related compounds. Tetrahed Lett 1975; 26: 2203–2206.

8. Menne T, Larsen K. Psoriasis treatment with vitamin D derivatives. Semin Dermatol 1992; 11:278–283.

9. Matsunaga T, Yamamoto M, Mimura H, Ohta T, Kiyoki M, Ohba T, Naruchi T, Hosoi J, Kuroki T. 1,24(R) dihydroxyvitamin D_3, a novel active form of vitamin D_3 with high activity for inducing epidermal differentiation but decreased hypercalcemic activity. J Dermatol 1990; 17:135–142.

10. Matsumoto K, Hashimoto K, Kiyoki, M, Yamamoto M, Yoshikawa K. Effect of 1,24R-dihydroxyvitamin D_3 on the growth of human keratinocytes. J Dermatol 1990; 17:97–103.

11. Kobayashi H, Fukaya T, Ogiso Y, Ohkawara A. Vitamin D_3 inhibits the mRNA expressions of fos and myc oncogenes in organ cultured skin (abstr). J Invest Dermatol 1991; 96:616.

12. Gerritsen MJP, Boezeman JBM, van Vlijmen-Willems IMJJ, van de Kerkhof PCM. The effect of tacalcitol $(1,24(OH)_2D_3)$ on cutaneous inflammation, epidermal proliferation and keratinization in psoriasis: A placebo-controlled, double-blind study. Br J Dermatol 1994; 131:57–63.

13. Sato H, Sugimoto I, Matsunaga T, Tsuchimoto M, Ohta T, Uno H, Kiyoki M. Tacalcitol $(1,24(OH)_2D_3,$ TV-02) inhibits phorbol ester-induced epidermal proliferation and cutaneous inflammation, and induces epidermal differentiation in mice. Arch Dermatol Res 1996; 288:656–663.

14. Ohta T, Mimura H, Kiyoki M. Effect of 1α, 24 dihydroxyvitamin D_3 on proliferation stimulated by epidermal growth factor in cultured mouse epidermal keratinocytes. Arch Dermatol Res 1996; 288:415–417.

15. Kato T, Terui T, Tagami H: Topically active vitamin D_3 analogue, 1 alpha, 24-dihydroxycholecalciferol, has an anti-proliferative effect on the epidermis of guinea pig skin. Br J Dermatol 1986; 115:431–433.

16. Kobayashi T, Okumura H, Azuma Y, Kiyoki M, Matsumoto K, Hashimoto K, Yoshikawa K. 1α, 24R dihydroxy vitamin D_3 has an ability comparable to that of 1α, 25 dihydroxyvitamin D_3 to induce keratinocyte differentiation. J Dermatol 1990; 17:707–709.

17. Danno K, Kiriyama T, Uehara M. Topical application of tacalcitol potentiates PUVA effectiveness in the initial treatment of psoriasis vulgaris (abstr). J Invest Dermatol 1995; 105:464.

18. Glade CP, van Erp PEJ, van Hooijdonk CAEM, Elbers ME, van de Kerkhof PCM. Topical treatment of psoriatic plaques with 1α, 24 dihydroxyvitamin D_3, a multiparameter flow cytometrical analysis of epidermal growth, differentiation and inflammation. Acta Derm Venereol 1995; 75:381–385.

19. Fukuoka M, Sato H, Ohta T, Kiyoki M. Pharmacological effects of $1,24(OH)_2D_3$ (tacalcitol) in vitro and in vivo (abstr). J Eur Acad Dermatol Venereol 1995; 5(suppl 1):S186.

20. Katayama I, Minatohara K, Yokozeki H, Nishioka K. Topical vitamin D_3 downregulates IgE-mediated murine biphasic cutaneous reactions. Int Arch Allergy Immunol 1996; 111:71–76.

21. Fukuoka M, Ogino Y, Sato H, Ohta T, Komoriya K, Nishioka K, Katayama I. Chemokine RANTES expression in psoriatic skin, and regulation of RANTES and IL-8 production in cultured epidermal keratinocyte by active vitamin D_3 (tacalcitol). Br J Dermatol 1998; 138:63–70.

22. Fukuoka M, Ogino Y, Sato H, Ohta T, Kiyoki M. Production of chemokines RANTES and IL-8 and its modulation by tacalcitol $(1,24(OH)_2D_3)$ in cultured human dermal fibroblast. J Eur Acad Dermatol Venereol 1996; 7(suppl 2):S182.

23. Kristensen M, Lund M, Larsen CG. Tacalcitol modulates the production of a leukocyte activating cytokine, interleukin-8: Tacalcitol Satellite Symposium. 3rd EADV Congress, Copenhagen, 1993.

24. Farkas B, Fujimura T, Tone T, Eto H, Matsuzawa M, Otani F, Nishiyama S. $1,24(OH)_2D_3$ enhances expression of GM-CSF mRNA and IL-8 mRNA in activated human dermal microvascular endothelial cells (abstr). J Invest Dermatol 1993; 101:490.

25. Komoriya K, Nagata M, Tsuchimoto K, Kunisawa K, Takeshita T, Naruchi T. 1,25-dihydroxyvitamin D_3 suppress in vitro antibody response to T cell-dependent antigen. Biochem Biophys Res Commun 1985; 127:753–758.

26. Sato H, Fukuoka M, Ohta T, Uno H, Kiyoki M. Tacalcitol inhibits the increase of trans-epidermal water loss induced by phorbolester in hairless mice (abstr). 25th Anniversary Meeting of the European Society for Dermatological Research, 1996:111.

27. Ohta T, Takada Y, Mimura H, Yamamoto M, Matsunaga T, Kiyoki M, Ohba T, Naruchi T. Pharmacokinetic studies of $1\alpha,24(R)-(OH)_2D_3$ (TV-02) (1): Plasma level distribution, metabolism and excretion after a single subcutaneous administration to rats. Xenobiot Metab Dispos 1990; 5:3–23.

28. Ohta T, Mimura H, Yamamoto M, Kiyoki M, Ohba M, Naruchi T. Pharmacokinetic studies of $1\alpha,24(R)-(OH)_2D_3$ (TV-02) (5): Plasma level and excretion in beagle dogs. Xenobiot Metab Dispos 1990; 5:63–69.

29. Ohta T, Ishii N, Yamamoto M, Kiyoki M, Ohba T, Naruchi T. Pharmacokinetic study of $1\alpha,24(R)-(OH)_2D_3$ (TV-02) in its intravenous administration to rats and dogs. Teijin Institute For Bio-Medical Research Report, 1989.

30. Ohta T, Yamamoto M, Mimura H, Matsunaga T, Kiyoki M, Ohba T, Naruchi T. Pharmacokinetic studies of $1\alpha,24(R)-(OH)_2D_3$ (TV-02) (2): Plasma level distribution metabolism and excretion after repeated subcutaneous administration to rats. Xenobiot Metab Dispos 1990; 5:25–37.

31. Ohta T, Yamamoto M, Takada Y, Mimura H, Matsunaga T, Kiyoki M, Ohba T, Naruchi T. Pharmacokinetic studies of $1\alpha,24(R)-(OH)_2D_3$ (TV-02) (3): Absorption, distribution excretion after a single or continuous transcutaneous application to rats. Xenobiot Metab Dispos 1990; 5:39–52.

32. Yamamoto M, Ohta T, Mimura H, Kiyoki M, Ohba T, Naruchi T. Pharmacokinetic studies of $1\alpha,24(R)-(OH)_2D_3$ (TV-02) (4): Plasma level facto-placental transfer and excretion into milk after subcutaneous administration to female rats. Xenobiot Metab Dispos 1990; 5:53–62.

33. Ohta T, Okabe K, Azuma Y. Kiyoki M. In vivo microautoradiography of [^{3}H] $1,24(OH)_2D_3$ (tacalcitol) following topical application to normal rats and in vitro metabolism in human ketatinocytes. Arch Dermatol Res 1996; 288:188–196.

34. Ohta T, Kiyoki M, Ohba T, Naruchi T. Pharmacokinetic study of $1\alpha,24(R)-(OH)_2D_3$ (TV-02). Excretion into urine and faeces and plasma protein in vitro and in vivo. Teijin Institute For Bio-Medical Research Report, 1989.

35. Ishizuka S, Honda A, Mori Y, Kurihara Tatsumi J, Anai K, Ikeda K. Effects of vitamin D-binding proteins on biological function of $1\alpha,25$-hydroxyvitamin D_3 ana-

logues. In: Norman AW, Bouillon R, Thomasset M, eds. Vitamin D-α Pluripotent Steroid Hormone: Structural Studies, Molecular Endocrinology and Clinical Applications. New York: de Gruyter, 1994:109–110.

36. Ohta T, Mimura H, Matsunaga T, Kiyoki M, Takeshita T, Kuroki T. Pharmacological action of 1,24(OH)$_2$D$_3$ in epidermal cells. In: Norman AW, Bouillon R, Thomasset M, eds. Vitamin D: Gene Regulation, Structure-Function Analysis and Clinical Application (Proceedings of the Eighth Workshop on Vitamin D, Paris, France, July 5-10, 1991). New York: de Gruyter, 1991:441–442.

37. Trasciatti S. Palumbo R, Paulumbo, Zeppa S. Pharmacokinetics of ^{3}H-tacalcitol in psoriatic patients. Tacalcitol Satellite Symposium, 3rd EADV Congress, Copenhagen, 1993.

38. Nishimura M, Makino Y, Matagi H. Tacalitol ointment for psoriasis. Acta Derm Venereol 1994; 186(suppl):166–168.

23
Japanese Experience with Tacalcitol

Masayuki Nishimura
Nishimura Dermatology Office, Usa, Oita, Japan

I. INTRODUCTION

The ointment containing tacalcitol, an active vitamin D_3 derivative, was confirmed to be effective and safe in the treatment of psoriasis, ichthyosis, pustulosis palmaris et plantaris, keratodermia palmaris et plantaris, and pityriasis rubra pilaris; this ointment has been available for clinical use in Japan since December 1993, following its approval by the Ministry of Health and Welfare. The results of premarketing clinical studies of tacalcitol ointment were reported in detail in a review article published by Nishimura et al. in 1993 [1]. This chapter summarizes the current state of antipsoriasis therapies in Japan, the position of topical tacalcitol in psoriasis treatment, and much accumulated clinical data with regard to this drug.

II. HISTORY OF TREATMENT FOR PSORIASIS IN JAPAN AND POSITION OF TACALCITOL

A very wide range of methods have been applied to the treatment of psoriasis, as shown in Table 1 [2], because of the lack of any established single basic treatment. However, actual treatment of psoriasis almost entirely relied on topical corticosteroids until the introduction of tacalcitol ointment, although psoralen plus ultraviolet A (PUVA) therapy or oral therapy with etretinate, etc., has also been used occasionally. Despite potential serious adverse effects of the long-term use of topical corticosteroids—such as adrenocortical hypofunction due to transdermal absorption, regional atrophy of skin, and a rebound phenomenon after discontinuation of the use—topical corticosteroids still have advantages in the treatment of

Table 1   Therapeutic Methods in the Treatment of Psoriasis

I. Drug therapy
A. Oral therapy
  1. Hormone preparations
     Adrenocortical hormone
     Pituitary hormone
     Thyroid hormone
  2. Central nervous system–acting
     anti-inflammatory drugs
     Antipyretic analgesic
     anti-inflammatory drugs,
     Psychoneurological drugs
  3. Antitumor drugs
     Cyclophosphamide
     MTX
     Ara-C
     BCNU
     5-FU
     Azaribine
     Actinomycin D
  4. Antibiotics
  5. Drugs for the cardiovascular
     system
  6. Vitamins
     A, B_2, B_6, B_{12}, D_2, D_3, and biotin
  7. Digestants
     Intestinal remedies
  8. Drugs for metabolism
     Remedies for gout
     Antidiabetic drugs
     Vitamin A acid derivatives
     Vitamin A acid analogs
  9. Immune suppressants
  10. Antiallergy drugs
  11. Biological preparations
     Interferon
     TNF γ-globulin
  12. Chinese medicines
  13. Others
B. External therapy
  1. Adrenocorticotropic hormone
     preparations (medium strong,
     very strong, strongest)

  2. Anti-inflammatory drugs
     Bufexamac
  3. Antitumor drugs
     Nitrogen mustard
     BCNU
     ACNU
     5FU
     Bleomycin
     Podophyllin
  4. Skin softeners
     Salicylic acid
     Urea preparations
     Sulfur preparations
  5. Chinese medicines
  6. Tars
  7. Anthraline
  8. Vitamin preparations
     vitamin D_3
     vitamin A
     acid preparations
  9. Hydrocolloid occlusion
  10. Arachidonic acid
  11. 5-HETE
II. Phototherapy
  1. Tarsplus ultraviolet
     Goeckerman treatment
  2. PUVA
  3. UVB
  4. Retinoid + PUVA
  5. Far-infrared radiation therapy
III. Dialysis
  1. Blood dialysis
  2. Plasma exchange
IV. Thermotherapy
V. Climatotherapy
VI. Diet therapy
  1. Fat-reduced diet
  2. Fish oil
  3. Starvation cure
VII. Others

Source: From Ref. 2.

psoriasis over other therapies because they are simple to use and have very high efficacy. Thus the dermatologist reluctantly uses topical corticosteroids through necessity.

To break away from the dependency on topical corticosteroids, the dermatologists have sought new therapeutic tools. Under these circumstances, tacalcitol ointment has attracted keen attention since its launch, since it is a novel topical antipsoriasis remedy that is also simple to use and effective, like as topical corticosteroids, but induces no serious adverse reactions, like those of topical corticosteroids. Tacalcitol ointment has generally shown excellent efficacy, as expected. In the postmarketing surveillance report including the third year after the launch of tacalcitol ointment, adverse reactions were observed in 83 (3.49%) of 2376 cases evaluated as to safety. Main adverse reactions were itching in 21 cases, pricking skin sensation in 14, and redness in 11. Additionally, allergic contact dermatitis, which was confirmed by patch testing and in vitro testing, occurred in one case [3]. Two cases developed erythema annulare–like eruption during treatment, probably as an allergic adverse reaction to tacalcitol ointment, although the causal relation to tacalcitol remained obscure [4]. Since many cases of allergic contact dermatitis have been reported as adverse reactions to some topical corticosteroids, the incidence of this adverse reaction is low in tacalcitol. As to systemic adverse reactions, although the effect of tacalcitol on calcium metabolism through transdermal absorption has been a matter of concern since its development, no such effect has not been observed based on measurement of the serum calcium level. Because of the absence of adverse reactions inherent in topical corticosteroids, as described above, tacalcitol is thought rather to have advantages over corticosteroids. Because the relative safety of tacalcitol ointment is higher than that of any of the other therapeutic methods used in Japan, this drug is now considered to be a first choice, not only for adults but also for children [5]. Because tacalcitol ointment is rated very high in both efficacy and safety and is increasingly used, it is now considered to be a first choice in the topical treatment of psoriasis.

III. SOME POINTS TO BE CONSIDERED ON CLINICAL APPLICATION OF TACALCITOL OINTMENT

However, the following precautions are necessary for clinical use of tacalcitol ointment. First, it should be kept in mind that symptoms may be exacerbated as a rebound phenomenon if a topical corticosteroid is abruptly replaced by tacalcitol ointment in cases pretreated with a strong topical corticosteroid. A case that I encountered after the launch of tacalcitol ointment is described here. This case was that of a 53-year-old man whose eruption was considerably worsened (Figure 1A and B) for a while after an ultrapotent topical corticosteroid was replaced by tacalcitol ointment, since there seems to be a tendency toward exacerbated eruptions during the use of a corti-

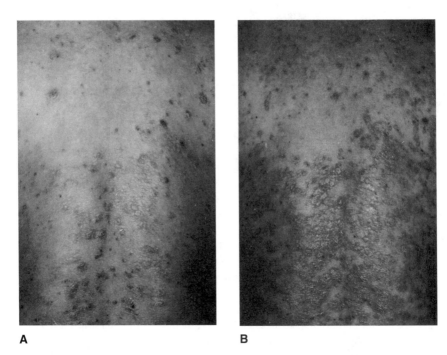

A   **B**

Figure 1 The eruption of this 53-year-old man was considerably worsened (A and B) when an ultrapotent topical corticosteroid was replaced by tacalcitol ointment because the corticosteroid had tended to exacerbate eruption. However, the patient's symptoms improved after continuous application of tacalcitol ointment (B, C, and D), remitting after 8 weeks of treatment (D). Under treatment (A) with a steroid preparation (ultrapotent topical corticosteroid), (B) 2 weeks after the steroid was replaced by tacalcitol ointment, (C) 4 weeks later, and (D) 8 weeks later.

costeroid. However, the patient's symptoms improved by continuous application of tacalcitol ointment (Figure 1B–D) and remitted after 8 weeks (Figure 1D) [6]. As mentioned previously, almost all cases of psoriasis had been treated with topical corticosteroids in Japan before the introduction of tacalcitol ointment.

Because psoriasis is generally treated over a long period of time, patients gradually become dependent on stronger topical corticosteroids. This is a cause of exacerbation at the time of a change to tacalcitol ointment. Although it was confirmed that psoriasis can be remitted by continuous application despite the initial exacerbation of symptoms (a rebound phenomenon), patients experience distress due to exacerbation even though it lasts for only a short period of time. Such a rebound phenomenon also influences the doctor-patient relationship. Thus a special

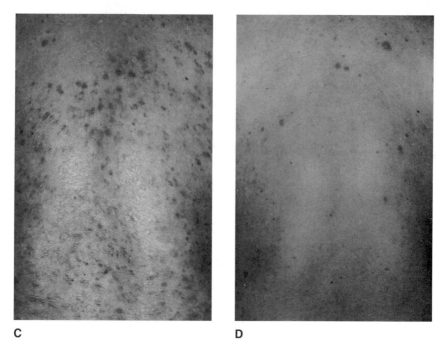

C   D

Figure 1 *(Continued)*

treatment regimen should be designed for the change from a strong topical corticosteroid to tacalcitol ointment. Second, because tacalcitol tends to manifest its effect slowly, tacalcitol ointment should sometimes be replaced by a topical corticosteroid at the request of patients who prefer fast-acting drugs after having switched over to tacalcitol. Therefore, particular care should be taken to watch for a rebound phenomenon at the time of shifting from a strong topical corticosteroid to this drug. It is also important to manage the situation when patients cannot wait for expression of the drug's effect. Against these problems, the concomitant use of a topical corticosteroid during an early period of the shift to tacalcitol has been attempted in Japan so as to avoid the rebound phenomenon and also to compensate for the slow onset of action of tacalcitol. As an actual technique, the number of corticosteroid applications and the degree of corticosteroid potency are gradually decreased by means of combined application, overlapping application, or morning and evening alternating application. At the time of occurrence of rebound—acute exacerbation, in other words—the concomitant use of appropriate therapy, such as cyclosporine, methotrexate, and PUVA, is also useful to prevent progression to a severer stage. However, care should be taken concerning compatibility for com-

Table 2 Compatibility and Incompatibility Between Tacalcitol Ointment and Steroid
External Preparations

Name of combination drug	Compatibility	Tacalcitol residue after 2 weeks	Tacalcitol residue after 4 weeks	Evaluation
Dermovate (clobetasol propionate) ointment	Satisfactory	97.4	98.5	○
Diflal (diflorasone diacetate) ointment	Satisfactory	73.4	39.9	×
Diacort (diflorasone diacetate) ointment	Satisfactory	94.7	96.4	○
Myser (difluprednate) ointment	Satisfactory	96.4	93.7	○
Nerisona (diflucortolone valerate) ointment	Satisfactory	100.2	100.7	○
Pandel (hydrocortisone butyrate propionate) ointment	Satisfactory	97.3	90.8	○
Budeson (budesonide) ointment	Satisfactory	91.4	73.3	△
Topsym (fluocinonide) ointment	Satisfactory	100.8	100.4	○
Rinderon-DP (betamethasone dipropionate) ointment	Satisfactory	101.5	99.6	○
Rinderon-VG (betamethasone valerate-gentamicin sulfate) ointment	Satisfactory	94.8	85.1	△
Fulmeta (mometasone furoate) ointment	Satisfactory	87.2	77.7	△
Methaderm (dexamethasone propionate) ointment	Satisfactory	104.3	102.5	○
Propaderm (beclometasone dipropionate) ointment	Satisfactory	71.3	28.4	×
Voalla (dexamethasone valerate) ointment	Satisfactory	98.7	87.1	△
Adcortin (halcinonide) ointment	Satisfactory	101.2	97.3	○
Lidomex Kowa (prednisolone valerate acetate) ointment	Satisfactory	100.0	101.1	○
Kindavate (clobetasone butyrate) ointment	Satisfactory	100.2	87.0	△
Almeta (alclometasone dipropionate) ointment	Satisfactory	94.8	75.7	△

Key: ○, Compatible; ×, Incompatible; △, Not-Incompatible.
Source: From Ref. 7.

bined application, because some topical corticosteroids affect the stability of tacalcitol while others do not (Table 2) [7]. By contrast, some investigators disagree with the concomitant use of tacalcitol with topical corticosteroids and recommend single therapy with tacalcitol. Their arguments are based on the view that it is unwise, in theory, to combine or concomitantly use drugs with reciprocal effects because differentiation of keratinocytes is inhibited by corticosteroids while it is stimulated by an active vitamin D_3 preparation such as tacalcitol. In a recent report of clinical evaluation, single therapy with tacalcitol is recommended. Abe et al. reported that tacalcitol ointment was used in 64 (61.0%) of 105 outpatients with psoriasis treated at Gumma University Hospital during the last year. When they retrospectively studied tacalcitol users, it was revealed that the efficacy rate of application of tacalcitol ointment alone was as high as 73% in patients also used no corticosteroid for more than 2 weeks prior to the use of tacalcitol, whereas the efficacy rate markedly dropped to 19% in patients who abruptly switched from a topical corticosteroid to tacalcitol (Figure 2). These results indicated the influences of topical corticosteroids on the manifestation of the effect of tacalcitol. In conclusion, they stated that it is practical to start application of tacalcitol ointment prior to the use of corticosteroid and to replace tacalcitol by a topical corticosteroid for nonresponders to tacalcitol [8]. Thorough explanation of the characteristic effects of both tacalcitol and corticosteroids should be given to patients before shifting from cor-

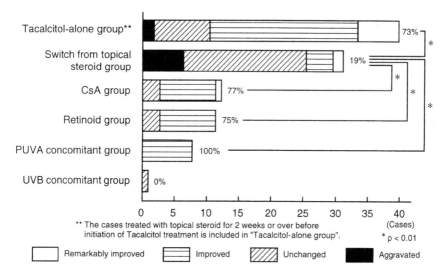

Figure 2 Difference in efficacy between tacalcitol alone group and concomitant therapy group. Each figure shows the percentage ratio of the sum of remarkable improvement versus improvement.

ticosteroids to single therapy with tacalcitol ointment. In general, the successful shift from topical corticosteroids to tacalcitol ointment largely depends on the degree of the potency of the topical corticosteroids that have been used.

IV. CLINICAL ADVANTAGES OF TACALCITOL OINTMENT

As for differences in clinical characteristics between corticosteroids and tacalcitol ointment, psoriasis recurs soon after the discontinuation of therapy in patients who have used corticosteroids ointments, sometimes in a severe state than the pretreatment state, because of a rebound phenomenon. For those treated with tacalcitol ointment, there is general agreement that the state of remission lasts longer, compared with corticosteroid users, after discontinuation following remission. In a report on the evaluation of tacalcitol and corticosteroids with regard to remission and recurrence [9], tacalcitol ointment and a steroid ointment (but not the ultrapotent class) were simply applied twice a day to one side each of the body in 11 selected psoriatic patients with symmetrical lesions until remission was achieved; then treatment was stopped and the lesions were observed until recurrence. The duration until remission was 67.5 ± 50.1 days in lesions treated with a corticosteroid ointment and 89.1 ± 46.8 days in those treated with tacalcitol ointment; there was no statistically significant difference between the two drugs. However, the duration between remission and recurrence was shorter in lesions treated with a topical corticosteroid in 10 patients; the remaining patient showed no recurrence on either side during the observation period. The mean duration until recurrence after discontinuation was 10.4 ± 12 days in corticosteroid-treated lesions and 32.1 ± 25.1 days in tacalcitol-treated lesions, showing a statistically significant difference between the two drugs. From these numerical data, the estimated numbers of eruption-free days per year can be estimated at 96.7 and 48.7 days in the use of tacalcitol ointment and a corticosteroid ointment, respectively. These results indicate that tacalcitol ointment takes a longer time to induce remission, but, compared with corticosteroid ointments, it maintains the state of remission for a longer period of time after it once induces remission.

V. CONCOMITANT THERAPY WITH TACALCITOL OINTMENT

Further, various attempts have been made to develop systemic therapies to support the antipsoriasis effect of tacalcitol. Danno treated symmetrical lesions in the same patients using PUVA plus tacalcitol ointment on one side of the body and PUVA plus corticosteroid ointment (betamethasone valerate) or white petrolatum on the other side. As PUVA therapy, UVA radiation was performed five times a week following the application of 0.1% methoxsalen. When the degree of eruption (erythema, dander, and infiltration) was scored and evaluated at 1 and 2 weeks after the start of treatment, PUVA plus tacalcitol ointment was found to be more effective in 3 of 5 cases and to be almost equal in the remaining 2 compared with PUVA plus corticosteroid ointment. PUVA plus tacalcitol ointment was also found to be more effective in 4 of 6 cases and to be almost equal in the remaining 2 compared with PUVA plus white petrolatum. The efficacy of PUVA plus tacalcitol ointment was higher than that of PUVA or tacalcitol ointment alone. Thus Danno concluded that combination therapy with PUVA and tacalcitol ointment can exert its effects more quickly and has a synergistic effect as compared with the use of either one alone [10]. Saito et al. evaluated the combination therapy with PUVA plus tacalcitol ointment according to a different protocol, and they reported that this combination was clearly superior to PUVA alone [11], although pigmentation due to PUVA tended to occur in regions treated with tacalcitol ointment. As to the concomitant use of tacalcitol ointment with UVB phototherapy, an opposing opinion has been elicited because the structure of active vitamin D_3 is easily destroyed by ultraviolet light— more strongly by ultraviolet B than by ultraviolet A—which also destroys active vitamin D_3, but only to a small extent. Aside from these opinions, there is a favorable view that this combination is effective in some cases. Oral therapy with cyclosporine has been used for severe psoriasis, and various attempts have been made to reduce adverse reactions to cyclosporine, such as renal dysfunction and blood pressure elevation, as much as possible by combining it with other therapy. When Nakagawa concomitantly used tacalcitol ointment or a topical corticosteroid (betamethasone valerate) in cases treated with cyclosporine at a reduced dose and compared changes in severity scores of eruption, he observed a higher degree of improvement of eruption in the tacalcitol ointment–combined group [12]. When oral therapy with methotrexate is combined with an external preparation, selection of an external preparation is of much importance, because methotrexate is administered only once a week. In other words, such an external preparation is a main medication, while methotrexate serves as an aid to compensate for the effect of the external preparation. When methotrexate therapy is combined with tacalcitol ointment, dose reduction and discontinuation of methotrexate can be done successfully, indicating that methotrexate is very compatible with tacalcitol ointment. Thus this combination is useful for adults who are not planning to have children and who maintain normal hepatic function. Methotrexate is thought to be an ideal drug that compensates for the slow onset of the action of tacalcitol ointment.

VI. EFFECT OF TACALCITOL OINTMENT ON SKIN DISEASES OTHER THAN PSORIASIS VULGARIS

Patients with pustular psoriasis are too few in number to compare the effect of tacalcitol ointment on this disease with that on psoriasis vulgaris. Based on clinical observation and genetic backgrounds of HLA types, Kobayashi et al. categorized generalized pustular psoriasis with acute inflammatory symptoms into the repeating type, in which psoriasis alternatively converted to psoriasis vulgaris with plaque-type lesions from pustular psoriasis, and the nonrepeating type without such conversion. After both types were treated with tacalcitol ointment, the investigators reached the conclusion that tacalcitol ointment is effective in the former type [13]. As for the effect of tacalcitol ointment on cutaneous diseases, other than psoriasis such as keratodermia, partial and complete responses have been reported in pityriasis rubra pilaris, pustulosis palmaris et plantaris, and Netherton's syndrome. Pityriasis rubra pilaris is a relatively rare form of inflammatory keratosis defined as an erythematous squamous disorder characterized by follicular plugging, perifollicular erythema tending to become confluent, and palmoplantar hyperkeratosis. This disease is classified into the following five types of Griffiths [14]: classical adult (type 1), atypical adult (type 2), classical juvenile (type 3), circumscribed juvenile (type 4), and atypical juvenile (type 5). A case with type 2 disease that had not been cured by oral administration of etretinate and application of a topical corticosteroid was completely cured by tacalcitol ointment alone within about 3 months [15]. In another case with type 2 disease, lesions treated with tacalcitol ointment were compared with those treated with a topical corticosteroid of the very strong class, and eruption in the tacalcitol-treated site was found to be definitely more improved at 1 month after the start of application compared with corticosteroid-treated lesions [16]. A pediatric case with this disease was also reported to be practically remitted at about 3 months after the start of application of tacalcitol ointment alone [17]. Partial and complete responses were also observed in keratosis follicularis squamosa [18,19]. As for pustulosis palmaris et plantaris, a case of complete response was reported [20]; sternoclavicular arthralgia and omarthralgia associated with this disease were also eliminated in another case [21]. Although seborrheic dermatitis worsened in 1 of 15 cases studied, no regional or systemic adverse reactions were observed in any of the other cases, and a complete response rate of 73% was obtained within 2 weeks [22]. These complete response cases did not recur for at least 4 weeks after the discontinuation of application. Further, tacalcitol ointment was also effective in the treatment of inflammatory linear verrucous epidermal nevus [23] and prurigo [24] even for topical corticosteroid–resistant cases.

VII. CONCLUSIONS

A cream containing tacalcitol at the same concentration as that of tacalcitol ointment was newly introduced to clinical practice in August 1997. The efficacy and safety of this cream have been reported to be comparable to those of the ointment [24,25].

The ointment may produce discomfort at use, such as a sticky feeling on the trunk and head and a greasy appearances on the face. The cream, however, has been highly rated because of the improvement of patients' quality of life by providing a better feeling at application. Only 4 years have passed since tacalcitol ointment was introduced to clinical practice, and only a limited number of reports on this drug have been published. Thus it was impossible to fulfill the purpose of this chapter based on the published data alone. Fortunately, because luncheon seminars concerning external preparations of active vitamin D_3 were held at conferences of the Japanese Dermatological Association in 1994–1997 (93d to 96th conferences) and at meetings of the Japanese Psoriasis Association in 1996 and 1997 (11th and 12th conferences), considerable data have been cited in this chapter from the reports presented at those seminars.

REFERENCES

1. Nishimura M, Yoshiaki H, Shigeo N, Yoshio N. Topical 1.24(OH)$_2$D$_3$ for the treatment of psoriasis: Review of the literature. Eur J Dermatol 1993; 3:255–261.
2. Ozawa, A. Up-to-date findings of the treatment of psoriasis. Nihon Iji Shinpo 1990; 3459:3–17 (in Japanese).
3. Kimura K, Katayama I, Nishioka K. Allergic contact dermatitis from tacalcitol. Contact Dermatitis 1995; 33:441–442.
4. Fukuda H, Imayama S. Erythma multiforme-like eruptions induced by topical tacalcitol ointment (abstr). Nishinihon J Derm 1995; 57:444–448 (in Japanese with English).
5. Yasuno Y. Psoriasis in childhood and its treatment. J Pediat Dermatol 1995; 14:1–6 (in Japanese).
6. Nishimura M. External therapy of psoriasis with active vitamin D_3. J Jpn Derm Assoc 1994; 104:1657–1661 (in Japanese).
7. Unpublished data (Biomedical General Laboratories, Teijin Co, Ltd).
8. Abe M, Ohnishi K, Warita S, Tamur´a A, Ishikawa O, Miyachi Y. External therapy with tacalcitol ointment for the treatment of psoriasis at the outpatient clinic of the Department of Dermatology, Gunma University School of Medicine. Hifuka Kiyo 1997; 92:395–402 (in Japanese).
9. Eto H. Recurrence after practical remission by tacalcitol ointment (part 2): Proceedings of the Luncheon Seminar at the 96th Conference of the Japanese Dermatological Association, 8–9, 1997 (in Japanese).
10. Kiriyama T, Danno K, Uehara M. Combination of topical tacalcitol and PUVA for psoriasis vulgaris. J Dermatol Treat 1997; 8:62–64.
11. Saito T, Kobayashi H, Ohkawara A. Treatment of psoriasis vulgaris with PUVA and topical vitamin D. Clin Dermatol 1996; 50:129–132 (in Japanese).
12. Nakagawa, H. Efficacy of the concomitant use with cyclosporine: Proceedings of the Satellite Seminar at the 11th Conference of the Japanese Psoriasis Association, 15–17, 1996 (in Japanese).

13. Kobayashi, H. Treatment of pustular psoriasis with an external active vitamin D_3 preparation: Proceedings of the Satellite Seminar at the 11th Conference of the Japanese Psoriasis Association, 18–20, 1996 (in Japanese).

14. Griffiths WAD. Pityriasis rubra pilaris. Clin Exp Dermatol 1980; 5:105–112.

15. Hirakawa T, Sato S, Okumoto Y, Yamamoto S. Successful treatment of pityriasis rubra pilaris with topical tacalcitol. Nishinihon J Dermatol 1995; 57:462–465 (in Japanese with English abstract).

16. Kikuchi S, Motoki Y, Nihei Y, Iwatuki K, Kaneko F. Complete response of pityriasis rubra pilaris associated with chronic renal failure to tacalcitol (Bonalfa®) ointment. Hifu Rinsho 1997; 39:1505–1508 (in Japanese).

17. Shukuwa T, Shimazaki K. A case of pityriasis rubra pilaris in childhood successfully treated with the topical application of $1\alpha,24$-dihydroxy vitamin D. Nishinihon J Derm 1995; 57:953–957 (in Japanese with English abstract).

18. Yamanaka K, Umeda Y, Mizutani H, Shimizu M. A case of keratosis follicularis squamosa with complete response to a vitamin D ointment. Hifu Rinsho 1996; 38:137–140 (in Japanese).

19. Oota T, Kubota Y, Oosuga Y, Sato Y, Mizoguchi M. A case of keratosis follicularis sqamosa. Hifu Rinsho 1996; 38:224–225 (in Japanese).

20. Mizutani H, Inachi S. Pustulosis palmoplantaris. Hifubyo Shinryou 1997; 19:617–618 (in Japanese).

21. Furue, M. A case of pustulosis palmaris et plantaris with complete response to tacalcitol ointment and elimination of sternoclavicular arthralgia and omarthralgia. Proc Med 1996; 16:1116–1118 (in Japanese).

22. Tadaki T, Kato T, Tagami H. Topical active vitamin D analogue, 1,24-dihydroxycholecalciferol, an effective new treatment for facial seborrhoeic dermatitis. J Dermatol Treat 1996; 7:139–141.

23. Mitsuhashi Y. Treatment of inflammatory linear verrucous epidermal naevus with topical vitamin D_3. Br J Dermatol 1997; 136:132–148.

24. Katayama I, Miyazaki Y, Nishioka K. Topical vitamin D (tacalcitol) for steroid-resistant prurigo. Br J Dermatol 1996; 135:237–240.

25. TV-02 Cream Psoriasis Research Group. Study of the efficacy of TV-02 cream on psoriasis an intergroup comparative study with TV-02 ointment. Nishinihon J Derm 1996; 58:144–153 (in Japanese).

26. TV-02 Cream Ichthyosis Research Group. Clinical results of the treatment of ichthyosis vulgaris with TV-02 cream. Nishinihon J Derm 1996; 58:154–158 (in Japanese).

24

European Experience with Tacalcitol

Niels K. Veien
The Dermatology Clinic, Aalborg, Denmark

I. INTRODUCTION

The vitamin D_3 analog 1,24-dihydroxycholecalciferol (tacalcitol), has been used as a systemic treatment for osteoporosis. In the course of this treatment it was seen that the psoriasis of some patients cleared. In an open study, Kato et al. [1] demonstrated that topical tacalcitol in concentrations of 1.2 or 4 $\mu g/g$ of ointment and occlusion was effective for the majority of 17 patients with psoriasis within approximately 3 weeks.

II. EUROPEAN STUDIES

Gerritsen et al. [2] studied the effects of once-daily treatment with 4 $\mu g/g$ tacalcitol ointment on epidermal proliferation, keratinization, and certain aspects of inflammation in a placebo-controlled, double-blind, right-left study of 10 patients with psoriasis vulgaris. Clinically, 8 of the 10 patients had statistically significantly greater improvement on the actively treated side than on the placebo-treated side. After 8 weeks, the psoriasis area and severity index (PASI) scores decreased from a mean of 3.7 to a mean of 1.9, compared with 3.8–2.8 for the placebo. Biopsies showed that markers of inflammation-and hyperproliferation-associated keratins returned to normal more rapidly on the actively treated than on the placebo-treated side. This difference was statistically significant.

A dose-finding study lasting 23 days was carried out by Baadsgaard et al. [3] in 50 patients who had stable psoriasis. Tacalcitol ointment containing concentrations of 0.25–16 $\mu g/g$ used once daily was compared with a placebo-treated site, an untreated site, and—as positive controls—sites treated with hydrocortisone butyrate, betamethasone dipropionate, and calcipotriol by applying each substance to a different test area on each of the 50 patients. The optimum concentration of tacalcitol was found to be 4 μg/g.

The overall scores for erythema, infiltration, and scaling decreased from a mean of 7.41 to 4.4 during the 23 days of the study, and the scores continued to decrease at the end of the study. In comparison, the mean score of sites treated only with the vehicle decreased from 7.4 to 6.0.

An 8-week multicenter, double-blind, placebo-controlled, right-left study with tacalcitol ointment 4 μg/g was carried out by van de Kerkhof et al. [4] in 122 patients with psoriasis vulgaris. After only 2 weeks of treatment, tacalcitol was seen to be statistically significantly more effective than the placebo, and it remained so throughout the study. The sum of the scores for desquamation, infiltration, and erythema decreased by a median of 5 points for the active treatment compared with 3 points for the placebo. The score for tacalcitol was still decreasing after 8 weeks of treatment. Of 122 patients, 30 had facial lesions. Only 2 patients reported skin irritation. Flexural lesions were also treated with tacalcitol, and the overall frequency of skin irritation was the same for tacalcitol and a placebo. Laboratory investigations showed no changes in calcium metabolism.

In an Italian multicenter study, once-daily treatment with 4 μg/g tacalcitol ointment was compared with betamethasone valerate ointment in a double-blind, right-left study lasting 6 weeks. Sixty-three patients with plaque-type psoriasis completed the study. During the 6 weeks, the mean score for erythema, thickness, and scaling decreased from 7.92 to 3.25 in the tacalcitol-treated group, compared with 7.92 to 2.65 in the bethamethasone valerate group. The difference was not statistically significant. There was no evidence that this treatment had any influence on calcium metabolism [5].

In a Scandinavian multicenter study [6], 287 patients with plaque-type psoriasis were treated once daily with 4 μg/g tacalcitol ointment, and they also applied the vehicle once daily. This was compared with twice-daily treatment with 50 μg/g calcipotriol ointment in an 8-week, double-blind study. The sum of the scores for severity of erythema, infiltration, and scaling was used to evaluate the severity of the disease before and during treatment. Whenever possible, three areas were evaluated: (1) elbows and/or knees, (2) an area distal to the knees, and (3) another area except the face or an intertriginous area.

Both treatments effectively reduced the severity of psoriasis. Twice-daily treatment with calcipotriol ointment was the most effective and reduced the sum score from a mean of 7.45 to 2.40, compared with a reduction of from 7.64 to 3.61 for tacalcitol. At the completion of the study, the severity scores for both treatments were still decreasing.

Both treatment schedules were safe with regard to calcium metabolism. There was no difference in irritancy, which was uncommon. Neither the face nor intertriginous areas were treated.

The results of the above studies are outlined in Table 1.

Table 1 European Tacalcitol Studies

Study	Number of patients	Type of study	Duration of treatment	Results	Side effects
Gerritsen et al. [2]	10	Cell-kinetics inflammation Placebo-controlled, double-blind, right-left One center	8 weeks	Tacalcitol normalized epidermal keratinization and proliferation and reduced inflammation Tacalcitol clinically superior to placebo	None No influence on calcium metabolism
Baadsgaard et al. [3]	58 enrolled 50 evaluated	Dose-finding, placebo-controlled, double-blind Limited areas Multiple concentrations and controls Two centers	23 days	Optimum concentration of tacalcitol $4\,\mu g/g$	13 had itching or irritation unrelated to concentration of tacalcitol 8 of the 13 had symptoms not necessarily related to treatment No laboratory data
Van de Kerkhof et al. [4]	122 (intention to treat) 103 (per protocol)	Clinical efficacy Placebo-controlled, double-blind, right-left Multicenter	8 weeks	Tacalcitol superior to placebo	15 had skin irritation—unilateral in 5 (3 tacalcitol, 2 placebo) Tolerance good in 95–99% No abnormal laboratory data

continued

Table 1 Continued

Study	Number of patients	Type of study	Duration of treatment	Results	Side effects
Scarpa [5]	76 enrolled 63 evaluated	Clinical efficacy compared with betamethasone valerate, double-blind, right-left Multicenter	6 weeks	No statistical difference between tacalcitol and betamethasone valerate	Itching in two treated with tacalcitol Folliculitis in one treated with betamethasone valerate No abnormality of calcium metabolism
Veien et al. [6]	287 (intention to treat) 226 (per protocol)	Clinical efficacy compared with calcipotriol Randomized, double-blind Multicenter	8 weeks	Twice-daily calcipotriol superior to once-daily tacalcitol	Minor in 12.7% treated with tacalcitol and 11.7% treated with calcipotriol Four treated with tacalcitol and five with calcipotriol dropped out due to local side effects No abnormality of calcium metabolism

III. DISCUSSION

The results of European trials show that topical tacalcitol treatment suppresses psoriasis vulgaris. In several of the studies cited here, scores for the severity of psoriasis continued to decrease at the completion of up to 8 weeks of treatment. This suggests that a longer treatment period would prove even more effective.

No direct comparisons of the efficacy of tacalcitol and calcipotriol, the only other vitamin D_3 derivative marketed for the topical treatment of psoriasis, have been made. Once-daily treatment with tacalcitol proved less effective than twice-daily treatment with calcipotriol [6]. This difference was marginal, and the clinical relevance of the difference is questionable, as a once-daily treatment regimen may be the most realistic for most patients. During a trial, patients are very loyal to treatment programs, as demonstrated in the Scandinavian multicenter study, where the mean amount of topical preparations used morning and evening was the same. Slightly less than twice the amount of calcipotriol (a mean of 189 g) was used compared with the amount of tacalcitol (a mean of 100 g) during the 8-week period of this trial. Such compliance cannot be expected outside the rigid regime of a well-conducted trial.

It has been suggested that tacalcitol is less of a skin irritant than calcipotriol. A comparison of the irritancy of calcipotriol, tacalcitol, and calcitriol carried out by patch testing on hairless guinea pigs showed no difference among the three compounds [7]. In this study, clinical readings as well as a histological examination, laser-Doppler image scanning, skin-color measurement, ultrasound determination of edema, and determination of transepidermal water loss were carried out.

Facial and intertriginous lesions were not treated in the Scandinavian multicenter study, which showed tacalcitol and calcipotriol to have an equal number of side effects. Only 2 of 30 patients with facial lesions in the study of van de Kerkhof et al. [4] had skin irritation following the use of tacalcitol, and the treatment of flexural psoriasis did not cause skin irritation either. Calcipotriol has been used successfully in an open study of intertriginous psoriasis, where 10 of 12 patients responded to the treatment. Five patients had slight perilesional irritation, and one had minimal burning [8].

A comparative study of calcipotriol and tacalcitol used for facial and flexural psoriasis would be useful in determining the relative skin irritancy of the two drugs.

The sensitizing potential of tacalcitol is not well documented. One patient developed allergic contact dermatitis from a tacalcitol ointment [9]. There have been only a few reports of sensitization to calcipotriol used extensively for a number of years as a topical treatment of psoriasis [10–12]. The scarcity of such reports suggests that these vitamin D_3 derivatives are weak sensitizers.

Most studies of the treatment of psoriasis with tacalcitol have included patients with stable plaque psoriasis. During treatment, PASI scores or total sum scores for erythema, infiltration, and scaling typically decrease for these patients to approximately half of the pretreatment levels. This indicates an effect of the drug but not necessarily that it is as effective as what patients expect from treatment. It may, therefore, be necessary to combine the use of tacalcitol with topical corticosteroids or ultraviolet light. Studies of such combination therapy have been carried out for calcipotriol but not for tacalcitol. It would also be of interest to study treatment results in less stable psoriasis, as such studies would reflect the needs of many psoriasis patients.

Another issue of interest to patients with chronic skin diseases like psoriasis is the long-term management of the disease. None of the studies published thus far has dealt with the usefulness of tacalcitol for maintenance therapy.

REFERENCES

1. Kato T, Rukugo M, Terui T, Tagami H. Successful treatment of psoriasis with topical application of active vitamin D_3 analogue, 1 alpha, 24-dihydroxycholecalciferol. Br J Dermatol 1986; 115:431–433.
2. Gerritsen MJP, Boezeman JBM, Van Vlijmen-Willems IMJJ, Van de Kerkhof PCM. The effect of tacalcitol (1,24(OH_2D_3) on cutaneous inflammation, epidermal proliferation and keratinization in psoriasis: A placebo-controlled, double-blind study. Br J Dermatol 1994; 131:57–63.
3. Baadsgaard O, Traulsen J, Roed-Petersen J, Jakobsen HB. Optimal concentration of tacalcitol in once-daily treatment of psoriasis. J Dermatol Treat 1995; 6:145–150.
4. Van de Kerkhof PCM, Werfel T, Haustein, UF, Luger T, Czarnetzki BM, Niemann R, Plänitz-Stenzel V. Tacalcitol ointment in the treatment of psoriasis vulgaris: A multicentre, placebo-controlled, double-blind study on efficacy and safety. Br J Dermatol 1996; 135:758–765.
5. Scarpa C. Tacalcitol ointment is an efficacious and well tolerated treatment for psoriasis. J Eur Acad Dermatol Venereol 1996; 6:142–146.
6. Veien NK, Bjerke JR, Rossmann-Ringdahl I, Jakobsen HB. Once daily treatment of psoriasis with tacalcitol compared with twice daily treatment with calcipotriol: A double-blind trial. Br J Dermatol 1997; 137:581–586.
7. Fullerton A, Serup J. Topical D-vitamins: Multiparametric comparison of the irritant potential of calcipotriol, tacalcitol and calcitriol in a hairless guinea pig model. Contact Dermatitis 1997; 36:184–190.
8. Kienbaum, S, Lehmann P, Ruzicka T. Topical calcipotriol in the treatment of intertriginous psoriasis. Br J Dermatol 1996; 135:647–650.
9. Kimura K, Katayma I, Nishioka K. Allergic contact dermatitis from tacalcitol. Contact Dermatitis 1995; 33:441–442.
10. De Groot AC. Contact allergy to calcipotriol. Contact Dermatitis 1994; 30:242–243.
11. Steinkjer B. Contact dermatitis from calcipotriol. Contact Dermatitis 1994; 31:122.
12. Garcia-Bravo B, Camacho F. Two cases of contact dermatitis caused by calcipotriol cream. Am J Contact Dermatitis 1996; 7:118–119.

25

Vitamin D Analogs in Ichthyosis and Other Disorders of Keratinization

Peter M. Steijlen and Peter C. M. van de Kerkhof
University Hospital Nijmegen, Nijmegen, The Netherlands

I. INTRODUCTION

The disorders of keratinization comprise a heterogenous group of diseases that include the different forms of ichthyosis, the various forms of palmoplantar keratodermas, Darier's disease, porokeratosis, pityriasis rubra pilaris, and verrucous epidermal nevus. Most of these diseases are genetically determined and require long-term therapy. Their treatment has not received the broad attention that has been dedicated to the more frequently occurring diseases, like psoriasis. Although each entity within the group of disorders of keratinization has a relatively low occurrence in itself, the total group is large. The general dermatologist is therefore often faced with the need to provide the patient suffering from a disorder of keratinization the most optimal treatment. The common treatment of these disorders with bland emolients containing keratolytics like urea, lactic acid, and salicylic acid can lead to some improvement, but in most cases this improvement is insufficient. Topical retinoids like all-trans-retinoic acid 0.1% can be effective, but their application has never been established owing to their irritative side effects. In many disorders of keratinization, systemic retinoids like etretinate and acitretin have proven to be very effective. As serious side effects may be associated with systemic retinoid treatment, the use of these drugs is limited. Therefore the development of vitamin D_3 analogs was and is very promising. The disorders of keratinization have in common a defect in cornification. The underlying pathogenesis is a disordered keratinocyte differentiation and/or proliferation. The effects of 1,25-dihydroxy vitamin D_3 on epidermal keratinocytes has been studied extensively. Although $1.25(OH)_2D_3$ promotes the differentiation of keratinocytes (1), the effect on keratinocyte proliferation is less clear. Apparently $1,25(OH)_2D_3$ and synthetic vitamin D3 analogs can stimulate the proliferation of normal epidermis (2,3). In contrast, the proliferation of hyperplastic epidermis is inhibited (4). Because of the modulating effect on epidermal growth and the enhancement of normal differentiation, a positive effect of vitamin D_3 analogs in the treatment of disorders of keratinization might be expected.

Several studies and case reports concerning the treatment of disorders of keratinization with vitamin D_3 analogs have been reported. This chapter reviews the disorders of keratinization in which vitamin D_3 analogs might be effective.

II. ICHTHYOSIS

This group comprises different etiological entities which have in common that they are all characterized by a generalized scaling involving the whole integument.

A. Autosomal Dominant Ichthyosis Vulgaris

Autosomal dominant ichthyosis vulgaris (ADIV) is the most common form of ichthyosis, with an estimated incidence of about 1:250. It usually starts during the first year of life and is characterized by white to light-gray scales covering mainly the trunk and extensor surfaces of the extremities. The severity can vary remarkably. Bland emollients are usually sufficient to control mild conditions. More severe forms require keratolytic treatment and in some cases even systemic treatment is needed with retinoids.

Vitamin D_3, or $1,25(OH)2D_3$, applied topically as 0.1 $\mu g/g$ in a Vaseline base three times daily, has been reported to be ineffective in five patients with ADIV after 4 weeks of treatment (5). Systemic treatment with $1(OH)D_3$ during 2 months appeared to be ineffective in patients with ADIV (6). In a randomized, double-blind, vehicle-controlled right/left comparative study, nine patients were treated with calcipotriol ointment 50 $\mu g/g$ for 12 weeks. In about 50% of the patients, a marked improvement was observed on the calcipotriol-treated side (7). Because in most patients a slight or moderate improvement could be observed on the vehicle side, the difference was not statistically significant. The ingredients of the vehicle were, among others, propylene glycol, petrolatum, and liquid paraffin. As is known, these ingredients can improve scaling, especially in milder forms of ichthyosis.

B. X-linked Recessive Ichthyosis Vulgaris

The frequency of X-linked recessive ichthyosis (XRI) is estimated at 1 in 2000 males. Although a slight scaling may often be visible during the first weeks after birth, the ichthyosis is clearly visible after about 2 to 6 months. The scales are often brown, thick, and rhombic and mainly located on the trunk and the extremities. The palms and soles are free. The underlying defect is a deficiency of the enzyme steroid sulfatase, which normally catalyzes the breakdown of cholesterol sulfate. Accumulation of cholesterol sulfate in the cornified cell layer causes increased cohesion between the corneocytes and therefore a retention hyperkeratosis. The gene coding for the enzyme is located on the X chromosome. Although patients may respond sufficiently to topical emollients, many require a more effective treatment. Sometimes systemic retinoids might be indicated. In a blind, vehicle-controlled, right/left comparative study, topical application of $1,25(OH)_2D_3$ as 0.1 $\mu g/g$ in a Vaseline base three times daily appeared to be ineffective in eight patients with XRI after 4 weeks of treatment (5). Also, systemic $1(OH)D_3$ was reported to be ineffective in patients with XRI (6). In a randomized, double-blind, vehicle-controlled right/left comparative study, eight patients were treated with calcipotriol ointment 50 $\mu g/g$ for 12 weeks (7). In about 50% of the patients, a marked improvement was observed on the calcipotriol-treated side. The difference between calcipotriol and vehicle appeared to be statistically significant. Irritation of the skin was common but didnot lead to discontinuation.

C. Lamellar Ichthyoses (LI)

Clinically and genetically, the lamellar ichthyoses form a heterogenous group. The frequency of LI has been estimated at about 1 in 100.000. One distinguishes an autosomal dominant type (ADLI) from the recessive forms, which can be subdivided into an erythrodermic form (ELI), also referred to as nonbullous congenital ichthyosiform erythroderma, and a nonerythrodermic form (NELI). The ELI type is characterized by the presence of an erythroderma since birth and often by a fine, translucent scaling. The NELI type has a rougher lamellar scaling. Palms and feet may be affected in both cases. In practice, it appeared that some patients could not be classified into either of the subgroups because they had characteristics of both forms. Molecular biological investigation has demonstrated that LI may be caused by a mutation in the gene that codes for transglutaminase 1 on chromosome 14. This enzyme is involved in the formation of the cornified envelope. Another locus situated on chromosome 2 has been identified. So far only systemic retinoids have been effective in these severe disorders (8).

In a randomized, double-blind, vehicle-controlled right/left comparative study, two patients with NELI and two with ELI were treated with calcipotriol ointment 50 $\mu g/g$ for 12 weeks (7). At the end of the study, all patients showed a statistically significant reduction of scaling and roughness on the calcipotriol-treated side (Figure 1).

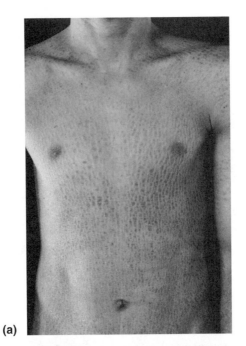

(a)

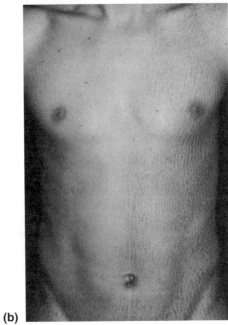

(b)

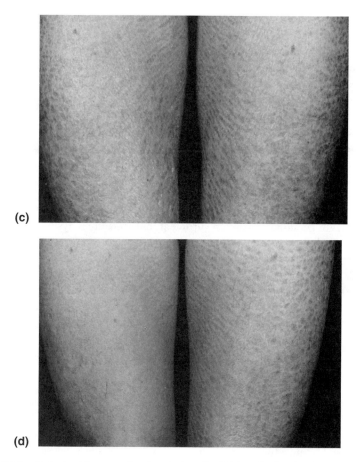

Figure 1 Patient with nonerythrodermic lamellar ichthyosis showing large brown scales on the trunk (a) and on the legs (c) before treatment. After 12 weeks of treatment, the calcipotriol-treated right side has improved markedly, whereas only slight improvement has occurred on the ointment base–treated left side (b) and (d).

D. Bullous Ichthyoses

The bullous ichthyoses form a heterogenous group characterized by the coexistence of blistering. Two types can be differentiated: bullous congenital ichthyosiform erythroderma of Brocq (BCIE) and ichthyosis bullosa of Siemens (IBS). BCIE is an autosomal dominant disease characterized by extensive erythroderma and considerable blister formation at birth. Nursing in an incubator is often necessary. The tendency to form blisters decreases during the first years but the hyperkeratosis increases substantially. The palms and soles may also be affected. Histological examination shows the picture of epidermolytic hyperkeratosis. Clumping of tonofilaments (keratins) and loosening of the desmosomes in the whole suprabasal region is observed upon electron microscopy. Molecular biology investigation has demonstrated that BCIE is based on a mutation in either the keratin 1 gene or keratin 10 gene. Systemic treatment of BCIE patients with retinoiods is limited because of the induction of blistering (9).

IBS is a milder disorder than BCIE. As such there is no congenital erythroderma and the tendency for blister formation and the hyperkeratosis is more limited. The histological findings that fit within the framework of epidermolytic hyperkeratosis are noted only in the upper layers of the stratum spinosum. Investigations showed that the disorder was based on a mutation in keratin 2e, a keratin that is expressed only in the upper layers of the stratum spinosum. Topical treatment with keratolytics is often sufficient, but sometimes systemic treatment with retinoids is required (9).

In a prospective, double-blind, bilaterally paired comparative study, one patient with BCIE and two patients with IBS were treated with calcipotriol ointment (50 $\mu g/g$) and the ointment vehicle (7). After 12 weeks, a marked improvement was observed on the calcipotriol-treated side in the patient with BCIE. In the two patients with IBS who displayed a milder hyperkeratosis, the difference between calcipotriol and vehicle was less clear.

E. Other Types of Ichthyoses

The Sjögren-Larsson syndrome (SLS) is a rare autosomal recessive disorder characterized by the triad of congenital ichthyosis, spastic bi-/quadriplegia, and mental retardation. The skin abnormalities are present at birth. Initially, they may consist of a slight scaling, but yellowish to dark brown wrinkled hyperkeratosis, often with a lichenoid aspect, develops after several months. The preferential locations are the flanks, abdomen and flexures. In this disease there is a disturbance in the fatty alcohol cycle. Mutations in the fatty aldehyde dehydrogenase gene situated on chromosome 17 have been demonstrated. So far only systemic treatment with retinoids has been effective to alleviate the ichthyosis. Two patients with SLS were treated with calcipotriol in ointment and the ointment base only for 12 weeks, using a double-blind bilaterally paired comparative study. Unilateral improvement was observed in both patients in favor of the calcipotriol-treated side (7). Comèl-Netherton syndrome is a very rare autosomal recessive disorder. Children are born with an erythroderma that requires nursing in an incubator. Later, migrating polycyclic scaling lesions develop. This form of ichthyosis is observed in association with hair-shaft anomalies. Treatment with bland emollients with or without keratolytics or systemic retinoids is disappointing. One patient, was treated with calcipotriol in ointment and the ointment base only for 12 weeks, using a double-blind, bilaterally paired comparative study (7). No improvement was observed in either the calcipotriol-treated side or the vehicle-treated side.

III. PALMOPLANTAR KERATODERMAS

About 20 different entities are differentiated in the group of the monogenic palmoplantar keratodermas. The hyperkeratosis can be diffuse or localized. The most frequent form is Vörner's disease.

Vörner's disease is an autosomal dominant palmoplantar keratoderma characterized by a diffuse hyperkeratosis located on the palms and soles. Knuckle-pad lesions can be present. Histological examination shows the features of epidermolytic hyperkeratosis, including perinuclear vacuolization and clumping of tonofilaments. The disorder is caused by point mutations in the gene coding for keratin 9, which lies on chromosome 17. Patients can be helped by the application of keratolytics. Systemic retinoids like acitretin are effective but may cause excessive peeling and even blistering. Using a bilaterally paired comparative approach, calcipotriol 50 µg/g and urea 40 mg/g, both in an ointment base, were applied twice daily to the right and left hands respectively (10). Within 4 weeks, focal reduction of hyperkeratosis was reached. As a result of increased tactile sensitivity, the application frequency was reduced to three applications per week. Clinical evaluation at 3 months revealed a marked improvement on the calcipotriol-treated side. In a randomized, double-blind, vehicle-controlled right/left comparative study, 22 patients with palmoplantar keratoderma were treated with calcipotriol ointment 50 µg/g for 12 weeks (7). There was no statistically significant difference between calcipotriol and vehicle.

IV. DARIER'S DISEASE

Darier's disease is an autosomal dominant trait with an estimated frequency ranging from 1:55,000 to 1:100,000. Skin-colored to reddish brown papules are found on the sites of predilection such as the chest, back, hairline, neck, scalp, and ears. The disease usually starts between the ages of 6 and 10 years. There is great interindividual variation in severity, from only a few lesions to widespread forms covering a substantial part of the body surface. On histological examination, acantholysis is found, due to disruption of the desmosome-keratin-filament complex as observed by electronmicroscopy. The underlying genetic defect is a mutation in a calcium 2+ pump coded for by a gene on chromosome 12. For widespread forms, the classic treatment is the administration of systemic retinoids. The dosage must be individualized. However side effects limit their use, especially in women of childbearing age. In a randomized, double-blind, vehicle-controlled right/left comparative study, 12 patients were treated with calcipotriol ointment 50 μg/g for 12 weeks (7). Seven patients withdrew because of lesional and perilesional irritation or worsening of the disease. Irritation was observed on both sides. There was no statistically significant difference between calcipotriol and vehicle in this study. Using a bilaterally paired comparative approach, calcipotriol 50 mg/g and emollient containing urea 40 mg/g were applied twice daily to the right and left sides of the back, respectively, in one patient with severe Darier's disease (11). In contrast to the first study, the typical keratotic lesions in this case began to regress after 1 month of therapy; a significant improvement was noted clinically and histologically after 3 months.

V. KERATOSIS PILARIS, DISSEMINATED SUPERFICIAL ACTINIC POROKERATOSIS, PITYRIASIS RUBRA PILARIS, INFLAMMATORY LINEAR VERRUCOUS NEVUS

Keratosis pilaris is a very common disorder of keratinization. The causative gene has so far not been identified. Small gray-white plugs obstruct the mouths of the hair follicles. Perifollicular erythema is often present. Sites of predilection include the extensor surfaces of the arms, thighs, and buttocks. Bland emollients are generally ineffective. In a randomized, double-blind, vehicle-controlled right/left comparative study, nine patients were treated with calcipotriol ointment 50 μg/g for 12 weeks. There was no statistically significant difference between calcipotriol and vehicle (7).

Disseminated superficial actinic porokeratosis is an autosomal dominant trait characterized by hyperkeratotic lesions in sun-exposed areas on the legs and arms. Histologically, the lesions show a column of parakeratosis (cornoid lamella) overlying an epidermal depression with dyskeratotic keratinocytes and an absent granular layer. Three patients were treated topically with calcipotriol once daily for a period of 6 to 8 weeks. Although there was minor skin irritation in two patients, there were no side effects and improvement was maintained for up to 6 months in two patients (12).

Pityriasis rubra pilaris is a rare polygenic disease comprising several varieties. The cause of the disease is unknown. Patients may show circumscribed follicular papular keratoses which can coalescence to plaques, palmoplantar keratoderma, and erythroderma. Histopathological examination shows follicular plugging, acanthosis, spotty parakeratosis, and a mild upper dermal infiltrate. The therapeutic options for patients with pityriasis rubra pilaris are limited. In three cases, calcipotriol ointment 50 μg/g used twice daily produced a substantial improvement (13). The long-term presence of the skin lesions and the prompt improvement within the first month of treatment strongly suggest that the improvement was induced by calcipotriol. However, it should be noted that the approach was not placebo-controlled. One patient experienced irritation, which necessitated discontinuation.

The Inflammatory linear verrucous epidermal nevus almost always occurs sporadically and has its onset during the first 5 years of life in most cases. The pruritic, scaly, confluent, erythematous papules are arranged in a linear pattern and are characterized histologically by a lymphohistiocytic inflammatory infiltrate with hypergranulosis and orthokeratosis alternating with agranulosis and parakeratotic hyperkeratosis. The most effective therapy is surgical excision. However, a surgical procedure will result in a permanent scar and is not always feasible. Zvulunov et al. treated a $2^1/_2$-year-old girl and a 10-year-old boy with calcipotriol ointment twice daily, achieving rapid relief of pruritus and marked regression of the lesions (14). A 20-year-old woman was treated with topical calcipotriol ointment twice daily. After 2 weeks, pruritus and erythema decreased. After 4 weeks, the hyperkeratosis was reduced, and after 8 weeks the lesions had almost completely resolved (15).

VI. CONCLUSIONS

Calcipotriol ointment has been applied in several disorders of keratinization. Much data had become available in the well-controlled multicenter study published by Kragballe et al (7). Additional findings were obtained from the published case histories reviewed in this chapter. It should be borne in mind that several of these case histories do not reflect a placebo-controlled approach. What has become clear is that calcipotriol ointment has a place in the treatment of the more severe disorders of keratinization, like X-linked recessive ichthyosis, lamellar ichthyosis, Sjögren-Larsson syndrome, pityriasis rubra pilaris, and inflammatory linear verrucous epidermal nevi. Although calcipotriol is well tolerated by patients with these disorders, it may worsen Darier's disease, probably due to its irritating capacity.

A major concern during treatment with calcipotriol is the theoretical risk of hypercalcemia. Most of the disorders of keratinization involve large areas. The recommended quantity of 100 g/week is easily reached when calcipotriol is applied twice daily. Another question is how much the abnormal epidermis might enhance or inhibit the absorption of calcipotriol. In the multicenter study, calcipotriol 120 g/week appeared to be safe (7). However, in this study, only half a side had been treated. Studies should be performed to determine whether once-daily application is as effective as twice-daily application. Further, it would be interesting to find out to what extent combination with topical or systemic treatment with retinoids might enhance effectiveness. Children with a severe disorder of keratinization need special attention. The dermatologist is often reluctant to use systemic retinoids to treat these patients. An alternative might be the use of calcipotriol ointment. Topical calcipotriol appeared to be safe in childhood psoriasis when the maximum amount was adjusted to the child's body surface (16).

REFERENCES

1. Hosomi J, Hosoi J, Abe E, Suda T, Kuroki T. Regulation of terminal differentiation of cultured mouse epidermal cells by 1 alpha,25-dihydroxyvitamin D3. Endocrinology 1983; 113:1950–1957.
2. Lutzow Holm C, De Angelis P, Grosvik H, Clausen OP. 1,25-Dihydroxyvitamin D3 and the vitamin D analogue KH1060 induce hyperproliferation in normal mouse epidermis: a BrdUrd/DNA flow cytometric study. Exp Dermatol 1993; 2:113–120.
3. Gniadecki R, Serup J. Stimulation of epidermal proliferation in mice with 1 alpha, 25-dihydroxyvitamin D3 and receptor-active 20-EPI analogues of 1 alpha, 25-dihydroxyvitamin D3. Biochem Pharmacol 1995; 49:621–624.
4. Kato T, Terui T, Tagami H. Topically active vitamin D3 analogue, 1 alpha,24-dihydroxy-cholecalciferol, has an anti-proliferative effect on the epidermis of guinea pig skin (letter). Br J Dermatol 1987; 117:528–530.
5. Okano M. 1 alpha,25-(OH)2D3 use on psoriasis and ichthyosis. Int J Dermatol 1991; 30:62–64.
6. Okano M, Kitano Y, Yoshikawa K. A trial of oral 1 alpha-hydroxyvitamin D3 for ichthyosis (letter). Dermatologica 1988; 177:23.
7. Kragballe K, Steijlen PM, Ibsen HH, van de Kerkhof PC, Esmann J, Sorensen LH, Axelsen MB. Efficacy, tolerability, and safety of calcipotriol ointment in disorders of keratinization: results of a randomized, double-blind, vehicle-controlled, right/left comparative study. Arch Dermatol 1995; 131:556–560.
8. Steijlen PM, van Dooren Greebe RJ, van de Kerkhof PC. Acitretin in the treatment of lamellar ichthyosis. Br J Dermatol 1994; 130:211–214.
9. Steijlen PM, van Dooren Greebe RJ, Happle R, van de Kerkhof PC. Ichthyosis bullosa of Siemens responds well to low-dosage oral retinoids. Br J Dermatol 1991; 125: 469–471.
10. Lucker GP, van de Kerkhof PC, Steijlen PM. Topical calcipotriol in the treatment of epidermolytic palmoplantar keratoderma of Vorner (letter). Br J Dermatol 1994; 130: 543–545.
11. Simonart T, Peny MO, Noel JC, De Dobbeleer G. Topical calcipotriol in the treatment of Darier's disease. Eur J Dermatol 1996; 6:36–38.
12. Harrison PV, Stollery N. Disseminated superficial actinic porokeratosis responding to calcipotriol [letter]. Clin Exp Dermatol 1994; 19:95.
13. van de Kerkhof PC, Steijlen PM. Topical treatment of pityriasis rubra pilaris with calcipotriol. Br J Dermatol 1994; 130:675–678.

14. Zvulunov A, Grunwald MH, Halvy S. Topical calcipotriol for treatment of inflammatory linear verrucous epidermal nevus. Arch Dermatol 1997; 133:567–568.
15. Gatti S, Carrozzo AM, Orlandi A, Nini G. Treatment of inflammatory linear verrucous epidermal naevus with calcipotriol (letter). Br J Dermatol 1995; 132:837–839.
16. Oranje AP, Marcoux D, Svensson A, Prendiville J, Krafchik B, Toole J, Rosenthal D, de Waard van der Spek FB, Molin L, Axelsen M. Topical calcipotriol in childhood psoriasis. J Am Acad Dermatol 1997; 36:203–208.

26
Role of Vitamin D and Analogs in Local and Systemic Scleroderma

Philippe G. Humbert
University Hospital St. Jacques, Besançon, France

I. INTRODUCTION

The treatment of progressive systemic sclerosis (PSS) as well as morphea is a difficult problem, since today there is little effective treatment. The principal therapies used in scleroderma are D-penicillamine, colchicine, penicillin G, aromatic retinoids, and interferon gamma (IFN-γ).

Some years ago, we reported the use of oral 1,25 dihydroxyvitamin D_3 [1,25(OH)$_2$D$_3$] in a patient with localized scleroderma [1]. The beneficial effects prompted us to treat other patients with morphea as well as patients with progressive systemic sclerosis.

II. HISTORY

Sixty years ago, scleroderma was considered by a French author to be a cutaneous expression of hyperparathyroidism [2]. Thus, parathyroidectomy was described as a successful treatment for certain type of scleroderma [3]. Nevertheless, Cornbleet and Struck [4] did not feel "that it has been proved that parathyroid dysfunction is the underlying cause of scleroderma." Therefore, they thought it of interest from a practical and a theoretical point of view to administer large amounts of vitamin D to subjects suffering from abnormal deposition of calcium in soft tissues. Accordingly 11 patients with scleroderma (systemic sclerosis and morphea) were treated with vitamin D. Only 2 patients did not respond to treatment.

Epidemiological evidence, such as the lesser prevalence of the condition in both Australian people and Eskimos (the first being exposed to sun, the second ingesting abundant vitamin D) led Norman to believe that vitamin D could be useful in the treatment of scleroderma. In his paper, Norman [5] reported on three patients suffering from scleroderma who were treated with vitamin D in amounts ranging from 50,000–100,000 U. These patients had serious skin manifestations and some muscle and tendon involvement. "In all three patients improvement to the point of complete rehabilitation occurred, with restoration of normal skin. . . . Joint involvement was markedly reduced, together with increase of active and passive movement and disappearance of pain." Maynard [6], as well, employed vitamin D therapy successfully in the treatment of scleroderma patches. Since then, no other papers on this subject have been published.

At our center, one patient with localized scleroderma experienced marked clinical improvement while receiving oral $1,25(OH)_2D_3$ [1]. This beneficial result prompted us to explore on the possible use of the hormone in the treatment of both localized scleroderma [7] and PSS [8]. The first group consisted in seven patients (mean age, 32.4 years) who suffered from localized scleroderma and whose duration of disease varied from 2–10 years. The mean dose of $1,25(OH)_2D_3$ administered orally was 1.75 μg/day. This dosage was progressively reached, beginning with 0.25 μg/day during the first week. All patients responded to treatment, four of them being cleared within 2–24 months. A quantitative assessment using a torsional device to measure skin extensibility and an echometer to measure skin thickness was performed. The intrinsic extensibility of the skin was enhanced from 1.51–3.67.

The second group consisted of 11 patients with systemic sclerosis who entered an open prospective trial during a 6-month to 3-year treatment period. Initial assessment and evaluation after the treatment period included clinical evaluation, oral aperture measurements, palmar flexion index, skin torsion measurements, and skin thickness. Oral aperture increased significantly from 28–33 mm, and the plamar flexion index decreased from 28.7–12 mm. The intrinsic skin extensibility was significantly enhanced during the treatment period. In October 1994, Hulshof et al. [9] described three patients with generalized morphea who were treated with calcitriol in an oral dose of 0.5–0.75 μg/day. After 3–7 months of treatment, the patients improved significantly in joint mobility and skin extensibility. These pilot studies suggest a beneficial effect of high dosages of vitamin D in patients with localized scleroderma and progressive systemic sclerosis.

III. SCLERODERMA AND VITAMIN D

A. Scleroderma

Scleroderma is a generalized fibrotic disorder of unknown etiology, but immunological factors play a role at some stage in the course of the disease [10]. It is characterized by excessive collagen synthesis and deposition in internal organs and the skin [11]. Disturbances of the fibroblast metabolism lead to fibrosis, with over-production and accumulation of matrix proteins in the involved connective tissue. Indeed, in scleroderma, a special functional subset of fibroblasts is able to over-produce collagen [12]. Overproduction of collagen seems to be mediated by cytokine dysregulation of the fibroblast function. It has been suggested that mediators from platelets or mononuclear infiltrating cells may be responsible for the activation of fibroblasts in these disorders, resulting in excessive deposition of connective tissue. To date, cytokines reported to stimulate fibroblast functions in vitro and to play an important role in the dysregulation of fibroblast metabolism, leading to fibrosis, include transforming growth factor beta (TGF-β) (which is produced by platelets, monocytes, macrophages and T lymphocytes), platelet-derived growth factor (PDGF) from platelets and monocytes/macrophages, tumor necrosis factor alpha (TNF-α), interferon gamma (IFN-γ), and other monokines from monocytes/macrophages. Most of these cytokines stimulate collagen synthesis [13].

B. Vitamin D

Calcitriol is 1,25-dihydroxycholecalciferol, the most potent form of vitamin D. Vitamin D controls calcium and phosphorus metabolism, and the natural supply of vitamin D in humans depends upon the ingestion of vitamin D_2 (ergocalciferol) or the ultraviolet rays of the sun for conversion of 7-dihydrocholesterol to vitamin D_3 (cholecalciferol). Vitamin D is biologically inert. Two successive hydroxylations (in the liver and in the kidney) are required to transform vitamin D into an active form [1,25(OH)$_2$D$_3$] [14].

Vitamin D must be viewed as a hormone that regulates calcium homeostasis and other cellular functions. The hormone exerts its effect via specific nuclear receptors belonging to the superfamily of steroid hormone receptors. These receptors have been identified in various organs and in cells including lymphocytes, macrophages, fibroblasts, and kératinocytes. Skin is a target organ for 1,25(OH)$_2$D$_3$ [15], which not only modulates epidermal proliferation and differentiation but also has an effect on the control of fibroblast function [16].

The discovery of new properties of this vitamin and effects on different targets prompted a renewed interest in some inflammatory conditions and especially in scleroderma. That is, it was felt that 1,25(OH)$_2$D$_3$ might be an immunomodulatory drug that could help to control collagen deposition in some tissues. Thus the physiological roles of this hormone are not limited only to calcium regulation. Indeed, 1,25(OH)$_2$D$_3$ promotes tissue differentiation and inhibits cellular proliferation in cell cultures.

The cell targets of vitamin D involved in scleroderma are thymocytes, T and B lymphocytes, monocytes, macrophages, neutrophils, and fibroblasts. These cells express vitamin D receptor, and thus can be affected by calcitriol.

IV. BIOLOGICAL EFFECTS OF VITAMIN D IN RELATION TO PATHOPHYSIOLOGICAL MECHANISMS OF SCLERODERMA

Cutaneous vitamin D_3 formation is not affected in progressive systemic sclerosis [17]. Nevertheless vitamin D may have immunoregulatory effects that ameliorate scleroderma. $1,25(OH)_2D_3$ has been shown to inhibit T lymphocyte mitogenesis [18] and to have varying effects on lymphokine production [19,20].

A. Involved Cells

Scleroderma is considered to be of autoimmune origin. Different autoantibodies are produced in scleroderma. Therefore, calcitriol regulates B-cell growth and differenciation and inhibits immunoglobulin production (IgG, IgM) in vitro [21]; it also inhibits immunoglobulin secretion in response to PWM and *Staphylococcus aureus* Cowen I in a dose-dependent manner [22]. Helper T-cell function is increased in systemic sclerosis [23], where an elevated ratio of T4/T8 lymphocytes has been detected [24]. Activated T-helper lymphocytes are observed in the skin in the early inflammatory stage of the disease. Stimulated T cells elaborate fibroblast chemotactic factors as well as factors that stimulate fibroblast proliferation and collagen synthesis. Picomolar concentrations of $1,25(OH)_2D_3$ inhibit the proliferation of T lymphocytes stimulated with antigens and mitogens [20,25]. The inhibitory effect of vitamin D on the rate of proliferation of the helper subset does not concern the suppressor subset [26]. Thus, suppressor cell activity is promoted and the generation of cytotoxic and natural killer cells is inhibited.

Monocytes constitutively express vitamin D receptors. Vitamin D enhances monocyte function in antigen presentation. Cytotoxicity of macrophages has been shown to be increased by vitamin D. Vitamin D regulates HLA-DR expression on human peripheral blood monocytes and potentiates the effects of IFN-γ [27].

A disturbed control of collagen synthesis has been found in fibroblasts derived from patients with PSS leading to an excessive overproduction of collagen types I and III [28]. Receptors for $1,25(OH)_2D_3$ have been demonstrated in human fibroblasts. At a high concentration, $1,25(OH)_2D_3$ is extremely potent in inhibiting fibroblast proliferation and collagen synthesis. The inhibition of fibroblast proliferation is maximal with a concentration of 10^{-9} mol/L and minimal with 10^{-12} mol/L of vitamin D. Moreover, cultured fibroblasts from biopsies of patients with morphea were inhibited by calcipotriol (a vitamin D analog) when compared with controls [29]. It can be concluded that morphea fibroblasts may have receptors that have increased sensitivity to vitamin D_3. In a study taking in account fibroblasts derived from the skin of scleroderma patients [30], it was demonstrated that calcitriol exerted an antiproliferative and antisynthetic effect on fibroblasts. Nevertheless, the inhibiting effect was not different between healthy fibroblasts and fibroblasts derived from scleroderma patients. In collagen type I gels, 1,25-dihydroxyvitamin D_3 inhibits contraction in a time- and concentration-dependent manner [31], probably by interfering with the expression of α_2 or the β_1 chain of integrins.

B. Cytokines

Enhanced production of interleukin-2 (IL-2) in phytohemaggutinin-stimulated peripheral lymphocytes [23] has been reported in patients with PSS. The lymphokine IL-2 and the soluble IL-2 receptor appear at high levels in scleroderma serum [13,32] and especially in patients with rapid skin progression. The production of IL-2 by T cells and CD4+ cells is inhibited by vitamin D. Calcitriol suppressed IL-2 production by phytohemagglutinin-stimulated peripheral mononuclear cells in a concentration-dependent manner and decreased IL-2 production in rat spleen cells stimulated with concanavalin A [33]. Moreover the release of IL-2 by mixed T lymphocytes activated by a mitogen is inhibited by $1,25(OH)_2D_3$ [34]. Besides, vitamin D inhibits IL-2 receptor expression on B cells and thus inhibits immunoglobulin production by B lymphocytes [22].

The action of IL-1 on fibroblasts results in the stimulation of their growth [35], enhancement of collagenase production [36,37], and inhibition of fibronectin synthesis [38]. Conversely, IL-1 activity in peripheral blood mononuclear cells from patients with PSS has been found to be low [39]; however, it has recently been proved that production of IL-1 by cultured peripheral blood monocytes from patients with scleroderma is enhanced [40]. The production of IL-1 inhibitor, which is mitogenic for fibroblasts, is significantly higher in scleroderma patients than in normal controls [41]. Vitamin D may be considered an inhibitor of IL-1 [42]. It inhibits IL-1–induced T-cell proliferation as well the production of both extracellular and cell-associated immunoreactive IL-1α and IL-1β by human monocytes [43].

Studies with a murine T-helper cell clone have shown that $1,25(OH)_2D_3$ inhibits the proliferative effect of IL-1 [44]. While $1,25(OH)_2D_3$ induced intracellular expression of IL-1, IFN-γ permitted release of the intracellular IL-1 activity after lipopolysaccharide stimulation [45].

IFN-γ has proved to have beneficial effects in the treatment of scleroderma [46] $1,25(OH)_2D_3$ and IFN-γ shared similar effects on immature monocyte lines. It is noteworthy that human macrophages activated by IFN-γ synthetize $1,25(OH)_2D_3$ [47,48].

PSS is characterized by an increased synthesis, deposition, and degradation of fibronectin [49]. The action of IL-1 (whose activity is increased in scleroderma) on fibroblasts results in the inhibition of fibronectin synthesis [37]. $1,25(OH)_2D_3$ stimulates fibronectin synthesis in different cells [50].

The collagenolytic activity measured in skin involved in systemic sclerosis was found to be mainly normal or decreased compared with that found in the skin of healthy controls. Surprisingly the activity of collagenase is lowered significantly in PSS skin [51]. Besides, osteoblasts grown on type I collagen films are stimulated by 1,25(OH)$_2$D$_3$ to degrade collagen and secrete latent collagenase [52]. Moreover, 1,25(OH)$_2$D$_3$ induces the differentiation of granulocyte colony forming units into macrophages and monocytes. These white blood cells may produce collagenase.

One other effect of vitamin D that could be useful in scleroderma, especially concerning microcirculation, could be mediated by monocytes. When they are treated with calcitriol, they may release increased amounts of prostaglandin E2 [53,54]. Prostaglandin E is a known suppressor of IL-2 production and lymphocyte proliferation.

V. CONCLUSION

The in vitro results as well as clinical experiments give grounds for optimism that vitamin D$_3$ or analogs might prove therapeutically useful in treatment of both progressive systemic sclerosis and localized scleroderma. Nevertheless, we must be aware of potential adverse reactions. Overdosage of vitamin D is dangerous. Decrease in serum alkaline phosphatase, weakness, headaches, muscle and bone pain, and gastrointestinal disturbances are early signs of vitamin D toxicity. Other signs may occur, such as dry mouth, constipation, metallic taste, nausea, and vomiting. The association of vitamin D with other drugs can lead to drug interactions. Thus, cholestyramine may decrease intestinal absorption of calcitriol. Digitalis toxicity due to calcitriol-induced hypercalcemia may occur. If antacids (especially magnesium-containing antacids) are given with calcitriol, hypermagnesemia may occur. Finally, phenobarbital, which is an enzyme inducer, may lower calcitriol levels.

The above data help to explain why oral calcitriol may be useful in the treatment of scleroderma [55]. These effects may be due to different properties of vitamin D on various cells or mechanisms involved in the pathogenesis of scleroderma. For the future, one must postulate safer and more potent vitamin D$_3$ analogs [56].

REFERENCES

1. Humbert P, Dupond JL, Rochefort A, Vasselet R, Lucas A, Laurent R, Agache P. Localized scleroderma: Response to 1,25-dihydroxyvitamin D$_3$. Clin Exp Dermatol 1990; 15:396–398.
2. Leriche R, Jung A. Thymectomy and parathyroidectomy in a case of dystrophy of the puny type and generalized calcinosis. Presse Med 1938; 46:809–811.

3. Liuzzo G. Parathyroidectomy in scleroderma. Policlinico 1940; 47:41.
4. Cornbleet T, Struck HC. Calcium metabolism in scleroderma. Arch Dermatol Syph 1937; 35:188–201.
5. Norman CF. Vitamin D therapy in the treatment of scleroderma and allied conditions: Three cases. Geriatrics 1946; 2:24–33.
6. Maynard MTR. Clinical note on scleroderma. California West Med 1939; 50:365.
7. Humbert P, Delaporte E, Dupond JL, Rochefort A, Laurent R, Drobacheff C, de Wazieres B, Bergoend H, Agache P. Treatment of localized scleroderma with oral 1,25-dihydroxyvitamin D_3. Eur J Dermatol 1994; 4:21–23.
8. Humbert P, Dupond JL, Agache P, Laurent R, Rochefort A, Drobacheff C, de Wazieres B, Aubin F. Treatment of scleroderma with oral 1,25-dihydroxyvitamin D_3: Evaluation of skin involvement using non-invasive techniques. Results of an open prospective trial. Acta Derm Venereol (Stockh) 1993; 73:449–451.
9. Hulshof MM, Pavel S, Breddveld FC, Dijkmans BAC, Vermeer BJ. Oral calcitriol as a new therapeutic modality for generalized morphea. Arch Dermatol 1994; 130:1290–1293.
10. Black C, Briggs D, Welsh K. The immunogenetic background of scleroderma: An overview. Clin Exp Dermatol 1992; 17:73–78.
11. Haustein UF, Herrmann K, Bruns M. Collagen metabolism in systemic sclerosis. J Eur Acad Dermatol Venereol 1992; 1:37–42.
12. Krieg T, Perlish JS, Mauch C, Fleischmajer R. Collagen synthesis by scleroderma fibroblasts. Ann NY Acad Sci 1985; 460:375–386.
13. Kahaleh MB, LeRoy EC. Interleukin-2 in scleroderma: Correlation of serum level with extent of skin involvement and disease duration. Ann Intern Med 1989; 110:446–450.
14. Texereau M, Viac J. Vitamin D, immune system and skin. Eur J Dermatol 1992; 2:258–264.
15. Holick MF, Smith E, Pincus S. Skin as the site of vitamin D synthesis and target tissue for 1,25-dihydroxyvitamin D_3. Arch Dermatol 1987; 123:1677–1683.
16. Clemens TL, Adamas JS, Horiuchi N, Gilchrest BA, Cho H, Tsuchiya Y. Interaction of 1,25-dihydroxyvitamin D_3 with keratinocytes and fibroblasts from skin of normal subjects and a subject with vitamin-D rickets, type II: A model for study the mode of action of 1,25-dihydroxyvitamin D_3. Clin Endocrinol Metab 1983; 56:824–830.
17. Matsuoka LY, Dannenberg MJ, Wortsman J, Hollis BW, Jimenez SA, Varga J. Cutaneous vitamin D_3 formation in progressive systemic sclerosis. J Rheumatol 1991; 18:1196–1198.
18. Rigby WFC, Denome S, Fanger MV. Regulation of lymphokine production and human T lymphocyte activation of 1,25-dihydroxyvitamin D_3. J Clin Invest 1987; 79:1659–1664.
19. Rigby WFC. The immunobiology of vitamin D. Immunol Today 1988; 9:54–58.
20. Bhalla AK, Amento EP, Krane SM. Differential effects of 1,25-dihydroxyvitamin D_3 on human lymphocytes and monocyte/macrophages: Inhibition of interleukin-2 and augmentation of interleukin-1 production. Cell Immunol 1986; 98:311–322.
21. Lemire JM, Adams JS, Sakai R, Jordan SC. 1-alpha,25-dihydroxyvitamin D_3 suppresses proliferation and immunoglobulin production by normal human peripheral blood mononuclear cells. J Clin Invest 1984; 74:657–661.

22. Chen WC, Vayuvegula B, Gupta S. 1,25-dihydroxyvitamin D$_3$-mediated inhibition of human B cell differentiation. Clin Exp Immunol 1987; 69:639–646.

23. Umehara H, Kumagai S, Ishida H, Suginoshita T, Maeda M, Imura H. Enhanced production of interleukin-2 in patients with progressive systemic sclerosis: Hyperactivity of CD4-positive T cells? Arthritis Rheum 1988; 31:401–407.

24. Whiteside T, Kumagai Y, Roumm A, Almendinger R, Rodnan GP. Suppressor cell function and T lymphocyte subpopulations in peripheral blood of patients with progressive systemic sclerosis. Arthritis Rheum 1983; 26:841–847.

25. Rigby WFC, Stacy T, Fanger MW. Inhibition of T lymphocyte mitogenesis by 1,25-dihydroxyvitamin D$_3$ (calcitriol). J Clin Invest 1984; 74:1451–1455.

26. Provvedini DM, Manolagas SC. 1-alpha, 25-dihydroxyvitamin D$_3$ receptor distribution and effects in subpopulations of normal human T lymphocytes. J Clin Endocrinol Metab 1989; 68:774–779.

27. Tamaki K, Nakamura K. Differential enhancement of interferon-gamma-induced MHC class II expression of Hep-2 cells by 1,25-dihydroxyvitamin D$_3$. Br J Dermatol 1990; 123:333–338.

28. Krieg T, Perlish JS, Fleischmajer R, Braun-Falco O. Collagen synthesis in scleroderma: Selection of fibroblast populations during subcultures. Arch Dermatol Res 1985; 277:373–376.

29. Bottomley WW, Jutley J, Wood EJ, Goodfield MDJ. The effect of calcipotriol on lesional fibroblasts from patients with active morphoea. Acta Derm Venereol (Stockh) 1995; 75:364–366.

30. Boelsma E, Pavel S, Ponec M. Effects of calcitriol on fibroblasts derived from skin of scleroderma patients. Dermatology 1995; 191:226–233.

31. Greiling D, Thieroff-Ekerdt R. 1-alpha,25-dihydroxyvitamin D$_3$ rapidly inhibits fibroblast-induced collagen gel contraction. J Invest Dermatol 1996; 106:1236–1241.

32. Degiannis D, Seibold JR, Czarnecki M, Raskova J, Raska K. Soluble interleukin-2 receptors in patients with systemic sclerosis. Arthritis Rheum 1990; 33:375–380.

33. Hodler B, Evequoz V, Trechsel U, Fleisch H, Stadler B. Influence of vitamin D$_3$ metabolites on the production of interleukins 1,2 and 3. Immunobiol 1985; 170:256–269.

34. Tsoukas CD, Provvedini DM, Manolagas SC. 1,25-dihydroxyvitamin D$_3$: A novel immunoregulatory hormone. Science 1984; 224:1438–1440.

35. Schmidt JA, Mizel SB, Cohen D, Green I. Interleukin 1: A potential regulator of fibroblast proliferation. J Immunol 1982; 128:2177–2182.

36. Dayer JM, De Rochemonteix B, Burrus R, et al. Human recombinant interleukin 1 stimulates collagenase and prostaglandin E2 production by human synovial cells. J Clin Invest 1986; 77:645–648.

37. Postlethwaite AE, Lachman LB, Mainardi CL, Kang AH. Interleukin 1 stimulation of collagenase production by cultured fibroblasts. J Exp Med 1983; 157:801–806.

38. Duncan MR, Berman B. Differential regulation of collagen, glycosaminoglycan, fibronectin and collagenase activity production in cultured human adult dermal fibroblasts by interleukin 1-alpha and beta and tumor necrosis factor alpha and beta. J Invest Dermatol 1989; 92:699–706.

39. Sandborg CI, Berman MA, Andrews BS, Friou GJ. Interleukin 1 production by mononuclear cells from patients with scleroderma. Clin Exp Immunol 1985; 60:294–302.

40. Umehara H, Kumagai S, Murakami M, Suginoshita T, Tanaka K, Hashida S, Ishikawa E, Imura H. Enhanced production of interleukin-1 and tumor necrosis factor alpha by cultured peripheral blood monocytes from patients with scleroderma. Arthritis Rheum 1990; 33:893–897.

41. Sandborg CI, Berman MA, Andrews BS, Mirick GR, Friou GJ. Increased production of an interleukin 1 (IL-1) inhibitor with fibroblast stimulating activity by mononuclear cells from patients with scleroderma. Clin Exp Immunol 1986; 66:312–319.

42. Muller K, Svenson M, Bendtzen K. 1-alpha,25-dihydroxyvitamin D_3 and a novel vitamin D analogue MC 903 are potent inhibitors of human interleukin 1 in vitro. Immunol Lett 1988; 17:361–366.

43. Tsoukas CD, Watry D, Escobar SS, Provvedini DM, Dinarello CA, Hustmyer FG, Manolagas SC. Inhibition of interleukin-1 production by 1,25-dihydroxyvitamin D_3. J Clin Endocrinol Metab 1989; 69:127–133.

44. Lacey DL, Axelrod J, Chappel JC, Kahn AJ, Teitelbaum SL. Vitamin D affects proliferation of a murine T helper cell clone. J Immunol 1987; 138:1680–1686.

45. Spear GT, Paulnock DM, Helgeson DO, Borden EC. Requirement of differentiative signals of both interferon-gamma and 1,25-dihydroxyvitamin D_3 for induction and secretion of interleukin-1 by HL-60 cells. Cancer Res 1988; 48:1740–1744.

46. Kahan A, Amor B, Menkes CJ, Strauch G. Recombinant interferon-gamma in the treatment of systemic sclerosis. Am J Med 1989; 87:273–277.

47. Adams JS, Gacad MA. Characterization of 1 alpha-hydroxylation of vitamin D_3 sterols by cultured alveolar macrophages from patients with sarcoidosis. J Exp Med 1985; 161:755–765.

48. Koeffler HP, Reichel H, Bishop JE, Norman AW. Gamma-interferon stimulates production of 1,25-dihydroxyvitamin D_3 by normal human macrophage. Biochem Biophys Res Commun 1985; 127:596–603.

49. LeRoy EC. The connective tissue in scleroderma. Collagen Rel Res 1981; 1:301–308.

50. Franceschi RT, Linson CJ, Peter TC, Romano PR. Regulation of cellular adhesion and fibronectin synthesis by 1-alpha,25-dihydroxyvitamin D_3. J Biol Chem 1987; 262:4165–4171.

51. Brady AH. Collagenase in scleroderma. J Clin Invest 1975; 56:1175–1180.

52. Thomson BM, Atkinson SJ, Reynolds JJ, Meikle MC. Degradation of type I collagen films by mouse osteoblasts is stimulated by 1,25-dihydroxyvitamin D_3 and inhibited by human recombinant TIMP (tissue inhibitor of metalloproteinases). Biochem Biophys Res Commun 1987; 148:596–602.

53. Rigby WFC, Noelle RG, Krause K, Fanger MW. The effects of 1,25 dihydroxyvitamin D_3 on human T lymphocyte activation and proliferation: A cell cycle analysis. J Immunol 1985; 135:2279–2286.

54. Koren R, Ravid A, Rotem C, Shohami E, Liberman UA, Novogrodsky A. 1,25 dihydroxyvitamin D_3 enhances prostaglandin E2 production by monocytes: A mechanism which partially accounts for the antiproliferative effect of $1,25(OH)_2D_3$ on lymphocytes. FEBS Lett 1986; 205:113–116.

27

Experience with Vitamin D Analogs in Cutaneous Malignancies

Slawomir Majewski and Stefania Jablonska
Warsaw School of Medicine, Warsaw, Poland

I. ANTITUMOR EFFECTS OF VITAMIN D (VD) ANALOGS

The antitumor activity of VD analogs is mainly dependent on inhibition of tumor-cell proliferation and stimulation of differentiation and apoptosis. In addition, VD analogs are capable of exerting immunomodulatory effects that could partially enhance some antitumor immune mechanisms. Finally, VD analogs were shown to inhibit tumor cell-induced angiogenesis (i.e. crucial step in tumor invasiveness and metastasis formation). Owing to these effects of VD, and especially because new analogs with slight effects on calcemia are presently available, they may find application in the treatment not only of benign proliferations but also of some malignant tumors.

A. Antiproliferative and Prodifferentiative Effects of VD Analogs on Tumor Cells In Vivo and In Vitro

Previous in vivo experimental studies have shown that in immunosuppressed mice bearing lung or colon melanoma carcinoma or human xenografts there was regression of transplanted tumors after treatment with calcitriol (1,2). Calcitriol was found also to inhibit in vivo growth of human retinoblastoma both in nude mice and in a heritable transgenic mouse model of retinoblastoma (3). Various VD analogs were shown to inhibit proliferation of cells isolated from neurofibromatosis of patients with von Recklinghausen's disease, which were xenografted into mouse skin in vivo (4,5). In addition, some VD analogs were shown to exert a marked antitumor effects in vivo and to decrease growth of breast (6,7), colon (8), and prostate cancer cells (9).

These data suggest that one of the antitumor effects of VD analogs may be due to their direct antiproliferative action upon tumor cells. Such a possibility was confirmed in various in vitro systems with the use of different tumor cell lines, including breast (10–13), prostate (13–15), colon (16), and pancreatic (17) cancer cells as well as neoplastic HPK1A-*ras* keratinocytes (18).

The antiproliferative effects of VD analogs seem to be mediated by specific nuclear receptors (VDR). In previous studies, it was shown that various human tumor cells—including breast, colon and lung cancers as well as melanoma cells—express VDR, and that high tumor–control sample ratios for VDR may be associated with a more favorable tumor stage (no or few metastases) (19). Findings on the correlation between growth inhibition and expression of VDR in gynecologic tumors suggest a possible therapeutic application of VD analogs in these tumors (20). VDR messenger RNA was found to be present in relatively high levels in well-differentiated breast carcinoma cells, which showed a lowered rate of proliferation and were sensitive to the antiproliferative effect of calcitriol (21). In contrast, breast carcinoma cell lines that had very low levels of VDR mRNA demonstrated no growth inhibition by calcitriol. From these data the authors conclude that VDR expression in breast cancer cells is lost with dedifferentiation and that this receptor is essential for the antiproliferative response to VD analogs (21). It seems also that suppression of the growth of ectocervical keratinocytes is mediated by VDR; this could be of significance for the treatment of the early stages of cervical disease (22). Thus regulatory mechanisms controlling the expression of VDR may determine antitumor efficacy of various VD analogs (23). Although autoregulation of VDR gene expression was found to occur in various tumor cells (24–26), molecular mechanisms responsible for the derangement of VDR expression during cancerogenesis are not clearly understood. In Pam212 keratinocytes (a transformed cell line derived from a mouse squamous cell carcinoma), it was found that the E1A gene product of adenoviruses induced resistance to the inhibition of cell growth by VD analogs owing to the blocking of autoregulated VDR gene expression (27). Moreover these authors showed that transfection of tumor cells with VDR restored the inhibitory action of calcitriol. Similarly, in breast (28) and in colon cancer cells (29), the resistance to VD analogs can be overcome by transfecting the VDR gene. These studies strongly suggest that overexpression (e.g., by transfection) of VDR in cancer cells may be of clinical significance. In human prostate cancer cells, it was found that VDR content and transcriptional activity do not fully predict antiproliferative effects of VD analogs (30), although it seems that polymorphism of VDR gene is associated with the risk of advanced prostate cancer (31). It has been speculated that in tumors showing low expression of VDR, a possibility of partial restoration of VDR-mediated inhibition of tumor cell growth might occur through overexpression of RXRa in cancer cells (32).

Molecular mechanisms of antiproliferative action of VD analogs is not completely known, but they may be related to induction of negative growth regulator

(TGFb) (33), suppression of the proto-oncogene c-*myc* and dephosphorylation of the retinoblastoma protein (34). More recently, it was shown that inhibition of cell proliferation by VD analogs was accompanied not only by accumulation of TGFB-1 and dephosphorylated retinoblastoma protein but also by induction of the cyclin-dependent kinase inhibitors CdkIs/WAF1, CIP1, and p27/KIP1 (35). Similar findings were reported for human breast cancer lines (36) and for prostate cancer cells (13). Moreover, induction of cdk inhibitors by VD analogs is responsible for growth arrest and stimulation of differentiation in retinoic acid–resistant neoplastic cells (37). Other mechanisms of growth inhibition of tumor cells by VD analogs might be related to their ability to increase expression of insulin-like growth factor–binding protein-3, as shown in breast cancer cells (38), and to inhibit production of parathyroid hormone–related protein, as reported for oral cancer cells (39).

Another important mechanism of antitumor action of VD analogs may involve the induction of apoptosis in cancer cells. This was shown for breast cancer cells (12,40,42) and for normal human keratinocytes (42) but not for leukemic cells (43). The molecular mechanisms of induction of apoptosis by VD analogs may be due to stimulation of sphingomyelin hydrolysis and to generation of ceramides (44) or to decreasing expression of bcl-2 protein (41). Analogs of VD are capable of stimulating differentiation of various tumor cells, including human breast cancer cells (21,41) and leukemic cells (45–47). Calcitriol was shown to induce transglutaminase activity in transformed epidermal PAM212 cells, and this was synergized by retinoic acid (48).

B. The Effects of VD Analogs on Human Nonmelanoma and Melanoma Cancer Cells

It was shown that normal keratinocytes and squamous cell carcinoma (SCC) lines synthesize VD and respond to exogenous VD; the latter are, however, less responsive than normal keratinocytes, probably because they have to the highest 1-hydroxylase activity (49). Thus VD had an inhibitory effect on linear growth but no prodifferentiating effect for these cell lines. The inhibition of growth was found in cell lines originating from head and neck cancers and was dose- and receptor-dependent (50). Specifically, in vitro, the strong dose-dependent effects on proliferation of SCC keratinocytes of VD analogs with low calcemic potency points to their potential usefulness in the treatment of cutaneous cancers (12).

The role of VDR in the effects of VD analogs in SCC is postulated by some researchers (50,51); however, it is not confirmed by others (52,53). SCC lines failed to respond to VD analogs despite normal levels of VDR and failed to differentiate under conditions favorable for the growth and differentiation of normal keratinocytes (52). These authors found that SCC had defective control of the expression of genes involved in differentiation despite the presence of functional

VDR in concentrations similar to those in normal keratinocytes. It was shown that sensitivity to growth inhibition does not correlate with VDR level and may be modulated by nonreceptor factors that are cell line–specific and/or due to promoter selectivity (54). However, the problem of the role of VDR in mediating antitumor effects of VD analogs in SCC is still not clear.

In basal cell carcinomas (BCC), strong expression of VDR and of some retinoid receptors (RARa/g and RXRa) would suggest that selective ligand of VD and retinoids may be useful for the chemoprevention and therapy of BCC (55).

Human melanoma cell lines that were shown to have widely disparate levels of VDR expression differed in growth inhibition by VD analogs. Lines that expressed lower levels of VDR did not show growth inhibition, which for these cells, appears to be receptor-mediated (56).

C. Inhibition of Tumor Angiogenesis by VD Analogs

Since VD analogs exert antitumor effects, not only in vitro but also in vivo, including various solid tumors (6–9,57,58), it seems possible that, in addition to their direct effects on tumor cell proliferation and differentiation, these compounds may indirectly inhibit the growth and progression of some solid tumors through host-related mechanisms (e.g., tumor cell-induced angiogenesis) (59–62).

Tumor-induced angiogenesis (TIA) is a prerequisite for tumor growth, invasion, and metastasis formation (63,64). Some clinical data indicate that the intensity of angiogenesis within the tumor masses correlates with the invasiveness of the neoplastic cells, and this parameter may be of an independent prognostic value, as shown for squamous cell carcinoma of the head and neck (65), breast cancer (66–68), cervical cancer (69), melanoma (70,71), cancer of prostate (72), and also cutaneous SCC (Majewski, in preparation).

In our recent studies, we found that VD analogs inhibit angiogenesis induced in the murine skin by xenografted human transformed keratinocyte lines, including SKV cell harboring HPV16 DNA and non-HPV-harboring breast cancer cells (60–62). Moreover, we found that preincubation of tumor cells in vitro with VD analogs decreased their angiogenic capability when they were injected intradermally into x-ray–immunosuppressed mice. These data suggest that VD analogs are capable of inhibiting production of angiogenic factors by tumor cells (e.g., vascular endothelial cell growth factor) (Majewski, in preparation). VD analogs may also decrease tumor angiogenesis owing to their ability to inhibit migration of microvascular endothelial cells (73) and to decrease extracellular plasminogen activator activity, which is known to be involved in new blood vessel formation (74). Most interestingly, it was reported that, in proliferating endothelial cells, there was 4.5-fold increase in VDR expression as compared with density-arrested cells (75), suggesting that rapidly growing endothelium during tumor angiogenesis could be preferentially inhibited by VD analogs.

D. Immunomodulatory Activity of VD Analogs

The immunomodulatory activities of VD analogs are described elsewhere in this monograph (see Chapter 8). It is generally accepted that VD analogs exert a slight immunosuppressive effect at various stages of development of immune reactions. However, some of the activities of VD analogs may contribute to the enhancement of immune reactions against virus-infected or transformed cells. Calcitriol was found to increase the IFN-γ–induced expression of HLA-DR on Hep-2 (human laryngeal carcinoma) cells (76) and on murine monocytic Wehi-3 cells (77); however, it exerted negative effects on PAM212 keratinocytes (78) and melanoma cells (79). VD analogs were found to increase ICAM-1 expression in renal carcinoma cell line, also after stimulation with IFN-γ (80). Since ICAM-1 is crucial for the adhesion of LFA-1–expressing lymphocytes, including cytotoxic T cells and natural killer (NK) cells, upregulation of this adhesion molecule on tumor cells may be of significance for lymphocyte lysis of neoplastic cells. Moreover, VD analogs were reported to increase stimulatory action of LPS and IFN-γ on production of TNF-α by bone marrow–derived macrophages (81); it is believed that the release of this cytokine by macrophages is a major mechanism by which these cells exert their tumoricidal function. TNF-α was also shown to stimulate calcitriol production by preconfluent (proliferating) keratinocytes in vitro (82), and IFN-γ and IL-1 were reported to upregulate VDR expression in transformed keratinocytes (HaCat cells) (83), suggesting a direct link between action of VD analogs and the cytokine network.

II. SYNERGISTIC ANTITUMOR EFFECTS OF VD ANALOGS AND OTHER BIOLOGICAL RESPONSE MODIFIERS

Owing to the interplay among VDR, RXRs, and RARs, several synergistic antitumor effects of VD analogs and retinoids have been described in various experimental systems (84–88). The antiproliferative and differentiative activities of VD analogs were also shown to be enhanced by various cytokines, including IFN-γ (89,90), TNF-α (91), TGF-β (92), epidermal growth factor (93), and GM-CSF (94).

Using a mouse model of cutaneous angiogenesis, we found a synergistic antiangiogenc effect of various retinoids (all-*trans* retinoic acid, 13-*cis* retinoic acid, 9-*cis* retinoic acid) and calcitriol in both HPV-harboring and non-HPV–harboring human cancer lines (60–62).

Most recently we investigated antineoplastic activity and specifically antiangiogenic effects of combined therapy with interleukin-12 (IL-12) and calcitriol in the murine L1 sarcoma system. We found that the growth of tumors induced by L1 sarcoma cells was decreased in all mice treated with IL-12 or calcitriol alone (Nowicka, in preparation). However, the best results were achieved in mice treated with both compounds applied simultaneously. The combined administration of IL-12 and calcitriol was found to have the strongest antiangiogenic effect in the experimental model of cutaneous angiogenesis induced by these cells. The molecular mechanism of the enhancement of angiogenic effect of calcitriol in this system may due to stimulation of the expression of VDR by IL-12–induced cytokines, as suggested for IFN-γ (83) and IFN-α (95). The enhanced antineoplastic and antiangiogenic effects of the combined application of IL-12 and calcitriol in mice may provide an experimental base for their use in human cutaneous malignancies. Such combination could make it possible to decrease the dosages and to limit the toxic effects of both compounds.

A possible potentiation of antitumor effect in a murine SCC model was achieved by combining VD analogs with retinoids and cisplastin (96) or with dexamethasone (51). This last modality is of special interest, since dexamethasone was found effective in the treatment of VD-induced hypercalcemia. By increasing VDR–ligand binding activity, it enhances the antitumor effect of VD analogs. Another combination that could be of clinical value is application of VD analogs with tamoxifen (97). The authors showed that the growth inhibition of breast cancer cells by VD analogs could be augmented by combination with tamoxifen, even when the compounds were used in small dosages. Recently, another interesting combination was reported (98) in which VD analogs were used simultaneously with suramin (i.e., a compound that shows a marked antitumor and antiangiogenic effects in vivo). These effects of suramin in a murine cell carcinoma model system were found to be significantly enhanced by VD analogs. Moreover, this combination was effective an in vitro system in which direct killing of tumor cells was observed.

III. USE OF VD ANALOGS IN CUTANEOUS TUMORS

A. VD Analogs in Monotherapy

In non-Hodgkin low-grade lymphoma, the response to VD therapy and clinical improvement in 10 patients was related to the amount of VDR in lymph nodes (99). These authors believe that the presence and levels of VDR should be used for predicting the response to therapy. However, this assumption is controversial.

Regression of cutaneous T-cell lymphoma under the topical treatment with the VD analog calcipotriol was reported in a single case (100) and has not been confirmed by others (101). The results in myelodysplastic syndromes and hematologic malignancies were also disappointing (102,103).

B. VD Analogs in Combined Therapy

In contrast to monotherapy, combined treatment with VD analogs and derivatives of vitamin A (retinoids) has been applied with success in various types of lymphoma (101,104) and acute promyelocytic leukemia (105). Such a combination was found to induce differentiation of myeloid leukemia cell lines and to promote growth inhibition (86,106).

In cutaneous low-grade T-cell lymphoma with widespread lesions, the treatment with calcitriol 0.5 μg every second day and acitretin 10 mg daily continued for over 9 months, producing complete clearance despite all previous unsuccessful therapies, including topical calcipotriol (101). Owing to the synergistic effects of both compounds, application of small doses of the drugs was effective, no side effects were observed, and the therapy was well tolerated.

With the use of cancer cells harboring HPV16 DNA (Skv) or HPV18 DNA (HeLa), and non HPV harboring cells (A431), we showed synergistic antiproliferative and antiangiogenic effects of VD analogs and retinoids (60,61). This prompted us to try a combination therapy in a small group of four patients with multiple precancerous skin lesions and early cancers. The dosages of calcitriol were 0.5–1.0 μg/day and of isotretinoin 0.4–0.5 mg/kg/day; the treatment lasted up to 12 months (107). The skin lesions started to improve 2–6 weeks after initiation of the therapy. Actinic keratoses regressed within several months in 40–80%, and small SCC and BCC decreased in size in 30–45%. Only one person was completely cleared within 1 year. In no patient had we seen any severe side effects. Calcium and triglyceride levels remained normal. Some dryness of the skin and mucosa due to isotretinoin was controlled by decreasing the dosage of the retinoid for a few days. This study showed that VD combined with retinoids has much stronger therapeutic effects than retinoids applied alone, which were found to be inefficacious in actinic keratoses (108). Small doses of both compounds were found not to be toxic in long-term application.

The further study was conducted in 11 patients with multiple early cancers and precancers and was found effective for all types of nonmelanoma cutaneous tumors. The tumors decreased in size for 50–85%; in two patients they regressed entirely after 15 months of the therapy (109). Worth stressing is that even a very large cancer, involving almost half of the face, which did not regress after this therapy did decreased in size, so that it could be removed surgically. The treatment was safe; hypercalcemia was not seen in any patient. However, several patients developed slight retinoid dermatitis and hyperlipidemia, which disappeared after the dosage of isotretinoin was reduced to 0.25–0.3 mg/kg/day. Only one 86-year-old female with multiple SCC and actinic keratoses discontinued the therapy due to a lack of response within 3 months. Thus this treatment is not invariably effective and in most patients is not sufficient for complete clearance. However, it is safe in the doses used in our study and makes it possible to avoid the severe undesirable effects of both calcitriol and isotretinoin.

The combined therapy is especially indicated in patients with numerous early carcinomas and precancers (e.g., those treated in the past with arsenic, those with severely sun-damaged skin, etc.), and in population at high risk for cancers (e.g., allograft recipients, patients with xeroderma pigmentosum, dystrophic epidermolysis bullosa hereditaria, and others).

REFERENCES

1. Sato T, Takusagawa K, Asoo N, Konno K, Antitumour effect of 1-hydroxyvitamin D3. Tohoku J Exp Med 1982; 138:445–446.
2. Eisman JA, Barkla DH, Tutton PJ. Suppression of in vivo growth of human cancer solid tumour xenografts by 1,25-dihydroxyvitamin D3. Cancer Res 1987; 47:21–25.
3. Albert DM, Marcus DM, Gallo JP, O'Brien JM. The antineoplastic effect of vitamin D in transgenic mice with retionoblastoma. Invest Ophthalmol Vis Sci 1992; 33: 2354–2364.
4. Nakayama J, Kokuba H, Terao H, Matsuo S, Ikebe H, Nakagava H, Hori Y. Inhibitory effects of various vitamin D3 analogues on the growth of cell isolated from neurofibromas in patients with von Recklinghausen's neurofibromatosis-1. Eur J Dermatol 1997; 7:169–172.
5. Nakayama J, Matsuo S, Rikihisa W, Hori Y. Inhibitory effect of a new vitamin D3 analogue, 22-oxacalcitriol, on the growth of neurofibroma cells xenografted into nude mouse skin in vivo. Eur J Dermatol 1997; 7:475–479.
6. Colston KW, Chander SK, Mackay AG, Coombes RC. Effects of synthetic vitamin D analogues on breast cancer cell proliferation in vivo and in vitro. Biochem Pharmacol 1992; 44:693–702.
7. Abe J, Nakano T, Nishii Y, Matsumoto T, Ogata E, Ikeda K. A novel vitamin D3 analog 22-oxa-1,25-dihydroxyvitamin D3, inhibits the growth of human breast cancer in vitro and in vivo without causing hypercalcemia. Endocrinology 1991; 129: 837–837.
8. Akhter J, Chen X, Bowrey P, Bolton EJ, Morris DL. Vitamin D3 analog, EB1089, inhibits growth of subcutaneous xenografts of the human colon cancer cell line, LoVo, in a nude mouse model. Dis Colon Rectum 1997; 40:317–321.
9. Schwartz GG, Hill CC, Oeler TA, Becich MJ, Bahnson RR. 1,25-dihydroxy-16-ene-23-yne-vitamin D3 and prostate cancer cell proliferation in vivo. Urology 1995; 46: 365–369.
10. Wu G, Fan RS, Li W, Ko TC, Brattain MG. Modulation of cell control by vitamin D3 and its analogue, EB 1089, in human breast cancer cells. Oncogene 1997; 15: 1555–1563.
11. Brenner RV, Shabahang M, Schumaker LM, Nauta RJ, Uskokovic MR, Evans SR, Buras RR. The antiproliferative effect of vitamin D analogs on MCF-7 human breast cancer cells. Cancer Lett 1995; 92:77–82.
12. Danielsson C, Mathiasen IS, James SY, Nayeri S, Bretting C, Hansen CM, Colston KW, Carlberg C. Sensitive induction of apoptosis in breast cancer cells by a novel 1,25-dihydroxyvitamin D3 analogue shows relation to promoter selectivity. J Cell Biochem 1997; 66:552–562.
13. Campbell MJ, Elstner E, Holden S, Uskokovic M, Koeffer HP. Inhibition of proliferation of prostate cancer cells by a 19-nor-hexafluoride vitamin D3 analogue in-

volves the inducation of p21 waf 1, p27kip1 and E-cadherin. J Mol Endocrinol 1997; 19:15–27.

14. de Vos S, Holden S, Heber D, Elstner E, Binderup L, Uskokovic M, Rude B, Chen DL, Le J, Cho SK, Koeffler HP. Effects of potent vitamin D3 analogs on clonal proliferation of human prostate cancer cell lines. Prostate 1997; 31:77–83.
15. Skowronski RJ, Peehl DM, Feldman D. Actions of vitamin D3, analogs of human prostate cancer cell lines: comparison with 1,25-dihydroxyvitamin D3. Endocrinology 1995; 136:20–26.
16. Akhter J, Goerdel M, Morris DL. Vitamin D3 analogue (EB 1089) inhibits in vitro cellular proliferation of human colon cancer cells. Br J Surg 1996; 83:229–230.
17. Kawa S, Yashizawa K, Tokoo M, Imai H, Kiyosawa K, Homma T, Nikaido T, Furihata K. Inhibitory effect of 22-oxa-1,25-dihydroxyvitamin D3 on the proliferation of pancreatic cancer cell lines. Gastroenterology 1996; 110:1605–1613.
18. Yu J, Papavasiliou V, Rhim J, Goltzman D, Kremer R. Vitamin D analogs new therapeutic agents for the treatment of squamous cancer and its associated hypercalcemia. Anticancer Drugs 1995; 6:101–118.
19. Sandgren M, Danforth L, Plasse TF, DeLuca HF. 1,25-dihydroxyvitamin D3 receptors in human carcinomas: a pilot study. Cancer Res 1991; 51:2021–2024.
20. Saunders DE, Christensen C, Lawrence WD, Malviya VK, Malone JM, Williams JR, Deppe G. Receptors for 1,25-dihydroxyvitamin D3 in gynecologic neoplasms. Gynecol Oncol 1992; 44:131–136.
21. Buras RR, Schumaker LM, Davoodi F, Brenner RV, Shabahang M, Nauta RJ, Evans SR. Vitamin D receptors in breast cancer cells. Breast Cancer Res Treat 1994; 31: 191–202.
22. Agarwal C, Chandraratna RAS, Rorke EA, Eckert RL. Vitamin D suppresses human ectocervical keratinocyte proliferation and increases insulin-like growth factor binding protein-3 (IGFBP-3) level. J Invest Dermatol 1997; 108–579.
23. Haussler MR. Vitamin D3 receptors: nature and function. Ann Rev Nutr 1986; 6: 527–562.
24. Pan LC, Price PA. Ligand dependent regulation of the 1,25-dihydroxyvitamin D3 receptor in rat osteosarcoma cells. J Biol Chem 1987; 262:4670–4675.
25. Mahnonen A, Pirskanen A, Keinanen R, Keinanen R, Maenpaa PH. Homologous and heterologous regulation of 1-dihydroxyvitamin D3 receptor mRNA levels in human osteosarcoma cells. Biochem Biophys Acta 1991; 1088:11–118.
26. Brehier A, Thomasset M. Human colon cell line HT-29: characterisation of 1,25-dihydroxyvitamin D3 receptor and induction of differentiation by the hormone. J Seroid Biochem 1988; 29:265–270.
27. Park K, Bae H, Heydemann A, Roberts AB, Dotto GP, Sporn MB, Kim SJ. The E1A oncogene induces resistance to the effect of 1-dihydroxyvitamin D3 on inhibition of growth of mouse keratinocytes. Cancer Res 1994; 54:6087–6089.
28. Lazzaro G, Agadir A, Mehta RG, Zhang RG, Zhang XK. Resistance to vitamin D action in HBL100 breast epithelial cells can be overcome by transfecting VDR gene. Proc Am Assoc Cancer Res 1997; 38:446.
29. Shabahang M, Danielsen M, Buras R, Nauta R, Evans S. The role of the vitamin D3 receptor (VDR) in mediating the antiproliferative effects of 1,25-(OH)2D3. Proc Am Assoc Cancer Res 1997; 38:456.

30. Zhuang SH, Schwartz GG, Cameron D, Burnstein KL. Vitamin D receptor content and transcription activity do not fully predict antiproliferative effects of vitamin D in human prostate cancer cell lines. Mol Cell Endocrinol 1997; 126:83–90.

31. Ingles S, Crocitto L, Diep A, Henderson B, Kolonel L, Coetzee G, Halle R. Vitamin D receptor polymorphisms and prostate cancer in African-Americans. Proc Am Assoc Cancer Res 1997; 38:212.

32. Shabahang M, Danielsen M, Buras R, Nauta R, Evans S. RXR-α overexpression plays a significant role in vitamin D receptor (VDR)-mediated growth inhibition. Proc Am Assoc Cancer Res 1997; 38:456.

33. Kim HJ, Abdelkader N, Katz M, Mc Lane JA. 1,25-dihydoxyvitamin D3 enhances antiproliferative effect and transcription of TGF-β1 on human keratinocytes in culture. J Cell Physiol 1992; 151:579–587.

34. Kobayashi T, Hashimoto K, Yoshikawa K. Growth inhibition of human keratinocytes by 1,25-dihydroxyvitamin D3 is linked to dephosphorylation of retinoblastoma gene product. Biochem Biophys Res Commun 1993; 196:487–493.

35. Segaert S, Garmyn M, Degreef H, Bouillon R. Retinoic acid modulates the anti-proliferative effect of 1,25-dihydroxyvitamin D3 in cultured human epidermal keratinocytes. J Invest Dermatol 1997; 109:46–54.

36. Koike M, Elstner E, Campbell MJ, Asou HA, Uskokovic M, Tsuruoka N, Koeffler HP. 19-nor-hexafluoride analogue of vitamin D3: a novel class of potent inhibitors of proliferation of human breast cell lines. Cancer Res 1997; 57:4545–4550.

37. Muto A, Kizaki M, Ueno H, Matsushita H, Awaya N, Takayama N, Kamata I, Hattori Y, Ikeda Y. Differentiation and growth arrest of retinoic acid-resistant APL cell line (UF-1) by 1,25-dihydroxyvitamin D3 through the activation of cdk inhibitors. Proc Am Assoc Cancer Res 1997; 38:86.

38. Colston KW, Perks CM, Xie SP, Holly JM. Growth inhibition of both MCF-7 and Hs578T human breast cancer cell lines by vitamin D analogue is associated with increased expression of inulin-like growth factor binding protein-3. J Mol Endocrinol 1998; 20:157–162.

39. Abe M, Akeno N, Ohida S, Horiuchi N. Inhibitory effects of 1,25-dihydroxyvitamin D3 and 9-cis-retinoic acid on parathyroid hormone-related protein expression by oral cancer cells (HSC-3). J Endocrinol 1998; 156:349–357.

40. Zhang TK, X-K Mehta, Mehta RG. Mechanism of action of a novel vitamin D analog 1α(OH)D5 in human breast cancer cells. Proc Am Assoc Cancer Res 1997; 38: 578.

41. Elstner E, Linker-Israeli M, Said J, Umiel J, de Vos S, Shintaku IP, Heber D, Binderup L, Uskokovic M, Koeffler HP. 20-epi-vitamin D3 analogues: a novel class of potent inhibitors of proliferation and inducers of differentiation of human breast cancer cell lines. Cancer Res 1995; 55:2822–2830.

42. Benassi L, Ottani D, Fantini F, Marconi A, Chiodino C, Gianneti A, Pincelli C. 1,25-dihydroxyvitamin D3, transforming growth factor β1, calcium, and ultraviolet B radiation induce apoptosis in cultured human keratinocytes. J Invest Dermatol 1997; 109:76–282.

43. Kleuser B, Cuvillier O, Spiegel S. 1α,25-dihydroxyvitamin D3 inhibits programmed cell death in HL-60 cells by activation of sphingosine kinase. Cancer Res 1998; 58: 1817–1824.

44. Geilen CC, Bektas M, Wieder Th, Orfanos CE. Increasing intracellular ceramides a possible mechanism underlying the antipsoriatic effect of vitamin D3 and its analogues. Br J Dermatol 1996; 135:836.

45. Murao SJ, Gemmell MA, Callaham MF, Anderson NL, Huberman E. Control of macrophage cell differentiation in human promyelocytic HL-60 leukemia cells by 1,25-dihydroxyvitamin D3 and phorbol-12-myristate-13-acetate. Cancer Res 1983; 43:4989–4996.

46. Olson J, Gullberg U, Ivbed I, Nilsson K. Induction of differentiation of the human histiocytic lymphoma cell line U-937 by 1,25-dihydroxycholecalciferol. Cancer Res 1983; 43:5862–5867.

47. Song X, Bishop JE, Okamura WH, Norman AW. Stimulation of phosphorylation of mitogen-activated protein kinase by 1 alpha,25-dihydroxyvitamin D3 in promyeloctic NB4 leukemia cells: a structure-function study. Endocrinology 1998; 139: 457–465.

48. Lee S.C., Ikai K, Ando Y, Imamura S. Effects of 1 alpha, 25-dihydroxyvitamin D3 on the transglutaminase activity of transformed mouse epidermal cells in culture. J Dermatol 1989; 16:7–11.

49. Bikle DD, Pillai S, Gee E. Tumor necrosis factor-α regulation of 1,25-dihydroxyvitamin D3 production by human keratinocytes. Endocrinology 1991; 129:33–38.

50. Kornfehl J, Formanek M, Temmel A, Knerer B, Willheim M. Antiproliferative effects of the biologically active metabolite of vitamin D3 (1,25 [0H]2D3) on head and neck squamous cell carcinoma cell lines. Eur Arch Otorhinolaryngol 1996; 253: 341–344.

51. Yu WD, McElwain MC, Modzelewski RA, Russell DM, Smith DC, Trump DL, Johnson CS. Enhancement of 1,25-dihydroxyvitamin D3-mediated antitumor activity with dexamethasone. J Natl Cancer Inst 1998; 90:134–141.

52. Ratnam AV, Bikle DD, Su MJ, Pillai S. Squamous carcinoma cell lines fail to respond to 1,25-dihydroxyvitamin D despite normal levels of the vitamin D receptor. J Invest Dermatol 1996; 106:522–525.

53. Chang PL., Lee TF, Garretson K, Prince CW. Calcitriol enhancement of TPA-induced tumorigenic transformation is mediated through vitamin D receptor-dependent and -independent pathways. Clin Exp Metastasis 1997; 15:580–592.

54. Nayeri S, Danielsson C, Kahlen JP, Schrader M, Mathiasen IS, Binderup L, Carlberg C. The anti-proliferative effect of vitamin D analogues is not mediated by inhibition of the AP-1 pathway, but may be related to promoter selectivity. Oncogene 1995; 11:1853–1858.

55. Kamradt J, Reichrath J, Zhue Z, Kong XF, Holick MF. Expression of 1-dihydroxyvitamin D3 receptor, retinoic acid receptor-α in basal cell carcinomas. J Invest Dermatol 1997; 108:604.

56. Evans SR, Houghton AM, Schumaker L, Brenner RV, Buras RR, Davoodi F, Nauta RJ, Shabahang M. Vitamin D3 receptor and growth inhibition by 1,25-dihydroxyvitamin D3 in human malignant melanoma cell lines. J Surg Res 1996; 61:127–133.

57. Young MR, Ihm J, Lozano Y, Wright MA, Prechel MM. Treating tumor-bearing mice with vitamin D3 diminishes tumor-induced myelopoiesis and associated immunosuppression, and reduces tumor metastasis and recurrence. Cancer Immunol Immunother 1995; 41:37–45.

58. Getzenberg RH, Light BW, Lapco PE, Konety BR, Nangia AK, Acierno JS, Dhir R, Shurin Z, Day RS, Trump DL, Johnson CS. Vitamin D inhibition of prostate adenocarcinoma growth and metastasis in the Dunning rat prostate model system. Urology 1997; 50:999–1006.

59. Oikawa T, Hirotani K, Ogasawara H, Katayama T, Nakamura O, Iwaguchi T, Hiragun A. Inhibition of angiogenesis by vitamin D3 analogues. Eur J Pharmacol 1990; 178:247–250.

60. Majewski S, Szmurlo A, Marczak M. Inhibition of tumor cell-induced angiogenesis by retinoids, 1,25-dihydroxyvitamin D3 and their combination. Cancer Lett 1993; 75:35–39.

61. Majewski S, Marczak M, Szmurlo A, Jablonska S, Bollag W. Retinoids, interferon α 1,25-dihydroxyvitamin D3 and their combination inhibit angiogenesis induced by non-HPV harboring tumor cell lines: RARα mediates the antiangiogenic effect of retinoid. Cancer Lett 1995; 89:117–124.

62. Majewski S, Skopinska M, Marczak M, Szmurlo A, Bollag W, Jablonska S. Vitamin D3 is a potent inhibitor of tumor cell-induced angiogenesis. J Invest Dermatol Symp Proc 1996; 1:97–101.

63. Folkman J. What is the evidence that tumors are angiogenesis-depondent? J Natl Cancer Inst 1990; 82:4–6.

64. Folkman J. Angiogenesis in cancer, vascular, rheumatoid and other diseases. Nature Med 1995; 1:27–31.

65. Gasparini G, Weidner N, Bevilacqua P, Maluta S, Boracchi P, Testolin A, Pozza F, Folkman J. Intratumoral microvessel density and p53 protein: correlation with metastasis in head-and-neck squamous cell carcinoma. Int J Cancer 1993; 55: 739–744.

66. Weidner N, Folkman J, Pozza F, Bevilacqua P, Allred EN, Moore DH, Meli S, Gasparini G. Tumor angiogenesis: a new significant and independent prognostic indicator in early-stage breast carcinoma. J Natl Cancer Inst 1992; 84:1875–1887.

67. Toi M, Kashitani J, Tominaga T. Tumor angiogenesis is an independent prognostic indicator of primary breast carcinoma. Int J Cancer 1993; 55:371–374.

68. Brown L, Berase B, Jackman R, Tognazzi K, Guidi A, Dvorak H, Senger D, Comnolly J, Schnitt S. Expression of vascular permeability factor (vascular endothelial growth factor) and its receptors in breast cancer. Hum Pathol 1995; 26:86–91.

69. Guidi AJ, Abu-Jawdeh G, Berse B, Jackman RW, Tognazzi K, Dvorak HF, Brown LF. Vascular permeability factor (vascular endothelial growth factor) expression and angiogenesis in cervical neoplasia. J Natl Cancer Inst 1995; 87:1237–1245.

70. Barnhil RL, Fandrey K, Levy MA, Mihm MC, Hymn B. Angiogenesis and tumor progression of melanoma quantitation of vascularity in melanocystic nevi and cutaneous melanoma. Lab Invest 1992; 67:331–337.

71. Graham CH, Rivers J, Kerbel RS, Stankiewicz KS, White WL. Extent of vascularization as a prognostic indicator in thin (<0,76 mm) malignant melanomas. Am J Pathol 1994; 145:510–514.

72. Weinder N, Carroll PR, Flax J. Blumenfeld W, Folkman J. Tumor angiogenesis correlates with metastasis in invasive prostate carcinoma. Am J Pathol 1993; 143: 401–409.

73. Hisa T, Taniguchi S, Tsuruta D, Hirachi Y. Vitamin D inhibits endothelial cell migration. Arch Dermatol Res 1996; 288:262–263.

74. Koli K, Keski-Oja J. Vitamin D3 calcipotriol decrease extracellular plasminogen activator activity in cultured keratinocytes. J Invest Dermatol 1993; 101:706–712.

75. Marke J, Milde P, Lewicka S. Identification and regulation of 1,25-dihydroxyvitamin D3 receptor activity and biosynthesis of 1,25-dihydroxyvitamin D3: studies in cultured bovine aortic endothelial cells and human dermal capillaries. J Clin Invest 1989; 83:1903–1915.

76. Tamaki K, Nakamura K. Differential enhancement of interferon-γ-induced MHC class II expression of HEp-2 cells by 1,25-dihydroxyvitamin D3. Br J Dermatol 1990; 123:333–338.

77. Morel PA, Manolagas SC, Provedini DM. Interferon-γ-induced IA expression in Wehi-3 cells is enhanced by the presence of 1,25-dihydroxyvitamin D3. J Immunol 1986; 136:2181–2186.

78. Tani M, Komura A, Horikawa T. 1,25-dihydroxyvitamin D3 modulates Ia antigen expression induced by interferon-γ and prostaglandin E_2 production in Pam 212 cells. Br J Dermatol 1992; 126:266–274.

79. Carrington MN, Tharp-Hiltbold B, Knoth J, Ward FE. 1,25-dihydroxyvitamin D3 decreases expression on HLA class II molecules in a melanoma cell line. J Immunol 1988; 140:4013–4018.

80. Kreft B, Brzoska S, Muller F, Doehn C, Sack K. 1,25-dihydroxycholecalciferol stimulates the expression of intercellular adhesion molecule-1 in renal carcinoma cells. Exp Nephrol 1995; 3:288–292.

81. Abu-Amer Y, bar-Savit Z. Regulation of TNF-alpha release from bone marrow–derived macrophages by vitamin D. J Cell Biochem 1994; 55:435–444.

82. Bikle DD, Pillai S, Gee E. Squamous carcinoma cell lines produce 1,25-dihydroxyvitamin D, but fail to respond to its prodifferentiating effect. J Invest Dermatol 1991; 97:435–441.

83. Reichrath J, Hugel U, Klaus G, Fusenig NE, Rauterberg EW. Modulation of 1,25-dihydroxyvitamin D3 receptor expression in HaCaT keratinocytes. In: A. Bernd et al, eds. Cell and Tissue Culture Models in Dermatological Research. 1993; pp. 37–43. Berlin: Springer-Verlag.

84. Koga M, Sutherland RL. Retinoic acid acts synergistically with 1,25-dihydroxyvitamin D3 or antioestrogen to inhibit T47D human breast cancer proliferation. J Steroid Biochem Mol Biol 1991; 39:455–460.

85. Nakaya K, Deguchi Y, Chon S, Nakamura Y. Combination differentiation-inducer therapy for leukemic cells in mice. Cancer J 1991; 4:108–113.

86. Defacque H, Dornand J, Commes T. Different combinations of retinoids and vitamin D3, analogs effeciently promote growth inhibition and differentiation of myelomonocytic leukemia cell lines. J Pharmacol Exp Ther 1994; 271:193–199.

87. Bollag W, Majewski S, Jablonska S. Biological interactions of retinoids with cytokines and vitamin D analogs as a basis for cancer combination chemotherapy. In: Livera MA, Vidaldi G, eds. Retinoids: From Basic Science to Clinical Application. Basel: Birkhauser Verlag, 1994, pp. 267–280.

88. Bollag W, Majewski S, Jablonska S. Cancer combination chemotherapy with retinoids: experimental rationale. Leukemia 1994; 8:1453–1457.

89. Gullberg U, Nilsson E, Einhorn S, Olsson I. Combinations of interferon gamma and retinoic acid or 1,25-dihydroxy-cholecalcitoferol induce differentiations of the human leukemia cell line U-937. Exp Hematol 1985; 13:675–679.

90. Kelsey SM, Makin HLJ, Macey MG, Newland AC. Gamma interferon augments functional and phenotypic characteristics of vitamin D3-induced monocytic differentiation in the U937 human leukemic cell line. Leukoc Res 1990; 14:1027–1033.

91. Trinchieri G, Rosen M, Perussia B. Induction of differentiation of human myeloid cell lines by tumor necrosis factor in cooperation with 1,25-dihydroxyvitamin D3. Cancer Res 1987; 47:2236–2242.

92. Testa U, Masciulli R, Tritarelli E, Pustorini G, Martucci R, Barberi T, Camagna A, Valteri M, Peschle C. Transforming growth factor-beta potentiates vitamin D3-induced terminal monocytic differentiation of human leukemic cell lines. J Immunol 1993; 150:2418–2430.

93. Chen TC, Persons K, Wen-Wei L, Chen ML, Holik MF. The antiproliferative and differentiative activities of 1-dihydroxyvitamin D3 are potentiated by epidermal growth factor and attenuated by insulin in cultured human keratinocytes. J Invest Dermatol 1995; 104:13–117.

94. Zuckerman SH, Surprenant YM, Tang J. Synergistic effect of granulocyte-macrophagus colony-stimulating factor and 1,25-dihydroxyvitamin D3 on the differentiation of the human monocytic cell line U937. Blood 1988; 71:619–624.

95. Petrini M, Dastoli G, Valentini P., Matth L, Trombi L, Ambrogi RT, Grassi B. Synergistic effects of alpha interferon and 1,25-dihydroxyvitamin D3: preliminary evidence suggesting that interferon induces expression of the vitamin receptor. Haematologica 1991; 76:467–471.

96. Light BW, Yu WD, McElwam MC, Russell DM, Trump DL, Johnson CS. Potentation of cisplatin antitumor activity using a vitamin D analogue in a murine squamous cell carcinoma model system. Cancer Res 1997; 57:3759–3764.

97. Vink van Wijngaarden T, Pols HA, Buurman CJ, van den Bemd GJ, Prossers LC, Birkenhager JC, van Leeuwen JP. Inhibition ob breast cell growth by combined treatment with vitamin D3 analogues and tamoxifen. Cancer Res 1994; 54: 5711–5717.

98. Mc Elwain MC, Modzelewski RA, Shurin ZR, Russell DM, Lapco PE, Trump DL, Johnson CS. Enhanced antitumor activity with the combination of suramin and vitamin D in a murine squamous cell carcinoma model system. Proc Am Assoc Cancer Res 1997; 38:321.

99. Cunningham D, Gilchrist NL, Cowan RA, Forrest GJ, McArdle C, Skoukop M. Alfacalcidol as a modulator of growth of low grade non Hodgkin's lymphomas. Br Med J 1985; 291:1153–1155.

100. Scott-Mackie P., Hickish T, Mortimer P., Slosne J, Cunningham D. Calcipotriol and regression in T-cell lymphoma of skin. Lancet 1993; 342:172.

101. French LE, Ramelet AA, Saureat JH. Remission of cutaneous T-cell lymphoma with combined calcitriol and acitretin. Lancet 1994; 344:686–687.

102. Pols HAP, Birkenhager JC, Foekens JA, Van Leeuwen JPTM. Vitamin D: a modulator of cell proliferation and differentiation. J Steroid Biochem Mol Biol 1990; 37: 873–876.

103. Koeffler HP, Hirji K, Itri L. 1,25-dihydroxyvitamin D3: in vivo and in vitro effects on human preleukemic and leukemic cells. Cancer Treat Rep 1985; 69:1399–1407.

104. Rains V, Cunningham D, Soukop M. Alfacalcidol is a nontoxic, effective treatment of follicular small-cleaved cell lymphoma. Br J Cancer 1991; 63:463–465.

105. Warrel RP, de The H, Wang ZY, Degos L. Acute promyelocytic leukemia. N Engl J Med 1993; 329:177–189.
106. Dore BT, Uskokovic MR, Momparler RL. Induction differentiation HL-60 myloid leukaemia cells by retinoic acid and vitamin D analogs. Proc Am Assoc Cancer Res 1992; 33:2640.
107. Majewski S, Skopinska M, Bollag W, Jablonska S. Combination of isotretinoin and calcitriol for precancerous and cancerous skin lesions. Lancet 1994; 344: 1510–1511.
108. Aliezai M, Dupuy P, Amblard P. Clinical evaluation of topical isotretinoin in the treatment of actinic keratoses. J Am Acad Dermatol 1994; 30:447–451.
109. Skopinska M, Majewski S, Bollag W. Jablonska S. Calcitriol and isotretinoin combined therapy for precancerous skin lesions. J Dermatol Treat 1997; 8:5–10.

Index